Communications in Computer and Information Science 2433

Series Editors

Gang Li⑩, *School of Information Technology, Deakin University, Burwood, VIC, Australia*
Joaquim Filipe⑩, *Polytechnic Institute of Setúbal, Setúbal, Portugal*
Zhiwei Xu, *Chinese Academy of Sciences, Beijing, China*

AF147636

Rationale

The CCIS series is devoted to the publication of proceedings of computer science conferences. Its aim is to efficiently disseminate original research results in informatics in printed and electronic form. While the focus is on publication of peer-reviewed full papers presenting mature work, inclusion of reviewed short papers reporting on work in progress is welcome, too. Besides globally relevant meetings with internationally representative program committees guaranteeing a strict peer-reviewing and paper selection process, conferences run by societies or of high regional or national relevance are also considered for publication.

Topics

The topical scope of CCIS spans the entire spectrum of informatics ranging from foundational topics in the theory of computing to information and communications science and technology and a broad variety of interdisciplinary application fields.

Information for Volume Editors and Authors

Publication in CCIS is free of charge. No royalties are paid, however, we offer registered conference participants temporary free access to the online version of the conference proceedings on SpringerLink (http://link.springer.com) by means of an http referrer from the conference website and/or a number of complimentary printed copies, as specified in the official acceptance email of the event.

CCIS proceedings can be published in time for distribution at conferences or as post-proceedings, and delivered in the form of printed books and/or electronically as USBs and/or e-content licenses for accessing proceedings at SpringerLink. Furthermore, CCIS proceedings are included in the CCIS electronic book series hosted in the SpringerLink digital library at http://link.springer.com/bookseries/7899. Conferences publishing in CCIS are allowed to use Online Conference Service (OCS) for managing the whole proceedings lifecycle (from submission and reviewing to preparing for publication) free of charge.

Publication process

The language of publication is exclusively English. Authors publishing in CCIS have to sign the Springer CCIS copyright transfer form, however, they are free to use their material published in CCIS for substantially changed, more elaborate subsequent publications elsewhere. For the preparation of the camera-ready papers/files, authors have to strictly adhere to the Springer CCIS Authors' Instructions and are strongly encouraged to use the CCIS LaTeX style files or templates.

Abstracting/Indexing

CCIS is abstracted/indexed in DBLP, Google Scholar, EI-Compendex, Mathematical Reviews, SCImago, Scopus. CCIS volumes are also submitted for the inclusion in ISI Proceedings.

How to start

To start the evaluation of your proposal for inclusion in the CCIS series, please send an e-mail to ccis@springer.com.

Yanchun Zhang · Qingcai Chen · Hongfei Lin ·
Lei Liu · Xiangwen Liao · Buzhou Tang ·
Tianyong Hao · Zhengxing Huang

Editors

Health Information Processing

10th China Health Information Processing Conference, CHIP 2024
Fuzhou, China, November 15–17, 2024
Proceedings, Part II

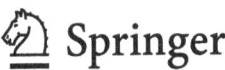

Editors
Yanchun Zhang
Zhejiang Normal University
Jinhua, China

Qingcai Chen
Harbin Institute of Technology
Shenzhen, China

Hongfei Lin
Dalian University of Technology
Dalian, China

Lei Liu
Fudan University
Shanghai, China

Xiangwen Liao
Fuzhou University
Fuzhou, China

Buzhou Tang
Harbin Institute of Technology
Shenzhen, China

Tianyong Hao
South China Normal University
Guangzhou, China

Zhengxing Huang
Zhejiang University
Hangzhou, China

ISSN 1865-0929   ISSN 1865-0937 (electronic)
Communications in Computer and Information Science
ISBN 978-981-96-3751-5   ISBN 978-981-96-3752-2 (eBook)
https://doi.org/10.1007/978-981-96-3752-2

© The Editor(s) (if applicable) and The Author(s), under exclusive license
to Springer Nature Singapore Pte Ltd. 2025

This work is subject to copyright. All rights are solely and exclusively licensed by the Publisher, whether the whole or part of the material is concerned, specifically the rights of translation, reprinting, reuse of illustrations, recitation, broadcasting, reproduction on microfilms or in any other physical way, and transmission or information storage and retrieval, electronic adaptation, computer software, or by similar or dissimilar methodology now known or hereafter developed.
The use of general descriptive names, registered names, trademarks, service marks, etc. in this publication does not imply, even in the absence of a specific statement, that such names are exempt from the relevant protective laws and regulations and therefore free for general use.
The publisher, the authors and the editors are safe to assume that the advice and information in this book are believed to be true and accurate at the date of publication. Neither the publisher nor the authors or the editors give a warranty, expressed or implied, with respect to the material contained herein or for any errors or omissions that may have been made. The publisher remains neutral with regard to jurisdictional claims in published maps and institutional affiliations.

This Springer imprint is published by the registered company Springer Nature Singapore Pte Ltd.
The registered company address is: 152 Beach Road, #21-01/04 Gateway East, Singapore 189721, Singapore

If disposing of this product, please recycle the paper.

Preface

Health information processing and applications is one of the essential fields in data-driven life health and clinical medicine and it has been highly active in recent decades. The China Health Information Processing Conference (CHIP) is an annual conference held by the Medical Health and Biological Information Processing Committee of the Chinese Information Processing Society (CIPS) of China, with the theme of "large models and smart healthcare". CHIP is one of the leading conferences in the field of health information processing in China and turned into an international event in 2022. It is also an important platform for researchers and practitioners from academia, business and government departments around the world to share ideas and further promote research and applications in this field. CHIP 2024 was organized by Fuzhou University and was held in hybrid mode, whereby people could attend face-to-face or freely connect to live broadcasts of the keynote speeches and presentations.

CHIP 2024 received 65 submissions, of which 32 high-quality papers were selected for publication in this volume after double-blind peer review with 3 reviews per submission, leading to an acceptance rate of just 49%. These papers have been categorized into 3 main topics: Biomedical data processing and model application, Mental health and disease prediction, and Drug prediction and Knowledge map.

The authors of each paper in this volume reported their novel results in computing methods or applications. The volume cannot cover all aspects of Medical Health and Biological Information Processing but may still inspire insightful thoughts for the readers. We hope that more secrets of Health Information Processing will be unveiled, and that academics will drive more practical developments and solutions.

November 2024

Zhou Fu
Yanchun Zhang
Qingcai Chen
Hongfei Lin
Lei Liu
Xiangwen Liao
Buzhou Tang
Tianyong Hao
Zhengxing Huang

Preface

Organization

Honorary Chairs

Yanchun Zhang   Zhejiang Normal University, China
Qingcai Chen   Harbin Institute of Technology (Shenzhen), China

General Co-chairs

Hongfei Lin   Dalian University of Technology, China
Lei Liu   Fudan University, China
Xiangwen Liao   Fuzhou University, China

Program Co-chairs

Buzhou Tang   Harbin Institute of Technology (Shenzhen) &
     Pengcheng Laboratory, China
Yanshan Wang   University of Pittsburgh, USA
Maggie Haitian Wang   Chinese University of Hong Kong, China

Young Scientists Forum Co-chairs

Zhengxing Huang   Zhejiang University, China
Yonghui Wu   University of Florida, USA

Publication Co-chairs

Tianyong Hao   South China Normal University, China
Xinyu He   Liaoning Normal University, China
Wenpeng Lu   Qilu University of Technology, China
Zhichang Zhang   Northwest Normal University, China
Ling Luo   Dalian University of Technology, China
Lu Xiang   Institute of Automation, Chinese Academy of
     Sciences, China
Yongxian Wu   South China University of Technology, China

Jiao Li   Institute of Medical Information, Chinese
                               Academy of Medical Sciences, China
Yongjun Zhu   Yonsei University, South Korea

Forum Co-chairs

Zhengxing Huang   Zhejiang University, China
Jun Yan   Yidu Cloud (Beijing) Technology Co., Ltd., China
Haofen Wang   Tongji University, China
Ming Feng   Peking Union Medical College Hospital, China
Zhumin Chen   Shandong University, China
Yi Zhou   Sun Yat-sen University, China
Sendong Zhao   Harbin Institute of Technology, China

Evaluation Co-chairs

Zuofeng Li   Takeda China, China
Jianbo Lei   Medical Informatics Center of Peking University,
                               China
Hui Zong   West China Hospital, Sichuan University, China

Publicity Co-chairs

Lishuang Li   Dalian University of Technology, China
Yinghui Jin   Zhongnan Hospital of Wuhan University, China
Ping Song   Children's Hospital Affiliated to Chongqing
                               Medical University, China

Sponsor Co-chairs

Siwei Yu   Guizhou Medical University, China
Yi Zhou   Sun Yat-sen University, China
Buyue Qian   Chaoyang Hospital Affiliated to Capital Medical
                               University, China
Yonghui Wu   University of Florida, USA

Web Chair

Kunli Zhang   Zhengzhou University, China

Program Committee

Wenping Guo   Taizhou University, China
Hongmin Cai   South China University of Technology, China
Chao Che   Dalian University, China
Mosha Chen   Alibaba, China
Qingcai Chen   Harbin Institute of Technology (Shenzhen), China
Xi Chen   Tencent Technology Co., Ltd., China
Yang Chen   Yidu Cloud (Beijing) Technology Co., Ltd., China
Zhumin Chen   Shandong University, China
Ming Cheng   Zhengzhou University, China
Ruoyao Ding   Guangdong University of Foreign Studies, China
Bin Dong   Ricoh Software Research Center (Beijing) Co.,
                              Ltd., China
Guohong Fu   Soochow University, China
Yan Gao   Central South University, China
Tianyong Hao   South China Normal University, China
Shizhu He   Institute of Automation, Chinese Academy of
                              Sciences, China
Zengyou He   Dalian University of Technology, China
Na Hong   Digital China Medical Technology Co., Ltd.,
                              China
Li Hou   Institute of Medical Information, Chinese
                              Academy of Medical Sciences, China
Yong Hu   Jinan University, China
Baotian Hu   Harbin University of Technology (Shenzhen),
                              China
Guimin Huang   Guilin University of Electronic Science and
                              Technology, China
Zhenghang Huang   Zhejiang University, China
Zhiwei Huang   Southwest Medical University, China
Bo Jin   Dalian University of Technology, China
Xiaoyu Kang   Southwest Medical University, China
Jianbo Lei   Peking University, China
Haomin Li   Children's Hospital of Zhejiang University
                              Medical College, China

Jiao Li	Institute of Medical Information, Chinese Academy of Medical Sciences, China
Jinghua Li	Chinese Academy of Traditional Chinese Medicine, China
Lishuang Li	Dalian University of Technology, China
Linfeng Li	Yidu Cloud (Beijing) Technology Co., Ltd., China
Ru Li	Shanxi University, China
Runzhi Li	Zhengzhou University, China
Shasha Li	National University of Defense Technology, China
Xing Li	Beijing Shenzhengyao Technology Co., Ltd., China
Xin Li	Zhongkang Physical Examination Technology Co., Ltd., China
Yuxi Li	Peking University First Hospital, China
Zuofeng Li	Takeda China, China
Xiangwen Liao	Fuzhou University, China
Hao Lin	University of Electronic Science and Technology, China
Hongfei Lin	Dalian University of Technology, China
Bangtao Liu	Southwest Medical University, China
Song Liu	Qilu University of Technology, China
Lei Liu	Fudan University, China
Shengping Liu	Unisound Co., Ltd., China
Xiaoming Liu	Zhongyuan University of Technology, China
Guan Luo	Institute of Automation, Chinese Academy of Sciences, China
Lingyun Luo	Nanhua University, China
Yamei Luo	Southwest Medical University, China
Hui Lv	Shanghai Jiao Tong University, China
Xudong Lv	Zhejiang University, China
Yao Meng	Lenovo Research Institute, China
Qingliang Miao	AI Speech Co., Ltd., China
Weihua Peng	Baidu Co., Ltd., China
Buyue Qian	Xi'an Jiaotong University, China
Longhua Qian	Suzhou University, China
Tong Ruan	East China University of Technology, China
Ying Shen	South China University of Technology, China
Xiaofeng Song	Nanjing University of Aeronautics and Astronautics, China
Chengjie Sun	Harbin University of Technology, China
Chuanji Tan	Alibaba Dharma Hall, China
Hongye Tan	Shanxi University, China

Jingyu Tan   Shenzhen Xinkaiyuan Information Technology
                              Development Co., Ltd., China
Binhua Tang   Hohai University, China
Buzhou Tang   Harbin Institute of Technology (Shenzhen), China
Jintao Tang   National Defense University of the People's
                              Liberation Army, China
Qian Tao   South China University of Technology, China
Fei Teng   Southwest Jiaotong University, China
Shengwei Tian   Xinjiang University, China
Dong Wang   Southern Medical University, China
Haitian Wang   Chinese University of Hong Kong, China
Haofen Wang   Tongji University, China
Xiaolei Wang   Hong Kong Institute of Sustainable Development
                              Education, China
Haolin Wang   Chongqing Medical University, China
Yehan Wang   Unisound Intelligent Technology, China
Zhenyu Wang   South China Institute of Technology Software,
                              China
Zhongmin Wang   Jiangsu Provincial People's Hospital, China
Leyi Wei   Shandong University, China
Heng Weng   Guangdong Hospital of Traditional Chinese
                              Medicine, China
Gang Wu   Beijing Knowledge Atlas Technology Co., Ltd.,
                              China
Xian Wu   Tencent Technology (Beijing) Co., Ltd., China
Jingbo Xia   Huazhong Agricultural University, China
Lu Xiang   Institute of Automation, Chinese Academy of
                              Sciences, China
Yang Xiang   Pengcheng Laboratory, China
Lei Xu   Shenzhen Polytechnic, China
Liang Xu   Ping An Technology (Shenzhen) Co., Ltd., China
Yan Xu   Beihang University, Microsoft Asia Research
                              Institute, China
Jun Yan   Yidu Cloud (Beijing) Technology Co., Ltd., China
Cheng Yang   Institute of Automation, Chinese Academy of
                              Sciences, China
Hai Yang   East China University of Technology, China
Meijie Yang   Chongqing Medical University, China
Muyun Yang   Harbin University of Technology, China
Zhihao Yang   Dalian University of Technology, China
Hui Ye   Guangzhou University of Traditional Chinese
                              Medicine, China
Dehui Yin   Southwest Medical University, China

Qing Yu	Xinjiang University, China
Liang Yu	Xi'an University of Electronic Science and Technology, China
Siwei Yu	Guizhou Provincial People's Hospital, China
Hongying Zan	Zhengzhou University, China
Hao Zhang	Jilin University, China
Kunli Zhang	Zhengzhou University, China
Weide Zhang	Zhongshan Hospital Affiliated to Fudan University, China
Xiaoyan Zhang	Tongji University, China
Yaoyun Zhang	Alibaba, China
Yijia Zhang	Dalian University of Technology, China
Yuanzhe Zhang	Institute of Automation, Chinese Academy of Sciences, China
Zhichang Zhang	Northwest Normal University, China
Qiuye Zhao	Beijing Big Data Research Institute, China
Sendong Zhao	Harbin Institute of Technology, China
Tiejun Zhao	Harbin Institute of Technology, China
Deyu Zhou	Southeast University, China
Fengfeng Zhou	Jilin University, China
Guangyou Zhou	Central China Normal University, China
Yi Zhou	Sun Yat-sen University, China
Conghui Zhu	Harbin Institute of Technology, China
Shanfeng Zhu	Fudan University, China
Yu Zhu	Sunshine Life Insurance Co., Ltd., China
Quan Zou	University of Electronic Science and Technology, China
Xi Chen	University of Electronic Science and Technology, China
Yansheng Li	Mediway Technology Co., Ltd., China
Daojing He	Harbin Institute of Technology (Shenzhen), China
Yupeng Liu	Harbin University of Science and Technology, China
Xinzhi Sun	First Affiliated Hospital of Zhengzhou University, China
Chuanchao Du	Third People's Hospital of Henan Province, China
Xien Liu	Beijing Huijizhiyi Technology Co., Ltd., China
Shan Nan	Hainan University, China
Xinyu He	Liaoning Normal University, China
Qianqian He	Chongqing Medical University, China
Xing Liu	Third Xiangya Hospital of Central South University, China
Jiayin Wang	Xi'an Jiaotong University, China

Ying Xu   Xi'an Jiaotong University, China
Xin Lai   Xi'an Jiaotong University, China

Contents – Part II

Contents – Part I

Mental Health and Disease Prediction

Mental Health and Disease Prediction

Data Augmentation and Instruction Fine-Tuning for ADR Detection

Weiru Fu[1], Hongfei Lin[1(✉)], Guangtao Xu[1], Yunzhi Qiu[1], Jian Wang[1], Yufeng Diao[2], and Puqi Zheng[1]

[1] School of Computer Science and Technology, Dalian University of Technology, Dalian, China
fuweiru0624@mail.dlut.edu.cn, hflin@dlut.edu.cn
[2] School of Computer Science and Technology, Inner Mongolia Minzu University, Tongliao, China

Abstract. With the rise of social media, users increasingly share their medication experiences online, offering a new data source for real-time ADR detection. However, ADR detection on social media faces two key challenges: limited labeled data and an imbalance between positive and negative samples. While previous studies have explored solutions like transfer learning, multi-source data fusion, joint task training, and loss function optimization, these approaches can introduce noise, increase annotation costs, or complicate training complexity. Moreover, despite the promising zero-shot and few-shot capabilities of large language models (LLMs) in natural language processing tasks, their performance in social media-based ADR detection remains below that of smaller, fine-tuned models. To tackle these challenges, we propose the Bal-LLaMA framework, comprising three modules: a data augmentation module to balance positive and negative samples as well as mitigating the challenge posed by limited annotated data, an instruction data construction module tailored for social media ADR detection, and a QLoRA-based module for efficient parameter fine-tuning. Experimental results demonstrate that Bal-LLaMA significantly outperforms existing state-of-the-art models on various social media ADR detection datasets, confirming the effectiveness of our approach.

Keywords: Adverse Drug Reactions · Social Media Data · Data Augmentation · Instruction Fine-tuning · Large Language Models

1 Introduction

Adverse Drug Reaction (ADR) refers to any harmful and unintended response that occurs during the clinical use of a medication. The accurate identification and monitoring of ADRs are critical to ensuring drug safety. Traditionally, ADR detection has relied on clinical trials, spontaneous reporting systems (e.g., the FDA's MedWatch[1]), medical literature, and pharmacovigilance databases (e.g.,

---

[1] https://www.fda.gov/safety/medwatch-fda-safety-information-and-adverse\penalty-\@M-event-reporting-program.

© The Author(s), under exclusive license to Springer Nature Singapore Pte Ltd. 2025
Y. Zhang et al. (Eds.): CHIP 2024, CCIS 2433, pp. 3–20, 2025.
https://doi.org/10.1007/978-981-96-3752-2_1

WHO's VigiBase[2]). However, these approaches have several significant limitations, particularly in terms of timeliness, the comprehensiveness of the information collected, and the coverage of diverse populations.

As social media continues to evolve, individuals increasingly share their health conditions and medication experiences on online platforms. These platforms have become valuable spaces for spontaneous discussions about drug use, providing a novel data source for detecting potential ADRs. Users frequently discuss drug reactions on platforms such as Twitter, presenting opportunities for real-time ADR collection and monitoring. Compared to traditional reporting systems, social media data is broader in scope and captures immediate feedback from diverse populations, thereby addressing limitations in timeliness, comprehensiveness, and population coverage.

However, ADR detection on social media often face two primary challenges: limited annotated data and imbalanced positive and negative samples. Lardon et al. [1] found that only 8.05% of 10,534 extracted tweets mentioned adverse reactions, underscoring the significant imbalance in social media data. The scarcity of annotated data further complicates model training. To address this, Li et al. [2] employed transfer learning by leveraging a larger source dataset to improve the generalization of a smaller target dataset. Sarker et al. [3] combined datasets from multiple sources, increasing the total amount of training data and mitigating the issue of limited annotations. Additionally, some studies have implemented joint training of named entity recognition (NER) and ADR detection models to facilitate information sharing between tasks, improving the model's adaptability to small annotated datasets [4,5]. Despite progress, these approaches may introduce other issues such as increased noise and additional annotation efforts. A line of studies have explored the use of weighted cross-entropy loss [6] and focal loss functions [7] to address the imbalance between positive and negative samples. Weighted cross-entropy increases the importance of minority class samples to reduce model bias toward the majority class. Focal loss down-weights easy examples, encouraging the model to focus on harder, misclassified instances. Both methods aim to improve model performance on imbalanced datasets, but they also introduce additional hyperparameters, such as the weight ratio or focusing parameter, which add complexity to the training process.

Generative large language models (LLMs) like GPT-3 [8] and LLaMA [9] have shown great potential in various natural language processing tasks. However, when applied directly to ADR detection, their performance still falls short of smaller, fine-tuned models trained on labeled datasets [10]. Additionally, with billions of parameters, fine-tuning LLMs on a single GPU is highly complex and resource-intensive, demanding higher hardware performance, increasing computation time, and complicating memory management. QLoRA [11] addresses this by adjusting low-rank model parameters and converting floating-point parameters into low-bit-width discrete values. Despite these advances, the performance of fine-tuned open-source LLMs in ADR detection on social media remains underexplored.

---

[2] https://who-umc.org/vigibase/.

To address these challenges, we propose the Bal-LLaMA framework, comprising three key components: a data augmentation module to balance the ratio of positive and negative samples in the training data, an instruction data construction module for adapting the model to ADR detection on social media, and a model training module using QLoRA for efficient parameter tuning. By incorporating positive samples from external data sources, we mitigate class imbalance and the lack of annotated data. We also developed a similarity-based augmentation strategy to minimize noise from external sources thus enhances the model's generalization and robustness. Additionally, we propose an instruction data construction approach tailored to social media ADR detection, leveraging role-playing and task descriptions to help the model better handle informal language commonly found in social media and to focus on ADR detection tasks. We utilize the LLaMA 3-8B-chat[3] model and apply QLoRA for efficient parameter fine-tuning, improving performance in resource-constrained environments.

The main contributions of this paper are as follows:

- We designed a similarity-based external positive sample selection strategy, which not only addresses the issue of class imbalance but also mitigates the impact of noise from external data.
- We proposed an instruction data construction method tailored for social media ADR detection, using role-playing and task descriptions to create specific instructions that enable the model to better adapt to the informal language used on social media and the task of adverse drug reaction detection.
- Experimental results demonstrate that the Bal-LLaMA model performs exceptionally well on multiple social media ADR detection datasets, significantly surpassing existing baseline models. Ablation studies further confirm the effectiveness of both the data augmentation and instruction data construction modules.

2   Related Work

2.1   ADR Detection on Social Media

The ADR detection task focuses on identifying whether a sentence mentions an adverse drug reaction, classifying it as either containing or not containing any ADRs. With the growth of social media, user-generated posts and comments about drug experiences have expanded the training corpus, prompting numerous studies on ADR detection on social media. These studies can be broadly categorized into three main approaches:

Sentiment-Based Methods. These approaches assume that when users describe adverse drug reactions, sentiment information (e.g., negative emotions) is closely linked to ADR mentions. As a result, many studies incorporate sentiment-related features or sentiment analysis techniques to improve ADR

---

[3] https://github.com/meta-llama/llama3.

detection [3,12–14]. For instance, Zhang et al. used a sentiment-aware attention mechanism to learn a compatibility matrix between sentences and sentiment words, extracting word-level sentiment features to enhance the model's focus on ADR mentions [15]. While these methods effectively capture emotional cues in text, their limitation lies in the non-linear relationship between sentiment and ADRs. In cases where sentiment is unclear, detection accuracy may be affected.

Graph Neural Network (GNN)-Based Methods. GNNs have gained popularity in ADR detection due to their ability to model complex relationships and structured data [16–18]. These methods create graph structures between entities like drugs and symptoms, using GNNs to capture relationships and global information. For instance, Gao et al. enhanced ADR detection by integrating graph embedding techniques with contextual information and medical knowledge [10]. Compared to traditional approaches, GNN-based methods excel at modeling complex entity relationships. However, constructing effective graphs often requires extensive annotated data or external knowledge bases (e.g., UMLS), which are time-consuming to annotate and may limit the model's generalization due to the coverage and update frequency of the knowledge bases.

Data Augmentation-Based Methods. Adversarial training, a form of data augmentation, improves model robustness by introducing perturbations during training. In ADR detection, adversarial methods typically apply small perturbations to text features or word embeddings to enhance the model's resilience to noise, spelling errors, and informal language common in social media data [15]. Additionally, some studies use synonym sets for augmentation to address limited annotated data [7]. While these methods improve robustness, they may not fully resolve issues related to data noise and expression diversity on social media, particularly when dealing with complex semantics or domain-specific terminology.

2.2   LLMs and Instruction Tuning

In recent years, LLMs have made significant strides in natural language processing. Pretrained on vast text corpora, these models learn extensive language patterns and knowledge, excelling across various tasks [8,9]. Two primary approaches for applying LLMs to downstream tasks are in-context learning [8] and instruction fine-tuning [19]. In-context learning enables the model to perform tasks using a few demonstration examples without adjusting parameters [20,21], making it particularly effective for larger models with hundreds of billions of parameters. Instruction fine-tuning, on the other hand, trains the model using explicit task instructions [22,23], adjusting pretrained parameters to help the model better understand and perform specific tasks. The key idea is to provide clear task descriptions and examples during the model's fine-tuning phase, guiding the model on how to handle task data. Research has shown that models fine-tuned with instructions tend to exhibit better generalization performance in downstream tasks [24,25].

3 Method

3.1 Overview of the Method

The overall framework of the proposed method is illustrated in Fig. 1. It consists of three main components: a data augmentation module designed to balance positive and negative samples, an instruction data construction module tailored for adapting the model to the task of adverse drug reaction detection, and a model training module.

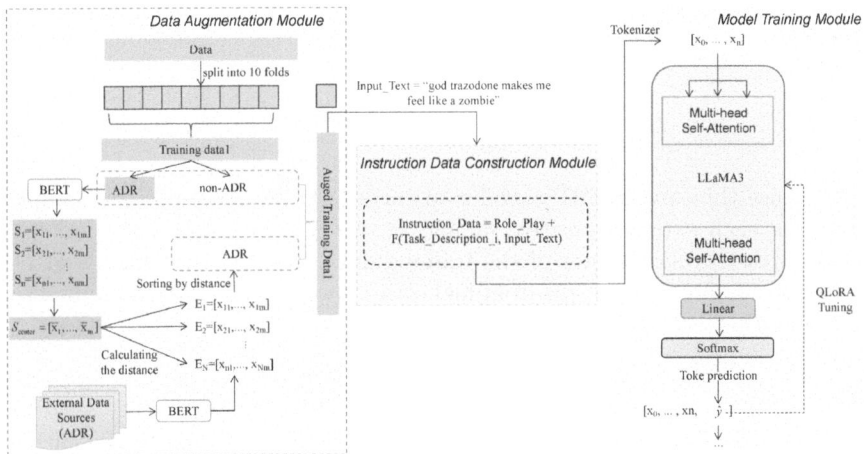

Fig. 1. The overall framework of our Bal-LLaMA model.

3.2 Data Augmentation Module

In the task of adverse drug reaction detection, there is often a significant imbalance between positive and negative samples, which can degrade model performance. To address this issue, we designed a data augmentation module. The core objective of this module is to balance the ratio of positive and negative samples in the training data by selectively introducing additional positive samples from external data sources, thereby enhancing model performance.

During the data augmentation process, we adopt a similarity-based strategy to select and filter external data, aiming to minimize noise interference. Let D_t denote the training dataset in the t-th fold, D_t^+ represent the set of positive samples in D_t, and D_t^- represent the set of negative samples in D_t. The number of samples in D_t^- and D_t^+ are denoted as N_t^- and N_t^+, respectively. Additionally, D_e^+ represents the set of positive samples from external data sources, n refers to the number of positive samples to be added, and $f_{\mathrm{BERT}}(\cdot)$ refers to the BERT encoder. Specifically, for the training dataset D_t in the t-th fold, we first calculate the number of positive samples N_t^+ and negative samples N_t^-, which allows us to determine the number of additional positive samples needed to balance the ratio of positive and negative samples.

$$n = N_t^+ - N_t^-. \tag{1}$$

We then extract the top n most similar positive samples from the external data source D_e^+ and add them to the current training dataset D_t. When selecting additional positive samples, we employ a class-center similarity metric. First, we use the BERT encoder $f_{\text{BERT}}(\cdot)$ to encode all positive samples in the training data. We then compute the centroid of these positive sample vectors c_t^+, serving as the class center for the positive samples in the current training data.

$$c_t^+ = \frac{1}{N_t^+} \sum_{x_i \in D_t^+} f_{\text{BERT}}(x_i). \tag{2}$$

Next, we use the same BERT encoder to encode the external positive samples in D_e^+. For each external positive sample x_j, we calculate its cosine similarity score s_j with the class center of the training data and sort the samples in D_e^+ based on their similarity scores from highest to lowest. The sorted sample set is denoted as $\tilde{D}_e^+$.

$$s_j = \frac{f_{\text{BERT}}(x_j) \cdot c_t^+}{\|f_{\text{BERT}}(x_j)\| \|c_t^+\|}, \quad x_j \in D_e^+. \tag{3}$$

Finally, we select the top n most similar samples and add them to the current training set D_t, resulting in the augmented training dataset D_t^{aug}.

$$D_t^{aug} = D_t \bigcup \left\{ x_j \mid x_j \in \tilde{D}_e^+[1:n] \right\}. \tag{4}$$

The proposed augmentation strategy effectively balances the ratio of positive and negative samples in the training data, helping to alleviate potential overfitting issues. Additionally, by introducing new positive samples from an external and independent data source, this approach improves the model's generalization ability and robustness. It is important to note that we only augment the training data, while the test data remains unchanged. This ensures that the distribution of the test set is consistent with the original dataset, providing a more accurate evaluation of the model's actual performance. Furthermore, during the cross-validation process, we apply the same data augmentation strategy to each fold's training data to ensure consistency and comparability across different folds. The selection of external data sources will be discussed in Sect. 4.1.

3.3 Instruction Data Construction Module

To enable the generative model to adapt effectively to the task of ADR detection based on social media, we constructed instruction data. The process of building this instruction data can be divided into the following three steps.

Step 1: Role-Playing Scenario. In this step, we provide the model with a role-playing scenario to help it better understand the context of the ADR detection task. On social media platforms, users often describe their medication experiences and adverse reactions in a more informal and colloquial manner. These descriptions may include a significant amount of slang, abbreviations, emojis, and other internet language, along with incomplete or grammatically incorrect expressions. Therefore, we designed the model to assume the role of a drug safety analysis expert who is well-versed in the language and communication styles of social media users. This helps the model better adapt to the nuances of social media data and improves its performance in detecting ADRs in social media-based tasks. The prompt of the instruction data includes the following role-playing template, Role_Play.

> *"Please assume the role of a drug safety analysis expert familiar with social media language. You possess extensive knowledge of drug safety and have a deep understanding of the language habits and expression styles of social media users."*

Step 2: Task Description. Once the model's role is defined, we need to describe the ADR detection task in detail. The purpose of this step is to clarify the input, output format, and evaluation criteria of the task for the model. The following task description template, Task_Description, is incorporated into the instruction data prompt.

> *"Identify adverse drug reactions (undesired, harmful effects resulting from a medication) from the following social media text. Output "yes" if the text contains any specific adverse drug reaction, and output "no" if side effects are mentioned but not specified, or no side effects are mentioned at all. No other outputs are required. Input: {}"*

Step 3: Inserting Input Text. Let the input text be denoted as Input_Text, and define the insertion function $F(\cdot)$ as the operation that inserts the input text into the placeholder position of the task description template. The construction of the instruction data can be outlined as follows:

$$\text{Instruction\_Data} = \text{Role\_Play} + F(\text{Task\_Description\_i}, \text{Input\_Text}) \quad (5)$$

Here, Task_Description_i represents the i-th task description template. We design a total of ten task instruction templates, and one is randomly selected each time to construct the instruction data. The task instruction templates we used in our experiments can be found in Appendix.

By following this method, the instruction data is built by inserting the input text into the appropriate task description template, thereby providing the generative model with the necessary contextual and task-specific information to perform ADR detection on social media data.

3.4   Model Training Module

In this study, we utilized the LLaMA-3 8B chat model[4] for training and pre-diction in the task of ADR detection. Due to limitations in computational resources, we employed Quantization-Aware Low-Rank Adaptation(QLoRA) [11] for parameter-efficient fine-tuning. QLoRA significantly reduces the computational resources required by applying a low-rank approximation to weight updates, making it well-suited for fine-tuning large-scale pre-trained models under constrained hardware conditions.

The loss function used during the model training phase is cross-entropy loss, and its formula is as follows:

$$Loss = -\sum_{t=1}^{T} \log p\left(y_t \mid x, y_{<t}\right). \tag{6}$$

where T is the length of the label sequence y and $y_{<t}$ denotes previously generated tokens. $p\left(y_t \mid x, y_{<t}\right)$ is the probability of the t-th word in the true label being generated by the model, given the previously generated words $y_{<t}$ and the instruction data x.

4   Experiments

4.1   Datasets and Metrics

Training Datasets. We evaluated the model's performance on three social media-based adverse drug reaction detection datasets. The statistical information for these datasets is shown in Table 1. As observed, the ratio of positive to negative samples is imbalanced across all three datasets, particularly in the Twitter dataset, where positive samples account for less than 15%. The ratio of positive to negative examples in each dataset after data augmentation is shown in Table 2.

Table 1. The statistical information for TwiMed-Twitter, Twitter, and CADEC.

Corpus	Total	ADR	non-ADR
TwiMed-Twitter	625	232	393
Twitter	6471	744	5727
CADEC	7474	2478	4996

1. **TwiMed-Twitter** [26] This dataset is part of the TwiMed dataset. TwiMed collects drug-related reports from both social media and formal scientific literature sources. The social media portion is referred to as TwiMed-Twitter. The original dataset is annotated at the entity level with drugs, diseases, symptoms, and their relationships. We consider a document to contain an ADR when any relationship in the document is labeled as a negative outcome.

---

[4] https://github.com/meta-llama/llama3.

Table 2. The ratio of positive to negative examples for TwiMed-Twitter, Twitter, and CADEC after data augmentation.

Corpus	ADR	non-ADR
TwiMed-Twitter	50%	50%
Twitter	27.8%	72.2%
CADEC	43.4%	56.6%

2. **Twitter** [27] This dataset is from the "Social Media Mining for Health (#SMM4H 2016) Shared Task." The dataset was annotated by domain experts, marking ADRs and their corresponding UMLS concept IDs. The dataset exhibits imbalance, with tweets containing spelling errors and informal language.
3. **CADEC** [28] This is an annotated corpus on adverse drug events. The dataset originates from patient reviews on the AskaPatient website[5], focusing on patient-reported ADRs. The text in the corpus is typically informal and conversational, often deviating from standard English grammar and punctuation rules.

Since none of these datasets were pre-divided into training and testing sets, we employed a ten-fold cross-validation approach to ensure a fair comparison with baseline models. We used macro F1, macro precision, and macro recall as evaluation metrics. To better simulate real-world scenarios, no preprocessing was applied to the raw data.

External Data Source. Additionally, we use positive samples from the training set of the "Social Media Mining for Health (#SMM4H 2021) Shared Task 1" as an external data source [29]. This dataset is highly relevant to our task. SMM4H 2021 Shared Task 1 focuses on identifying ADRs from social media text, aligning closely with our goal of social media-based ADR detection. Thus, the dataset provides directly applicable positive examples for our research. Furthermore, the source and nature of this dataset are quite similar to the training datasets we use, ensuring contextual consistency between the external data and our training data, thereby minimizing bias due to contextual differences. It is important to note that when using this dataset as an external data source, the total number of external samples is 1209. If the number of additional positive samples needed exceeds the number of samples in the external data source, we include all available samples from the external dataset in the training set.

---

[5] https://www.askapatient.com.

4.2   Baselines

Discriminative Models

- **CNN+Transfer** [2]: This framework is based on adversarial transfer learning and uses Convolutional Neural Networks (CNNs) as a shared feature extractor. It simultaneously learns both shared features across corpora and corpus-specific features.
- **ATL** [2]: This framework is also based on adversarial transfer learning and designs shared-private feature extractors to capture global features shared between source and target datasets.
- **ANNSA** [15]: By employing an emotion-aware attention mechanism, ANNSA learns a compatibility matrix between sentences and emotional words, extracting word-level emotional features and enhancing the model's focus on ADR mentions.
- **CGEM** [18]: CGEM constructs a heterogeneous graph representing words and documents as nodes and utilizes graph neural networks (such as GCN and GAT) to learn complex relationships between nodes, effectively improving the accuracy and robustness of ADR detection.
- **KESDT** [7]: KESDT achieves more effective ADR detection through shallow and deep fusion strategies. Shallow fusion integrates domain-specific keywords into the model, enhancing interactions between keywords and other words in the sentence. Deep fusion introduces synonym sets to expand the dataset size and improve performance on low-annotated datasets.
- **SEDGCN** [14]: SEDGCN redefines the ADR detection task as an aspect-level sentiment analysis task by combining sentiment information with global information to enhance the Graph Convolutional Network (GCN).
- **KnowCAGE** [10]: Building upon the CGEM model, KnowCAGE incorporates UMLS medical knowledge to enhance the representational ability of graph embedding models and proposes a concept-aware self-attention mechanism to improve feature differentiation. The model has achieved state-of-the-art results in ADR detection tasks across multiple public datasets.

Generative Models

- **GPT-4**[6]: GPT-4 is a large-scale language model based on the Transformer architecture. We conducted our experiments on the gpt-4o-2024-05-13 model with the default parameters.
- **LlaMA-3**[7]: LLaMA-3 is an open-source family of large language models based on a decoder-only transformer architecture, trained on 15 trillion tokens with an 8k token context window. The currently released versions of LLaMA-3 come in 8B and 70B parameter sizes. We carried out experiments using the LLaMA-3-8B-chat model.

---

[6] https://openai.com/api.
[7] https://github.com/meta-llama/llama3.

4.3   Experimental Setups

Data Construction Phase. In the process of constructing a balanced dataset, we utilized the bert-base-uncased model[8] to tokenize and encode positive examples from both the training data and the external data source. The maximum token length was set to 128.

Training Phase. We chose the LLaMA-3-8B-chat model as our base model and applied the QLoRA method for parameter-efficient fine-tuning to develop the ADR detection model. In the QLoRA configuration, we set the dropout rate, lora_alpha, and lora_rank to 0.3, 16, and 64, respectively, and used 16-bit floating-point precision (FP16) to enhance training efficiency. During training, we used a batch size of 16 for the Twitter and CADEC datasets and a batch size of 8 for the Twimed-Twitter dataset. Gradient accumulation was set to 2 steps, and the maximum sequence length was configured to 1024 tokens. We employed a constant learning rate scheduler with an initial learning rate of 2e-4 and a warm-up ratio of 0.1 to help the model better adapt to the training data.

Inference Phase. To ensure the stability of inference results, we set the following values during inference: top_p to 1, top_k to 1, temperature to 0.1, and repetition_penalty to 1.0. We performed model training and inference on the three datasets using a single RTX 4090 GPU. The experimental environment included Python version 3.10.0 and PyTorch version 2.0.0.

4.4   Main Results

Table 3 presents the predictive performance of the proposed Bal-LLaMA model on three social media ADR detection datasets, compared with baseline models. The results for all discriminative models are reported values from the original papers, while the results for generative models were obtained through our experiments.

The experimental results demonstrate that the Bal-LLaMA model achieves the best performance across all datasets. On the Twitter dataset, Bal-LLaMA achieved precision, recall, and F1 scores of 86.8%, 88.2%, and 87.4%, respectively, surpassing the previous best discriminative method, SEDGCN, by 10.7, 13.0, and 12.0% points. On the TwiMed-Twitter dataset, Bal-LLaMA obtained an F1 score of 85.5%, which is an improvement of 1.6 and 1.1% points over CGEM and KnowCAGE, respectively. On the CADEC dataset, Bal-LLaMA achieved an F1 score of 92.4%, outperforming the previous best discriminative method, KnowCAGE, by 2% points.

Additionally, we compared Bal-LLaMA with two powerful large language models, GPT-4o and LLaMA-3-8B-chat, in a zero-shot setting. GPT-4o zero-shot performance surpassed some earlier discriminative methods across all three datasets, while LLaMA-3-8B-chat zero-shot performance was relatively weaker.

---

[8] https://huggingface.co/google-bert/bert-base-uncased.

Table 3. Experimental results on tree benchmark datasets (%). The best results are in bold, and the second-best results are underlined.

Model	Twitter			TwiMed-Twitter			CADEC		
	P	R	F1	P	R	F1	P	R	F1
CNN+Transfer (2020)	60.2	35.6	44.76	61.8	60.0	60.9	84.8	79.4	82.0
ATL (2020)	56.3	39.3	46.2	63.7	63.4	63.5	84.3	81.3	82.8
ANNSA (2021)	49.1	50.5	48.8	58.8	73.3	64.2	82.7	83.5	83.1
CGEM (2022)	-	-	-	84.2	83.7	83.9	-	-	-
KESDT (2023)	70.4	75.6	72.2	-	-	-	<u>88.2</u>	87.6	87.8
SEDGCN (2023)	76.1	75.2	75.4	-	-	-	-	-	-
KnowCAGE (2024)	-	-	-	<u>84.8</u>	<u>84.1</u>	<u>84.4</u>	87.1	**93.9**	<u>90.4</u>
GPT-4o (0-shot) (2024)	<u>80.9</u>	78.3	<u>79.5</u>	82.1	79.6	80.2	84.7	83.8	84.2
LLaMA3-8B (0-shot) (2024)	63.4	<u>78.4</u>	64.0	71.2	71.0	66.4	59.5	57.7	57.7
Bal-LLaMA (ours)	**86.8**	**88.2**	**87.4**	**85.9**	**86.3**	**85.5**	**92.0**	<u>93.0</u>	**92.4**

However, by constructing a balanced dataset and fine-tuning, Bal-LLaMA showed significant performance improvements, outperforming both GPT-4o and LLaMA in zero-shot settings across all datasets. This highlights the effectiveness of data augmentation and model fine-tuning.

4.5   Ablation Study

To explore the impact of data augmentation and prompt tuning on the performance of the proposed Bal-LLaMA model, we designed and conducted a series of ablation experiments. We evaluated the performance of Bal-LLaMA and its variants on the Twitter, TwiMed-Twitter, and CADEC datasets, comparing their precision (P), recall (R), and F1 scores. The results are presented in Tables 4, Tables 5, and Tables 6.

Table 4. Experimental results on Twitter (%).

Model	P	R	F1	Δ F1
Bal-LLaMA	86.8	88.2	87.4	-
w/o aug	84.3	88.9	86.3	−1.1
w/o prompt	84.2	90.9	87.2	−0.2
w/o prompt, aug	86.1	86.4	86.2	−1.2

On the Twitter dataset (Table 4), Bal-LLaMA achieved an F1 score of 87.4%. Removing data augmentation (w/o aug) led to a 1.1% point decrease in F1 score, while removing prompt tuning (w/o prompt) resulted in a 0.2% point decrease.

In comparison, the baseline model(w/o prompt, aug), which did not use either technique, experienced a more significant drop of 1.2% points in F1 score. These results indicate that data augmentation plays a dominant role in improving model performance on the Twitter dataset, while prompt tuning, although beneficial, has a relatively smaller impact.

Table 5. Experimental results on TwiMed-Twitter (%).

Model	P	R	F1	Δ F1
Bal-LLaMA	85.9	86.3	85.5	-
w/o aug	84.8	85.0	84.7	−0.8
w/o prompt	83.6	82.4	82.9	−2.7
w/o prompt, aug	82.0	82.6	81.9	-3.6

On the TwiMed-Twitter dataset (Table 5), Bal-LLaMA outperformed its variants with an F1 score of 85.5%. The absence of data augmentation (w/o aug) and prompt tuning (w/o prompt) resulted in F1 score reductions of 0.8 and 2.7% points, respectively. These findings suggest that prompt tuning is crucial for enhancing model performance on the TwiMed-Twitter dataset, likely due to the smaller sample size which limits the amount of learnable knowledge and information. In such cases, prompt tuning introduces additional task-related knowledge and guidance, effectively compensating for the lack of data and helping the model better understand the task objectives and optimization directions. The baseline model(w/o prompt, aug) showed a more pronounced performance decline with a 3.6% point drop in F1 score. This suggests that while data augmentation's contribution is relatively smaller on the TwiMed-Twitter dataset, its combination with prompt tuning remains a key factor in improving model performance.

Table 6. Experimental results on CADEC (%).

Model	P	R	F1	Δ F1
Bal-LLaMA	92.0	93.0	92.4	-
w/o aug	92.0	92.8	92.3	−0.1
w/o prompt	91.5	92.9	92.3	−0.1
w/o prompt,aug	92.3	92.2	92.2	−0.2

For the CADEC dataset (Table 6), the effects of data augmentation and prompt tuning were less pronounced. Bal-LLaMA achieved an F1 score of 92.4%, with only a minor decrease of 0.1% points for variants without data augmentation (w/o aug) and prompt tuning (w/o prompt). The baseline model's(w/o prompt, aug) performance was comparable, with an F1 score of 92.2%. A possible reason for this could be that the CADEC dataset, being a high-quality medical patient review dataset, inherently contains well-defined domain-specific patterns and regularities. This allows the model to perform well even without data augmentation and prompt tuning. In contrast, for datasets like Twitter and TwiMed-Twitter, which have smaller sample sizes and more noise, data augmentation and prompt tuning techniques significantly enhance model performance. Despite the relatively minor impact of these techniques on the CADEC dataset, Bal-LLaMA still achieved a slightly higher F1 score compared to the baseline model(w/o prompt, aug) and other variants. This suggests that even with a sufficiently large sample size, the judicious application of data augmentation and prompt tuning techniques can still contribute to improved model performance.

5   Conclusion

This work presents a novel framework, Bal-LLaMA, designed for detecting adverse drug reactions (ADR) in social media texts. The framework consists of three main components: the data augmentation module, the instruction data construction module, and the model training module.

In the data augmentation module, positive examples from external datasets are leveraged, using a similarity-based strategy to balance the ratio of positive and negative samples in the training set. This approach enhances the model's generalization and robustness. The instruction data construction module employs role-playing and task descriptions to create tailored prompts, enabling the model to better handle informal language commonly found in social media and to focus on ADR detection tasks. For training, the LLaMA-3-8B-chat model is fine-tuned using the QLoRA method, which facilitates efficient parameter optimization while operating under constrained computational resources.

Experimental results show that the Bal-LLaMA model outperforms traditional discriminative models and zero-shot generative models across the Twitter, TwiMed-Twitter, and CADEC datasets, achieving state-of-the-art performance. Ablation studies further demonstrate the significant contributions of data augmentation and instruction tuning, especially on the imbalanced and small-scale Twitter and TwiMed-Twitter datasets. Overall, the Bal-LLaMA model effectively addresses data imbalance and enhances the robustness and generalizability of ADR detection in the noisy social media environment through data augmentation and prompt tuning techniques.

Acknowledgements. This work is partially supported by grant from the Natural Science Foundation of China (No. 62366040, 62006130), Inner Mongolia Science Foundation (No. 2022MS06028). This work is supported by Program for Young Talents of Science and Technology in Universities of Inner Mongolia Autonomous Region.

Appendix

The Task Instruction Templates

Task_Description_1 = "Identify any adverse drug reactions (unwanted, harmful effects caused by a medication) in the following social media post. Respond with "yes" if a specific adverse drug reaction is mentioned. Respond with "no" if there are no specific adverse drug reactions mentioned or if side effects are discussed but remain vague. No other output is required. Input: {}"

Task_Description_2 = "Identify adverse drug reactions (undesired, harmful effects resulting from a medication) from the following social media text. Output "yes" if the text contains any specific adverse drug reaction, and output "no" if side effects are mentioned but not specified, or no side effects are mentioned at all. No other outputs are required. Input: {}"

Task_Description_3 = "From the given social media text, determine if there is any reference to adverse drug reactions (negative, harmful consequences from medication use). If a specific adverse drug reaction is mentioned, respond with "yes". If the side effects are not clearly specified or no side effects are discussed, respond with "no". No other output is necessary. Input: {}"

Task_Description_4 = "Your task is to identify whether the following social media post describes any specific adverse drug reactions (undesirable effects from medication). If any specific adverse drug reaction is mentioned, answer with "yes". If no specific side effects are noted or no adverse reactions are mentioned, answer "no". No additional information is needed. Input: {}"

Task_Description_5 = "Analyze the following social media text to check for any adverse drug reactions (harmful effects caused by medication). If a specific adverse drug reaction is mentioned, respond "yes". If side effects are discussed in general or no side effects are mentioned, respond "no". No further details are required. Input: {}"

Task_Description_6 = "Determine whether the given social media text contains any specific adverse drug reactions (harmful outcomes resulting from medication). If a specific adverse reaction is mentioned, respond with "yes". If no specific reactions are discussed or if only general side effects are mentioned, respond with "no". Input: {}"

Task_ Description_ 7 = "In the provided social media text, identify whether any specific adverse drug reactions (unintended, negative effects from medication) are mentioned. If any are present, respond "yes". If side effects are vague or no adverse reactions are referenced, respond "no". No additional response is required. Input: {}"

Task_ Description_ 8 = "Evaluate the following social media text to detect any specific adverse drug reactions (unwanted effects caused by medication). Answer "yes" if a specific adverse reaction is identified. If no specific reactions are mentioned, or side effects are discussed in a general way, answer "no". No further explanation is needed. Input: {}"

Task_ Description_ 9 = "Your task is to determine whether the given social media text contains any specific adverse drug reactions (negative effects of a drug). If a specific adverse reaction is mentioned, respond "yes". If no adverse reactions are specified or if the side effects are general, respond "no". No other details are necessary. Input: {}"

Task_ Description_ 10 = "From the provided social media text, identify whether any specific adverse drug reactions (harmful effects from a medication) are described. If specific adverse reactions are present, answer "yes". If side effects are discussed generally or not mentioned, answer "no". Input: {}"

References

1. Lardon, J., et al.: Evaluating Twitter as a complementary data source for pharmacovigilance. Expert Opinion Drug Saf. **17**(8), 763–774 (2018)
2. Li, Z., et al.: Exploiting adversarial transfer learning for adverse drug reaction detection from texts. J. Biomed. Inform. **106**, 103431 (2020)
3. Sarker, A., Gonzalez, G.: Portable automatic text classification for adverse drug reaction detection via multi-corpus training. J. Biomed. Inform. **53**, 196–207 (2015)
4. Yadav, S., et al.: A unified multi-task adversarial learning framework for pharmacovigilance mining. In: Proceedings of the 57th Annual Meeting of the Association for Computational Linguistics, pp. 5234–5245 (2019)
5. Chowdhury, S., Zhang, C., Yu, P.S.: Multi-task pharmacovigilance mining from social media posts. In: Proceedings of the 2018 World Wide Web Conference, pp. 117–126 (2018)
6. Huang, J.-Y., Lee, W.-P., Lee, K.-D.: Predicting adverse drug reactions from social media posts: data balance, feature selection and deep learning. Healthcare **10**(4), 618. MDPI (2022)
7. Qiu, Y., et al.: Kesdt: knowledge enhanced shallow and deep transformer for detecting adverse drug reactions. In: CCF International Conference on Natural Language Processing and Chinese Computing, pp. 601–613. Springer, Cham (2023)

8. Brown, T.B.: Language models are few-shot learners. arXiv preprint arXiv:2005.14165 (2020)
9. Touvron, H., et al.: Llama: open and efficient foundation language models. arXiv preprint arXiv:2302.13971 (2023)
10. Gao, Y., Ji, S., Marttinen, P.: Knowledge-augmented graph neural networks with concept-aware attention for adverse drug event detection. In: LREC/COLING (2024)
11. Dettmers, T., et al.: QLoRA: efficient finetuning of quantized LLMs. In: Oh, A., et al. (eds.) Advances in Neural Information Processing Systems 36: Annual Conference on Neural Information Processing Systems 2023, NeurIPS 2023, New Orleans, LA, USA, 10–16 December 2023 (2023). http://papers.nips.cc/paper
12. Li, Z., Lin, H., Zheng, W.: An effective emotional expression and knowledge-enhanced method for detecting adverse drug reactions. IEEE Access **8**, 87083–87093 (2020)
13. Shen, C., et al.: Detecting adverse drug reactions from social media based on multi-channel convolutional neural networks. Neural Comput. Appl. **31**, 4799–4808 (2019)
14. Qiu, Y., et al.: SEDGCN: sentiment enhanced dual graph convolutional networks for detecting adverse drug reactions. In: 2023 IEEE International Conference on Bioinformatics and Biomedicine (BIBM). pp. 2183–2186. IEEE (2023)
15. Zhang, T., et al.: Adversarial neural network with sentiment-aware attention for detecting adverse drug reactions. J. Biomed. Inform. **123**, 103896 (2021)
16. Kwak, H., Lee, M., Yoon, S., Chang, J., Park, S., Jung, K.: Drug-disease graph: predicting adverse drug reaction signals via graph neural network with clinical data. In: Lauw, H.W., Wong, R.C.-W., Ntoulas, A., Lim, E.-P., Ng, S.-K., Pan, S.J. (eds.) PAKDD 2020. LNCS (LNAI), vol. 12085, pp. 633–644. Springer, Cham (2020). https://doi.org/10.1007/978-3-030-47436-2_48
17. Shen, C., et al.: GAR: graph adversarial representation for adverse drug event detection on Twitter. Appl. Soft Comput. **106**, 107324 (2021)
18. Gao, Y., et al.: Contextualized graph embeddings for adverse drug event detection. In: Joint European Conference on Machine Learning and Knowledge Discovery in Databases, pp. 605–620. Springer, Cham (2022)
19. Wei, J., et al.: Finetuned language models are zero-shot learners. arXiv preprint arXiv:2109.01652 (2021)
20. Zhao, Z., et al.: Calibrate before use: improving few-shot performance of language models. In: International Conference on Machine Learning, pp. 12697–12706. PMLR (2021)
21. Reynolds, L., McDonell, K.: Prompt programming for large language models: beyond the few-shot paradigm. In: Extended Abstracts of the 2021 CHI Conference on Human Factors in Computing Systems, pp. 1–7 (2021)
22. Sanh, V., et al.: Multitask prompted training enables zero-shot task generalization. arXiv preprint arXiv:2110.08207 (2021)
23. Wang, Y., et al.: Super-natural instructions: generalization via declarative instructions on 1600+ NLP tasks. arXiv preprint arXiv:2204.07705 (2022)
24. Peng, B., et al.: Instruction tuning with GPT-4. arXiv preprint arXiv:2304.03277 (2023)
25. Phang, J., et al.: Hypertuning: toward adapting large language models without back-propagation. In: International Conference on Machine Learning, pp. 27854–27875. PMLR (2023)

26. Alvaro, N., Miyao, Y., Collier, N., et al.: TwiMed: Twitter and PubMed compara-
    ble corpus of drugs, diseases, symptoms, and their relations. JMIR Publ. Health
    Surveill. **3**(2), e6396 (2017)
27. Sarker, A., Nikfarjam, A., Gonzalez, G.: Social media mining shared task workshop.
    In: Biocomputing 2016: Proceedings of the Pacific Symposium, pp. 581–592. World
    Scientific (2016)
28. Karimi, S., et al.: Cadec: a corpus of adverse drug event annotations. J. Biomed.
    Inform. **55**, 73–81 (2015)
29. Magge, A., et al.: Overview of the sixth social media mining for health applications
    (# SMM4H) shared tasks at NAACL 2021. In: Proceedings of the Sixth Social
    Media Mining for Health (# SMM4H) Workshop and Shared Task, pp. 21–32
    (2021)

Deep Fusion Network with Feature Engineering for Discharge Risk Assessment

Leyan Wang[1(✉)], Runzhi Li[2], Shuo Wang[1], Siyu Yan[3], Lihong Ma[3], and Yunli Xing[4]

[1] School of Computer and Artificial Intelligence, Zhengzhou University, Zhengzhou, China
leyanw@gs.zzu.edu.cn
[2] Cooperative Innovation Center of Internet Healthcare, Zhengzhou University, Zhengzhou, China
rzli@ha.edu.cn
[3] Fuwai Hospital, National Center for Cardiovascular Diseases, Chinese Academy of Medical Sciences and Peking Union Medical College San Antonio, Beijing, China
[4] Department of Geriatrics, Beijing Friendship Hospital, Capital Medical University, Beijing, People's Republic of China

Abstract. Assessing discharge conditions for elderly coronary patients, especially those with serious or complex disease symptoms, is a crucial task for physicians. Clinical evaluations need to consider demographic information, physiological monitoring, diagnoses, and vital signs, which are multi-dimensional, multi-source, and heterogeneous data. While machine learning models can predict discharge risk based on these data, challenges remain in dealing with redundant features and extracting key features to enhance prediction performance.

In this work, we restructured patients' comprehensive characteristics into a data sequence according to multiple vital clinical stages. Through feature engineering, we constructed steady-state indexes (SSIs), which are generated features that track the patient's condition changes and the stability of vital signs. Additionally, we standardized variable-length biochemical test data to a fixed-length to address the issue of inconsistent data lengths. Then, we proposed a two-stage multi-module deep fusion network for discharge risk assessment. In the first stage, the data was divided into modules and we extracted features from biochemical test data, SSIs, and comprehensive clinical data using a transformer encoder, CNN, and BiLSTM, respectively. In the second stage, we designed a dual-layer attention fusion network, where dual pooling channel attention was applied to biochemical test data to capture more relevant relationships for discharge results, and sparse attention combining local and simple global information was used on aggregated features to reduce computational complexity.

Experiments were conducted on datasets collected from three local 3A hospitals, and the results demonstrated that our method outperformed other methods in the evaluated metrics. Ablation experiments further verified the benefits of segmenting different types or sources of data into different modules for clinical data analysis.

© The Author(s), under exclusive license to Springer Nature Singapore Pte Ltd. 2025
Y. Zhang et al. (Eds.): CHIP 2024, CCIS 2433, pp. 21–36, 2025.
https://doi.org/10.1007/978-981-96-3752-2_2

Keywords: Deep fusion network · Discharge risk assessment · Feature engineering · Steady-state indexes

1   Introduction

In recent years, the issue of population ageing has become increasingly severe [5], with Coronary Heart Disease (CHD) posing a major threat among the elderly population. The successful management of elderly CHD patients includes not only timely and effective interventions during hospitalization but also a comprehensive assessment of risk factors before discharge. The purpose of this assessment is to predict the extent of discharge risk and prognosis of the patients, thereby providing a basis for clinical decision-making.

Currently, disease risk assessment has gradually shifted from traditional statistical analysis [3] and rule-based models [20] to leveraging machine learning techniques, such as Multilayer Perceptron (MLP) [19], Logistic Regression [1], Random Forest (RF) [23], and deep learning technologies including Convolutional Neural Networks (CNN) [17], Long Short-Term Memory Networks (LSTM) [25], and Recurrent Neural Networks (RNN) [8]. These technologies have shown their prowess not only in general risk assessments but also in specific disease risk assessments, particularly in the discharge risk evaluation for elderly CHD patients, where they offer substantial potential and value. Discharge risk assessment for elderly patients with CHD is significantly supported by risk factor analysis and post-discharge risk monitoring. Risk factor analysis aids in identifying characteristics that substantially impact CHD. For instance, Malakar, A.K., et al. [16] have conducted a comprehensive review of CHD-related risk factors, and El-Bialy, et al. [4] have analyzed important features within CHD datasets. These studies have greatly advanced our ability to accurately evaluate the discharge risks for CHD patients. Post-discharge risk monitoring focuses on predicting the risk of patient readmission or other adverse health outcomes, enabling us to analyze risk factors based on post-discharge conditions and construct predictive models. For example, Li, Y., et al. [11] investigated the readmission of CHD patients within one year after discharge, using Logistic regression to analyze risk factors and build a predictive model. Xi Rui han [18], through a literature review, identified key factors affecting the onset of frailty in patients after discharge from CHD and developed a nomogram risk prediction model for patient risk prediction.

Although the analysis of risk factors and post-discharge risk monitoring have propelled the development of discharge risk assessment for CHD patients, there are still deficiencies in this area of research. Current research often focuses on a few known risk factors, neglecting the diversity of data sources. Additionally, existing evaluation processes frequently overlook the dynamic fluctuations in patients' physiological indicators, disregarding the significance of these indicators' stability for discharge risk assessment. Moreover, combining medical knowledge with clinical data can uncover deeper implicit information in the data, which can improve the accuracy and interpretability of the assessment, but research in this area is still far from adequate.

To overcome the limitations of existing research, this study selects multi-source data that significantly impacts the discharge risk assessment of elderly patients with CHD. By feature engineering [2], we construct steady-state indexes and process biochemical test data to a fixed length, achieving stability assessment and integrating medical prior knowledge. Employing a multi-module strategy, we segment the data into three modules and apply Bi-directional Long Short-Term Memory (BiLSTM), CNN, and Transformer Encoder to extract features. Features are then fused using an enhanced dual-layer attention network, yielding the output through a fully connected layer. We summarize the contributions as follows:

1. We propose a two-stage deep fusion network that includes feature extraction and feature fusion. During feature extraction, data is modularized based on its source and type to accomplish modular feature extraction. In the feature fusion stage, a dual-layer attention fusion network is designed for intra-module and inter-module feature fusion.
2. In the preprocessing, we utilize feature engineering to generate steady-state indexes and fixed-length biochemical test data. Steady-state indexes represent the changes in a patient's condition and the stability of vital signs. Transforming variable-length biochemical test data into a fixed-length not only solves the problem of inconsistent data lengths but also incorporates medical prior knowledge.
3. We construct a local dataset from three 3A hospitals, in which we finish the reconstruction of patients' comprehensive characteristics in a data queue by multiple vital clinical stages.

2 Feature Engineering

2.1 Construction of Steady-State Indexes

During discharge risk assessment, the changes in the patient's condition throughout the disease often serve as a crucial basis for medical decision-making by physicians. To intuitively evaluate these variations, we have introduced the novel concept of the "steady-state index." We have developed a function known as $f(\cdot)$ that generates these steady-state indexes, which takes as input a feature matrix 'x' composed of clinical data from various time points. The output of $f(\cdot)$ is the steady-state index, providing a metric for the patient's condition stability. Among clinical indicators, the return to and maintenance of normal ranges for vital signs, such as body temperature and blood pressure, as well as the relief or disappearance of clinical symptoms, are key points when physicians assess the discharge risk. Based on this practical basis, we select corresponding indicators and construct steady-state indexes according to the type of data. For symptoms described textually, like headache and nausea, we convert them into binary data indicating presence or absence and establish rules for generating an n-level stability index. For continuous data like body temperature, we calculate the variance to assess the stability of the patient's condition.

Textual Data. For textual descriptive data, we first discretize it, and then obtain the corresponding discrete values according to different stages such as stage 1, stage 2, stage 3, etc. As depicted in Fig. 1, these discrete values are taken as a set of input data $X = [X_{S1}, X_{S2}, X_{S3}, \ldots, X_{Sn}]$, which are input into the n-level steady-state index generation function $f(\cdot)$. The function $f(\cdot)$ is formulated based on the experience of doctors in judging the stability of a patient's condition, and its output y represents the stability of the input features.

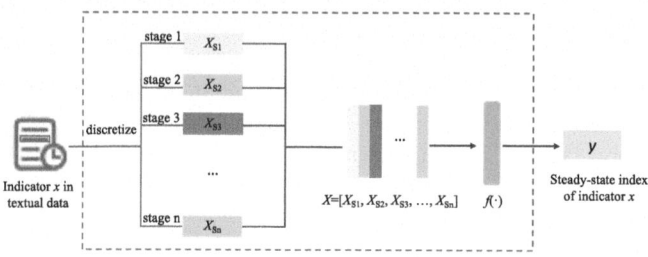

Fig. 1. The flowchart on generating of steady-state index for textual data

In our work, we have converted features such as clinical symptoms, consciousness state, and clinical signs from a descriptive text format into binary discrete data. We use '1' to indicate symptom presence, '0' to indicate absence and have formulated a steady-state indicator generation function $f(\cdot)$ as shown in Eq. 1 to construct a three-level stability index. In Eq. 1, X_{S_1} represents the value of the admission stage, X_{S_n} represents the value of the discharge stage, and $X_{S_{n-1}}$ represents the value of the stage immediately preceding discharge. When the state of both the discharge stage and the stage before discharge are asymptomatic, the steady-state index value is set to 3, which is relatively stable. When admission stage is asymptomatic, and the state values of either the discharge stage or the stage before discharge show symptoms, the steady-state index value is set to 1, which is relatively unstable. In other cases, the steady-state index takes a value of 2, which is relatively stable. A higher index indicates greater stability and a lower discharge risk.

$$f(\cdot) = \begin{cases} 3 & \text{if } X_{S_{n-1}} = 0 \text{ and } X_{S_n} = 0 \\ 1 & \text{if } X_{S_1} = 0 \text{ and } (X_{S_{n-1}} = 1 \text{ or } X_{S_n} = 1) \\ 2 & \text{else} \end{cases} \tag{1}$$

Continuous Data. For continuous data like body temperature and blood pressure, we calculate variance to generate steady-state indexes. By calculating the variance of multiple measurements of a patient's examination indicator, we can gain an intuitive understanding of the fluctuation of the examination data in relation to the μ. In Eq. 2, x_i represents the value of indicator x during the i-th inspection, n represents the number of inspections, μ represents the medical expected value, and the variance obtained, denoted as σ^2, is the steady-state index for the indicator x. When the variance is small, it indicates that the difference between the indicator and the μ is minor and the patient is in a relatively stable state. Conversely, when the variance is large, it suggests that the patient's examination data for this indicator are scattered, which may imply some unstable factors or potential health risks. This steady-state index helps physicians assess the patient's health status more accurately and adjust treatment plans promptly.

$$\sigma^2 = \frac{1}{n} \sum_{i=1}^{n} (x_i - \mu)^2 \tag{2}$$

2.2   Fixed-Length Processing for Biochemical Test Data

During the patient's hospitalization, the number of biochemical tests varies depending on the severity of their condition and postoperative recovery, resulting in variable-length biochemical test data. To address this, we use an innovative method of feature engineering to standardize this data into a fixed-length format. First, we calculate the maximum, minimum, and average values across the multiple data. Then, we qualitatively assess and categorize these values as 'up' for above standard range, 'down' for below standard range, and 'normal' for within the standard range. We then use One-Hot encoding to represent these categories and finally get a 3×4 fixed-length dataset. The calculated value is one-dimensional, and the tags are three-dimensional, making a total of four dimensions.

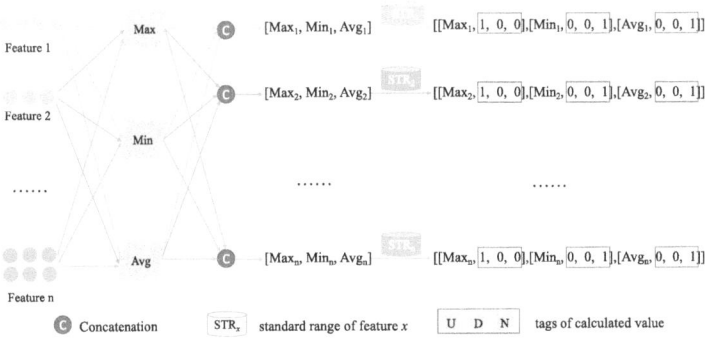

Fig. 2. This is the fixed-length processing for biochemical test data. We first compute the maximum, minimum, and average values across the multiple data. Next, the calculated values are concatenated and compared with the standard ranges (STR) of corresponding features to obtain qualitative analysis results of 'up', 'down', and 'normal'. To represent these categories, we apply One-Hot encoding, assigning a unique code to each. Ultimately, we obtain a 3×4 fixed-length dataset.

Figure 2 illustrates the process of converting variable-length data into fixed-length data. We begin by calculating the maximum value(V_{Max}), minimum value(V_{Min}), and average value(V_{Avg}) for each feature, and concatenate them to obtain [V_{Max}, V_{Min}, V_{Avg}] as preliminary fixed-length data. Then, we perform a qualitative analysis, comparing each of these values to the standard range for the feature. Depending on these comparisons and using One-Hot encoding, the tags up, down, and normal are assigned accordingly, culminating in the creation of structured fixed-length dataset. Assuming Feature 1's V_{Max1} surpasses the standard range while both the V_{Min1} and V_{Avg1} remain within it. Then, the V_{Max1} is labeled as [1, 0, 0], and both the V_{Min1} and V_{Avg1} are labeled as [0, 0, 1]. Finally, we transform the four data points for Feature 1 into a 3×4 fixed-length format like [[V_{Max1},1,0,0],[V_{Min1},0,0,1],[V_{Avg1},0,0,1]].

3   Method

We propose a deep fusion network for discharge risk assessment, in which we divide features into modules for feature extraction and then fuse features by dual-layer attention network. The overall architecture is shown in Fig. 3. Firstly, based on feature engineering, we generate steady-state indexes and finish fixed-length processing for biochemical test data. Secondly, There are three modules for feature extraction, consisting of BiLSTM for the comprehensive clinical data, CNN for state-steady indexes, and transformer encoder for biochemical test data. In the dual-layer attention fusion network, one is a dual-pooling channel attention mechanism for biochemical test data. The other is the sparse attention combining local and simple global information for all the integrated features. Finally, a fully connected layer is employed to produce the predicted output.

3.1   BiLSTM for the Comprehensive Clinical Data

The comprehensive clinical data provides a detailed record, detailing their initial condition and all subsequent diagnoses and treatments during hospitalization. To analyze the intricate patterns and interdependencies within this extensive data, we have chosen the BiLSTM [9]. It processes both forward and backward information of the input data simultaneously and concatenates or merges the obtained forward and backward hidden information as feature representation, thereby capturing global dependencies in the sequence. This bidirectional analysis significantly enhances the model's depth of understanding, yielding a richer and more nuanced set of features, which helps the model perform the discharge assessment task more effectively.

3.2   CNN for Steady-State Indexes

In the process of feature extraction for steady-state indexes, we skillfully harness the power of CNN and introduce an innovative layer known as learned_Softmax which is used to dynamically weight and fuse multi-scale convolutional features.

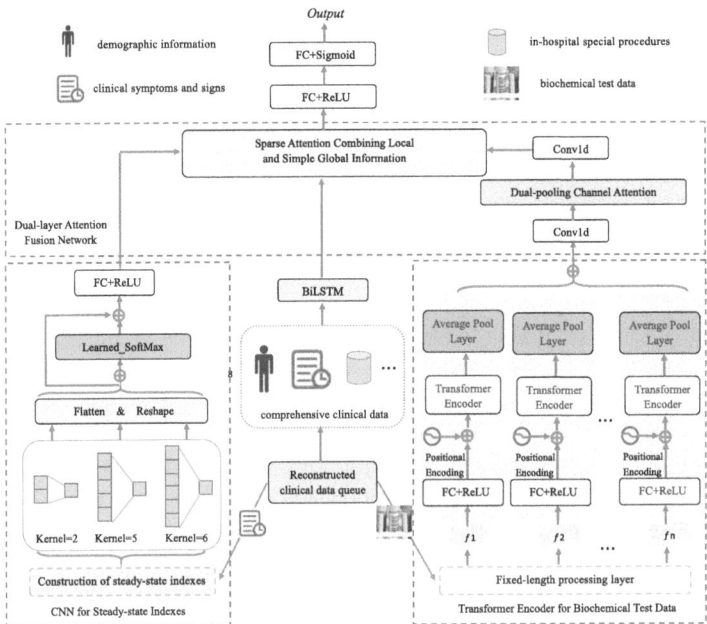

Fig. 3. We propose a multi-module feature extraction with dual-layer attention fusion deep architecture for discharge risk assessment. We select certain features from the reconstructed clinical data queue and generate steady-state indexes and fixed-length biochemical test data using specialized processing layers. Then we divide the data into three modules based on its source and type and design different methods for feature extraction. These features are fed into a dual-layer attention fusion network, culminating in outputs from a fully connected layer.

This layer normalizes the trainable weights W_s through the softmax function, thereby amplifying their impact and achieving dynamic weighting of features. Initially, we capture a variety of features from the input data using three 1D convolution kernels of varying sizes. The network's nonlinear capabilities are then boosted with the Rectified Linear Unit (ReLU) activation function. Then the extracted features are flattened, reshaped, and concatenated to form a comprehensive feature matrix. Following this, the learned_Softmax layer applies the softmax-normalized weights to fuse the concatenated features, which significantly enhances the model's adaptability to the input data. The fused features, now weighted, are added back to the original features and processed through a fully connected layer to produce the output. This design fully exploits the information in the original features and, through the dynamic weighting by the learned_Softmax layer, enriches the hierarchy and depth of the features, providing robust support for subsequent discharge risk assessments.

3.3   Transformer Encoder for Biochemical Test Data

Through feature engineering, we transform each variable-length sequence of biochemical test data into a 3×4 matrix as the input feature. For multiple biochemical test items, we construct a multi-channel [10] feature extraction framework. Each channel corresponds to a feature, and the channels are independent of each other. For each channel internally, the Encoder part in the Transformer [21] is used for extraction, fully exploring the correlation information between different nodes within each feature and maximizing the retention of the feature representation. The feature extraction process is as follows, where d_i represents the embedding dimension of this feature.

Firstly, the fixed-length biochemical test data within a channel is enhanced by a fully connected layer and ReLU activation function, resulting in the feature sequence representation E_i. Then, sequence position information is embedded using trigonometric position encoding [6]. Here, pos is the sequence position, i is the embedding dimension, P is the position encoding matrix, and P^i is the matrix after adding position data. The formulas are shown in (3) to (5).

$$PE(pos, 2i) = \sin(pos/1000^{2i/d_{\text{model}}}) \tag{3}$$

$$PE(pos, 2i + 1) = \cos(pos/1000^{2i/d_{\text{model}}}) \tag{4}$$

$$P^i = P + E^i \tag{5}$$

Subsequently, the obtained matrix P^i is fed into the Encoder for feature extraction, utilizing a multi-head self-attention mechanism [24] to capture the inter-node information. After generating the output M_i, P^i is subsequently incorporated and subjected to normalization through the method of layer normalization [14]. Then the normalized M_i' is fed into a feedforward neural network, goes through a fully connected layer, ReLU activation function and layer normalization to obtain one layer of Encoder output $\overline{M}_i$. The formulas are as follows.

$$M_i' = LayerNormalizantion(M_i + P^i) \tag{6}$$

$$\widetilde{M}_i = \text{ReLU}\,(M_i' W_1 + b_1)W_2 + b_2 \tag{7}$$

$$\overline{M}_i = LayerNormalizantion(M_i' + \widetilde{M}_i) \tag{8}$$

The above is a processing method inside an Encoder, which can extract deeper features of the patient by stacking multiple Encoders to obtain the final output M^{final}, then perform average pooling on the node dimension to obtain the characterization of the biochemical test data.

3.4   Dual-Layer Attention Fusion Network

Dual-Pooling Channel Attention. Based on a multi-channel feature extraction strategy and the assessment of feature importance, the initial layer employs a dual-pooling channel attention mechanism for biochemical features, as depicted in Fig. 4. This framework combines global average pooling with global maximum pooling, enabling the model to analyze data characteristics from various angles. The pooled features are then concatenated, passed through a sequence of fully connected layers, and merged with the original input to generate the final output. To enhance the model's generalization capability and reduce parameter count, a parameter called *reduction_ratio* is introduced in the fully connected layer, and set to 4 in the experiment based on experimental results and accumulated experience. This ensures that while reducing parameters and computational load, essential information is preserved. Furthermore, the feature representation is enhanced by applying 1D convolutional layers before and after the dual-pooling channel attention, which enriches and refines the features.

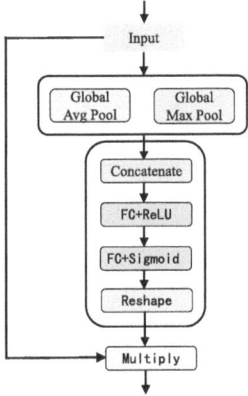

Fig. 4. Dual-pooling Channel Attention Fusion Module

Sparse Attention Combing Local and Simple Global Information. Traditional attention mechanisms often suffer from high computational complexity and poor interpretability. To tackle these issues, we have taken inspiration from sparse attention mechanisms [7], integrating both local and simple global information, as shown in Fig. 5. When calculating local information, we perform a linear transformation on the input tensor using parameters W_q, W_k, and W_v to generate queries (Q), keys (K), and values (V). Then, the dot product of Q and K is used to measure the local similarity in the sequence. The larger the dot product value, the higher the similarity between certain parts of the input sequence and the query vector, thus achieving local attention. Subsequently, a threshold-based sparsification operation is performed on the local weight matrix, preserving important local correlations and ultimately obtaining local information A_local. As for global information, this paper adopts the method of calculating the average of Q to capture simple global context information. Then, Combine them and multiply them with the value V to obtain the final output. By integrating dot product similarity with average background knowledge, our method achieves a robust feature representation. This approach not only improves computational efficiency but also enhances the interpretability of the attention mechanism.

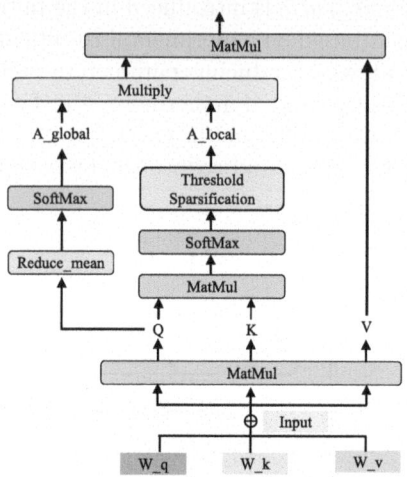

Fig. 5. Sparse Attention Mechanism Combining Local and Simple Global Information

4   Experiments

4.1   Dateset

The experimental dataset is collected from three local 3A hospitals, focusing on the elderly population suffering from coronary heart disease. With the guidance of medical experts, we select 148 key features that are significantly correlated with the assessment of post-discharge risks, constructing a comprehensive dataset. This dataset includes the full cycle of diagnostic data from admission to discharge, as well as prognostic feedback from a subsequent period, thereby capturing the physiological status and health indicators of patients at various time stages.

Specifically, we reconstruct the clinical data queue according to multiple vital clinical stages from 1007 elderly patients with coronary heart disease. It includes crucial information for clinical decision-making, such as patient's gender, age [13], medical history, and other admission details, as well as in-hospital data like biochemical tests and special procedures. Furthermore, the dataset encompasses detailed discharge information, including diagnoses and symptoms. It also extends to comprehensive follow-up data, tracking occurrences of adverse events, deaths, and instances of re-admission. In the reconstructed clinical data queue, we choose 93 features such as demographics, clinical symptoms and signs, and in-hospital special procedures as comprehensive clinical data. Based on feature engineering, we select clinical symptoms and signs to generate 43-dimensional steady-state indexes and transform 14 types of variable-length biochemical test data into 168-dimensional fixed-length data. Ultimately, we form a 304-dimensional, patient-centered, timeline-based, multi-source heterogeneous [22], and multidimensional clinical dataset. Additionally, the target variable in our experiment is the discharge risk, which is derived from the follow-up records that include adverse events, deaths, and re-admissions, categorized into two types: risk-free and risky. It is noteworthy that the proportion of risk-free cases is significantly higher than that of risky cases, with a ratio of 8:1.

4.2 Experimental Settings

In the process of discharge risk assessment, we select certain specific features and generate steady-state indexes and fixed-length biochemical test data through feature engineering. Based on the data's source and type, we segment the data into three modules and design different methods for feature extraction. Module 1(M1) employs the BiLSTM to extract features across the comprehensive clinical data, Module 2 (M2) utilizes the CNN to process features from steady-state indexes, and Module 3 (M3) applies the Transformer Encoder to feature extraction on fixed-length biochemical test data. Subsequently, we employ a dual-layer attention fusion network for feature integration. The first layer utilizes a dual-pooling channel attention mechanism (DCAM) to fuse the biochemical test data, and we apply the 1D conventional layer before and after the DCAM to enrich and refine the features. The second layer conducts the sparse attention mechanism that combines local and simple global information (LGSPAM) on the modular data.

During data processing, an 8:2 ratio is used to divide the training set and test set, and training is conducted using a five-fold cross-validation method [15]. Encountering imbalanced data issues, we use the stratify parameter during data partitioning to maintain a consistent ratio of positive and negative samples. The experiment selects the Adam optimizer, sets the learning rate to 0.001, uses mini-batch gradient descent with a sample size of 32 for each iteration, and sets the number of training rounds to 150. Additionally, five evaluation metrics are selected to assess the model: accuracy (Acc), precision (P), recall (R), F1 score (F), and the area under the ROC curve (AUC).

4.3 Results and Analysis

Comparison Experiments. To demonstrate the superiority of our proposed model, we select four deep learning models, namely BiLSTM, CNN, Gate Recurrent Unit (GRU), Transformer Encoder, as well as a Random Forest (RF) model, for comparative experiments. All four deep learning models employ multi-head attention mechanisms (MHAM) for feature fusion. The results of these comparative experiments are presented in Table 1, highlighting the strengths of our model.

Table 1. Results of the Comparison Experiments

Model	Acc	P	R	AUC	F
BiLSTM	0.931	0.700	0.636	0.828	0.67
CNN	0.941	0.813	0.591	0.884	0.68
GRU	0.941	0.750	0.682	0.866	0.71
Transformer Encoder	0.931	0.654	0.773	0.886	0.71
RF	0.916	0.957	0.614	0.885	0.74
Our model	0.965	0.941	0.727	0.855	0.82

The data presented in Table 1 reveals that all four deep learning approaches achieved commendable accuracy. However, the CNN method had a significantly low recall, scoring only 0.591. While the Transformer Encoder method boasted a high recall, it achieved the lowest precision. Both the BiLSTM and GRU methods performed well across all evaluation metrics, yet they did not match our model's performance in terms of accuracy, precision, and recall. In the application of a random forest for discharge risk assessment, precision reached its peak. However, the method was hindered by a low recall rate. Additionally, the model's accuracy, at 91.6%, did not meet expectations. In contrast, our model excelled with an accuracy rate of 96.5%, the highest among all models. It also scored high in both precision and recall, achieving a remarkable balance between the two. Upon reviewing all metrics, our model's superior performance in discharge risk assessment is evident. However, we also found some issues. Although our model's recall rate is second-highest at 0.727 among all models, it still leaves room for enhancement. In future work, we will continue to explore small sample and adaptive learning, researching different model adjustments and data augmentation techniques to improve the model's recall rate while maintaining precision and accuracy.

The Ablation Study of Modules. In the experimental process, we generate steady-state indexes and fixed-length biochemical test data. Then we segment the data into three modules based on its source and type, and adopt different feature extraction methods for modular feature extraction. To elucidate the distinct contributions of each module and to showcase the merits of our dual-layer attention fusion network, we undertake a series of ablation studies. The first group uses M1 as the basic control, employing the MHAM for feature fusion. The second group utilizes M1 and M2 to explore the role of M2, with the fusion method remaining unchanged. The third group combines all three modules, still using the MHAM for fusion. The fourth group changes the feature fusion method of the third group to the dual-layer attention fusion network.

Table 2 records the outcomes of these ablation studies. The analysis of Experiment 1 and Experiment 2 indicates that the introduction of steady-state indexes significantly improved the model's precision by 7.8% and recall by 4.6%. Exper-

Table 2. Experimental Results of Ablation Study on Modules

Module	Feature Fusion	Acc	P	R	AUC	F
M1	MHAM	0.921	0.636	0.636	0.885	0.64
M1 M2	MHAM	0.936	0.714	0.682	0.909	0.70
M1 M2 M3	MHAM	0.946	0.790	0.682	0.902	0.73
M1 M2 M3	DCAM LGSPAM	0.965	0.941	0.727	0.855	0.82

iment 3, which included fixed-length biochemical test data, further enhanced precision by 7.6%, raising the model's accuracy to 94.6% while other metrics remained stable. Experiment 4 achieved the highest scores in accuracy, precision, recall, and F1 scores by employing a dual-layer attention fusion network for feature integration. The analysis reveals that M2 and M3 excavate more complex and comprehensive feature information by establishing associations across multiple stages and incorporating medical prior knowledge through tagging. The dual-layer attention fusion network first retains key feature information and then fuses it with all features to refine critical information, enabling the model to perform more accurate risk assessments. Each module contributes to the model's outstanding performance in the discharge assessment task for elderly patients with coronary heart disease.

Interpretability of Steady-State Indexes Generation and Fixed-Length Processing. In our study, we design a series of meticulous operations to ensure the interpretability of data processing. First, we select clinical symptoms, vital signs, and functional scores as features and combine them with the admission and discharge stages to construct the steady-state indexes. These indexes reflect the comprehensive evaluation that doctors conduct to assess a patient's health status over time, providing a holistic view of the patient's condition and treatment progress. Next, to address the issue of variable-length biochemical test data, we employ feature engineering to transform it into fixed-length data. During this process, we consider not only the statistical properties of the data but also integrate prior medical knowledge. This standardization is akin to how doctors organize and interpret test results to identify patterns and make informed judgments about a patient's biochemical health. Both operations are designed to distill complex medical data into a form that is not only analytically robust but also transparent and understandable.

Interpretability of Dual-Layer Attention Fusion Network. This study introduces a dual-layer attention fusion network to enhance the interpretability and predictive performance of medical data. Initially, we utilize a random forest to assess the feature importance within the dataset. We rank the features from high to low based on their importance scores and find that biochemical test data accounted for 80% of the top 20% of features. This discovery has made us fully aware of the significant role that biochemical test data plays in the assessment of discharge risks. Leveraging this insight, we embed an innovative DCAM in the network's first layer, tailored for the multi-channel characteristics of biochemical test data. And we apply the 1D conventional layer before and after the DCAM to enrich and refine the features. In the network's second layer, we implement an LGSPAM, facilitating feature fusion across diverse data sources.

Table 3. Contributions of Each Layer of the Dual-layer Attention Network

Feature Fusion	Acc	P	R	AUC	F
MHAM	0.946	0.790	0.682	0.902	0.73
DCAM MHAM	0.951	0.833	0.682	0.895	0.75
DCAM LGSPAM	0.965	0.941	0.727	0.855	0.82

Table 3 represents the impact of each attention layer on the model's evaluative efficacy. When adding the DCAM for feature fusion in biochemical features, combining different pooling operations makes the model more flexible in learning and utilizing the relationships between features, resulting in a 4.3% increase in precision. After replacing the MHAM with LGSPAM, we achieved a significant improvement, with precision rising by 10.8% and accuracy peaking at 96.5%. This is because there is a strong correlation between input features, such as using the reconstructed clinical data queue to generate steady-state indexes. The LGSPAM can better capture this correlation information, reduce the introduction of redundant information, and improve fusion efficiency. By analyzing the results in Table 3, we confirm that each layer of the dual-layer attention fusion network contributes to enhancing the model's performance in risk assessment.

5   Conclusion

This study aims to address the discharge risk assessment issues for patients. Based on feature engineering, we have generated steady-state indexes representing the stability of patients' vital signs and transformed the biochemical test data into fixed-length. We construct a multi-module feature extraction prediction model with dual-layer attention fusion, which has achieved outstanding performance in assessing discharge risks, specifically demonstrated by high accuracy and precision rates. Notably, the dual-layer attention fusion network module we designed not only conducts in-depth feature extraction for features strongly related to discharge results but also reduces computational complexity. Despite making some progress, the study still has limitations and room for improvement. For example, considering the difficulty in acquiring medical data and the imbalance issue in the dataset used in this study, we will continue to explore few-shot learning to enhance the model's generalizability. Furthermore, we anticipate that future research will integrate multi-modal information [12], including images and audio, which will help to further enhance the accuracy and practicality of the model. We believe that these efforts will have a more profound impact on research in the fields of medicine and health.

Acknowledgments. This work was supported in part by National Science and Technology Major Project under Grant No. 2021ZD0111000, in part by the Science and Technology Project of Henan Province under Grant No. 232102311232.

References

1. Bao, N., et al.: A risk prediction model for hemorrhagic events in elderly patients with coronary artery disease and malignant gastrointestinal tumors. Circulation **140**(Suppl_1), A9556–A9556 (2019)
2. Chicco, D., Oneto, L., Tavazzi, E.: Eleven quick tips for data cleaning and feature engineering. PLoS Comput. Biol. **18**(12), e1010718 (2022)
3. Choi, S.G., et al.: Comparisons of the prediction models for undiagnosed diabetes between machine learning versus traditional statistical methods. Sci. Rep. **13**(1), 13101 (2023)
4. El-Bialy, R., Salamay, M.A., Karam, O.H., Khalifa, M.E.: Feature analysis of coronary artery heart disease data sets. Procedia Comput. Sci. **65**, 459–468 (2015)
5. Feng, Z., et al.: Long-term care system for older adults in china: policy landscape, challenges, and future prospects. Lancet **396**(10259), 1362–1372 (2020)
6. Gehring, J., Auli, M., Grangier, D., Yarats, D., Dauphin, Y.N.: Convolutional sequence to sequence learning. In: International Conference on Machine Learning, pp. 1243–1252. PMLR (2017)
7. Jiang, Q., Bao, B., Hou, X., Huang, A., Jiang, J., Mao, Z.: Feature mining and sensitivity analysis with adaptive sparse attention for bearing fault diagnosis. Appl. Sci. **13**(2), 718 (2023)
8. Li, D., Lyons, P., Klaus, J., Gage, B., Kollef, M., Lu, C.: Integrating static and time-series data in deep recurrent models for oncology early warning systems. In: Proceedings of the 30th ACM International Conference on Information and Knowledge Management, pp. 913–936 (2021)
9. Li, F., et al.: Medium-term load forecasting of power system based on BiLSTM and parallel feature extraction network. IET Gener. Transm. Distrib. **18**(1), 190–201 (2024)
10. Li, P., Wang, Q.: A multichannel model for microbial key event extraction based on feature fusion and attention mechanism. Secur. Commun. Netw. (2021). https://api.semanticscholar.org/CorpusID:245619777
11. Li, Y.L., et al.: A readmission risk prediction model for elderly patients with coronary heart disease. J. Clin. Nurs. Res. **6**(2), 126–133 (2022)
12. Liu, H., Shi, Y., Li, A., Wang, M.: Multi-modal fusion network with intra-and inter-modality attention for prognosis prediction in breast cancer. Comput. Biol. Med. **168**, 107796 (2024)
13. Liu, K., Chen, Y., Lin, R., Han, K.: Clinical features of COVID-19 in elderly patients: a comparison with young and middle-aged patients. J. Infect. **80**(6), e14–e18 (2020)
14. Liu, T., Zhang, P., Huang, W., Zha, Y., You, T., Zhang, Y.: How does layer normalization improve batch normalization in self-supervised sound source localization? Neurocomputing **567**, 127040 (2024)

15. Mahesh, T., Geman, O., Margala, M., Guduri, M., et al.: The stratified k-folds cross-validation and class-balancing methods with high-performance ensemble classifiers for breast cancer classification. Healthc. Anal. **4**, 100247 (2023)

16. Malakar, A.K., Choudhury, D., Halder, B., Paul, P., Uddin, A., Chakraborty, S.: A review on coronary artery disease, its risk factors, and therapeutics. J. Cell. Physiol. **234**(10), 16812–16823 (2019)

17. Morid, M.A., Sheng, O.R.L., Kawamoto, K., Abdelrahman, S.: Learning hidden patterns from patient multivariate time series data using convolutional neural networks: a case study of healthcare cost prediction. J. Biomed. Inform. **111**, 103565 (2020)

18. Ruihan, X.: Developing a risk prediction model for frailty among coronary heart disease patients after discharge (2024)

19. Song, X., et al.: Predicting 7-day unplanned readmission in elderly patients with coronary heart disease using machine learning. Front. Cardiovascu. Med. **10** (2023)

20. Staff, P.O.: Correction: a rule-based prognostic model for type 1 diabetes by identifying and synthesizing baseline profile patterns. PLoS ONE **9**(9), e109514 (2014)

21. Vaswani, A., et al.: Attention is all you need. In: Advances in Neural Information Processing Systems, vol. 30 (2017)

22. Wang, M., et al.: Big data health care platform with multisource heterogeneous data integration and massive high-dimensional data governance for large hospitals: design, development, and application. JMIR Med. Inform. **10**(4), e36481 (2022)

23. Xu, Q., Peng, Y., Tan, J., Zhao, W., Yang, M., Tian, J.: Prediction of atrial fibrillation in hospitalized elderly patients with coronary heart disease and type 2 diabetes mellitus using machine learning: a multicenter retrospective study. Front. Publ. Health **10**, 842104 (2022)

24. Yao, L., Liu, L.: Air quality index prediction model integrating multi-head self-attention mechanism. In: 5th International Conference on Information Science, Electrical, and Automation Engineering (ISEAE 2023), vol. 12748, pp. 289–295. SPIE (2023)

25. Zhao, A., Qi, L., Dong, J., Yu, H.: Dual channel LSTM based multi-feature extraction in gait for diagnosis of neurodegenerative diseases. Knowl.-Based Syst. **145**, 91–97 (2018)

Analysis of Risk Factors for Hemorrhagic Complications in Pediatric Acute Liver Failure

Qiang Xiong[1], Li Xiao[2(✉)], Ruijue Wang[1,3], Wenlong Li[4], Songhua Hu[5], Qinshi Hu[2], Zhuangcheng Wang[3], and Ximing Xu[2]

[1] Department of Hepatobiliary Surgery, Children's Hospital of Chongqing Medical University, National Clinical Research Center for Child Health and Disorders, Ministry of Education Key Laboratory of Child Development and Disorders, Chongqing Key Laboratory of Pediatrics, Chongqing, China
[2] Big Data Engineering Center, Children's Hospital of Chongqing Medical University, National Clinical Research Center for Child Health and Disorders, Ministry of Education Key Laboratory of Child Development and Disorders, Chongqing, China
feeceebee@hospital.cqmu.edu.cn
[3] Department of Pediatric Surgery, Yibin Hospital Affiliated to Children's Hospital of Chongqing Medical University, Chongqing, China
[4] Department of Epidemiology and Health Statistics, School of Public Health, Chongqing Medical University, Yixue Road, Chongqing 400016, China
[5] Department of Epidemiology and Health Statistics, School of Public Health, Wannan Medical College, Wuhu, China

Abstract. Objective: To analyze the clinical data of children with acute liver failure to identify risk factors for hemorrhagic complications, thereby providing a basis for clinical diagnosis and treatment decisions in pediatric acute liver failure (PALF). Methods: Clinical data from children diagnosed with acute liver failure and hospitalized at the Children's Hospital affiliated with Chongqing Medical University from January 2014 to June 2024 were collected. Data included general information, laboratory indicators, and hemorrhagic complications. Patients were categorized into hemorrhagic and non-hemorrhagic complication groups for comparative analysis. Results: A total of 663 cases were analyzed, with 239 cases (36.05%) having hemorrhagic complications and 424 cases (63.95%) without. Only 21 cases (3.17%) had spontaneous bleeding. Multivariate analysis identified infection ($OR = 4.05$, 95%CI: 2.47~6.64, $p < 0.001$), hepatorenal syndrome (HRS) ($OR = 2.95$, 95%CI: 1.82~4.77, $p < 0.001$), multiple organ dysfunction syndrome (MODS) ($OR = 2.47$, 95%CI: 1.57~3.88, $p < 0.001$), low platelet count ($\leq 50 \times 10\text{^}9/L$) ($OR = 2.51$, 95%CI: 1.58~3.99, $p < 0.001$), and low fibrinogen (≤ 1 mg/dL) ($OR = 1.73$, 95%CI: 1.12~2.69, $p = 0.014$) as independent risk factors for hemorrhagic complications in children with acute liver failure. Conclusion: Spontaneous bleeding in PALF is relatively rare, with infection, HRS, MODS, thrombocytopenia, and hypofibrinogenemia being high-risk factors for bleeding. Active prevention and control of infections and maintenance of organ function are crucial in preventing bleeding in PALF. Routine coagulation tests like prothrombin time and international normalized ratio are not sufficient to predict bleeding risk in PALF, necessitating a more comprehensive coagulation evaluation system.

© The Author(s), under exclusive license to Springer Nature Singapore Pte Ltd. 2025
Y. Zhang et al. (Eds.): CHIP 2024, CCIS 2433, pp. 37–49, 2025.
https://doi.org/10.1007/978-981-96-3752-2_3

Keywords: Children · Acute Liver Failure · Coagulation Function · Bleeding

Pediatric acute liver failure (PALF) is a complex, rapidly progressive clinical syndrome that is prone to complications in other organ systems and multiple organ failure [1]. Coagulopathy based on liver failure is an important characteristic of acute liver failure [2]. It was previously believed that the prolongation of prothrombin time (PT) and international normalized ratio (INR) indicated a higher bleeding risk in children with liver failure, and the occurrence of bleeding in the clinic often predicted poor prognosis and a high risk of death [3–5]. In recent years, with the deepening understanding of the relationship between liver disease and coagulopathy, it has been found that the spontaneous bleeding in patients with acute liver failure is much lower than expected [5], and the prolongation of PT and INR does not well predict the bleeding risk in children with acute liver failure [5–7]. This study retrospectively analyzed the clinical data of children with acute liver failure to explore the risk factors for hemorrhagic complications in pediatric acute liver failure, to provide a basis for the clinical diagnosis and treatment decisions of PALF.

1   Materials and Methods

Our retrospective study called "Analysis of efficacy and prognostic risk factors for acute liver failure in children" was approved by the institutional review board of Children's Hospital of Chongqing Medical University (approval number 2022-3) on February 23, 2022, with a waiver of the informed consent requirement. The study has been registered with the Chinese Clinical Trial Registry under ChiCTR2200058970. Data were deidentified and entered an encrypted Excel (Microsoft Corp) worksheet. The study procedures were conducted in accordance with the declaration of Helsinki and followed the Strengthening the Reporting of Observational Studies in Epidemiology (STROBE) reporting guideline for cross-sectional studies.

1.1   Study Population

We conducted an observational retrospective cohort study at the Children's Hospital of Chongqing Medical University. It is one of China's two National Clinical Research Centers for Children's Health and Diseases. The hospital built the Clinical Science Research Big Data Platform (CSRBDP) in 2021 and made it available to clinical researchers. As of June 2024, the platform contains medical information on over 8.5 million pediatric outpatients and inpatients. Patients from birth to 18 years of age were eligible for enrollment in the PALF study if they met the following entry criteria between January 2014 and June 2024. The diagnostic criteria for acute liver failure were established according to the "Guideline for Diagnosis and Treatment of Liver Failure (2024 version)" [8] and the "Diagnosis and Management of Acute Liver Failure" published by the American Gastroenterological Association [9]. The patients were screened by the CSRBDP in the following logical manner (meeting either condition 1 or 2 for inclusion): 1. Patients whose discharge diagnosis contains "liver failure"; 2. One or more of the following conditions: (1) Alanine aminotransferase (ALT) or aspartate aminotransferase (AST) ≥ 500

U/L; (2) Prothrombin time (PT) $\geq$ 15s and INR $\geq$ 1.5; (3) 1.5 < INR < 2 and presence of an International Classification of Diseases (ICD) code containing encephalopathy at discharge diagnosis. (4) PT $\geq$ 20s or INR $\geq$ 2.0. Following electronic medical record review by the attending physician, we excluded patients with less than 48 h of hospitalization or incomplete data; pre-existing liver disease within 8 weeks of admission; surgery (including LT).

1.2 Data Collection

Clinical data were extracted from CSRBDP, encompassing: (1) General information: age at diagnosis, gender, complications, comorbidities, and invasive procedures; (2) Laboratory indicators: primarily encompassing complete blood count, liver and kidney function, coagulation function, and infection markers. (3) Hemorrhagic complications mainly included: gastrointestinal bleeding, pulmonary bleeding, intracranial bleeding, urinary system bleeding, and skin and mucous membrane bleeding.

1.3 Statistical Methods

Statistical analyses were performed utilizing R software, version 4.4.1. Categorical data were presented as frequencies or percentages, and comparisons between groups were conducted using the chi-squared (χ^2) test. A multivariate logistic regression model was employed to ascertain the independent risk factors, with statistical significance defined by p-values less than 0.05.

2 Results

2.1 General Information

From January 2014 to June 2024, a total of 964 children's with liver failure were hospitalized in our hospital. After excluding 146 cases with hospitalization of less than 48 h or incomplete data, 112 cases with pre-existing liver disease within 8 weeks of admission, and 43 cases who underwent surgery, a final total of 663 cases were analyzed. Among them, there were 239 cases (36.05%) with hemorrhagic complications and 424 cases (63.95%) without hemorrhagic complications; 377 males (56.86%) and 286 females (43.14%); ages ranged from 1 month to 17 years, with 169 cases (25.49%) aged $\leq$ 7 months, 239 cases (36.05%) aged between 7 months and 5 years, and 255 cases (38.64%) aged $\geq$ 5 years. In children with bleeding, we defined bleeding events that did not occur with other complications during the disease as spontaneous bleeding, and the results showed that only 21 cases (3.17%) had spontaneous bleeding.

2.2 Univariate Analysis of Hemorrhagic Complications in Children with Acute Liver Failure

The univariate analysis comparing children with acute liver failure with hemorrhagic complications to those without showed that infection, hepatorenal syndrome (HRS), multiple organ dysfunction syndrome (MODS), utilization of plasma or cryoprecipitate, platelet count, activated partial thromboplastin time (APTT), fibrinogen, D-dimer, Indirect Bilirubin, ALT, absolute neutrophil count, hemoglobin, total protein, albumin, lactate dehydrogenase (LDH), alkaline phosphatase (ALP), uric acid, plasma creatinine, creatine kinase (CK) and total calcium had statistically significant differences between the two groups ($P < 0.05$). There were no statistically significant differences in gender, age, INR, thrombin time (TT), total bilirubin, direct bilirubin, AST, gamma-glutamyl transferase (GGT), globulin, ammonia, lactic acid, c-reactive protein (CRP), procalcitonin and creatine kinase-MB (CKMB) ($P > 0.05$), see Table 1.

2.3 Multivariate Analysis of Hemorrhagic Complications in Children with Acute Liver Failure

Using the occurrence of bleeding in children as the dependent variable and including all variables in a multivariate Logistic regression analysis, the results indicated that infection (OR = 4.05, 95%CI: 2.47~6.64, p < 0.001), HRS (OR = 2.95, 95%CI: 1.82~4.77, p < 0.001), MODS (OR = 2.47, 95%CI: 1.57~3.88, p < 0.001), low platelet count ($\leq$50 × 10^9/L) (OR = 2.51, 95%CI: 1.58~3.99, p < 0.001), and low fibrinogen ($\leq$1 mg/dL) (OR = 1.73, 95%CI: 1.12~2.69, p = 0.014) are independent risk factors for hemorrhagic complications in children with acute liver failure, see Table 2.

3 Discussion

PALF is a rapidly progressive clinical syndrome in pediatric critical care that can quickly evolve into multi-organ dysfunction, sometimes leading to life-threatening cerebral edema and internal bleeding. Coagulopathy in PALF is the result of the interaction of multiple factors. In patients with acute liver failure, assessing the occurrence of coagulopathy requires a deeper understanding of the balance between anticoagulation and procoagulation. Although an INR value > 1.5 is recognized as evidence of coagulopathy and has been considered a prognostic risk factor for PALF [6], it only assesses procoagulant factors and does not take into account the effects of anticoagulants in liver failure, and thus may not accurately reflect the bleeding risk in PALF [10–13].

In our study, we found that the proportion of children with PALF who experienced spontaneous bleeding was relatively low. Most cases of bleeding were associated with infection, HRS, and MODS. Therefore, despite causing a series of coagulation abnormalities, PALF did not result in significant spontaneous bleeding. The analysis suggests that procoagulants, anticoagulants, and the fragile lytic system change simultaneously, leading to "rebalanced hemostasis." Since the liver is involved in the synthesis of both procoagulant (factors II, V, IX, X, XI, and fibrinogen) and anticoagulant (protein C, protein S, and antithrombin) proteins, PALF leads to "hemostatic rebalancing," which

Table 1. Univariate Analysis of Hemorrhagic Complications in Children with Acute Liver Failure

Variables	Total	Non-Bleeding	Bleeding	P
N	663	424	239	
Gender, n (%)				0.756
Female	286 (43.14)	181 (42.69)	105 (43.93)	
Male	377 (56.86)	243 (57.31)	134 (56.07)	
Age, n (%)				0.353
5 years to 18 years	255 (38.46)	156 (36.79)	99 (41.42)	
7 months to 5 years	239 (36.05)	153 (36.08)	86 (35.98)	
Less than 7 months	169 (25.49)	115 (27.12)	54 (22.59)	
Infection, n (%)				**<0.001**
No	245 (36.95)	215 (50.71)	30 (12.55)	
Yes	418 (63.05)	209 (49.29)	209 (87.45)	
HRS, n (%)				**<.001**
No	430 (64.86)	321 (75.71)	109 (45.61)	
Yes	233 (35.14)	103 (24.29)	130 (54.39)	
MODS, n (%)				**<.001**
No	457 (68.93)	346 (81.60)	111 (46.44)	
Yes	206 (31.07)	78 (18.40)	128 (53.56)	
Utilization of plasma or cryoprecipitate, n (%)				**0.019**
No	326 (49.17)	223 (52.59)	103 (43.10)	
Yes	337 (50.83)	201 (47.41)	136 (56.90)	
Platelet count, $\times$ 10^9/L, n (%)				**<.001**
>50	491 (74.06)	351 (82.78)	140 (58.58)	
$\leq$50	172 (25.94)	73 (17.22)	99 (41.42)	
APTT, seconds, n (%)				**0.029**
<47	298 (44.95)	204 (48.11)	94 (39.33)	
$\geq$47	365 (55.05)	220 (51.89)	145 (60.67)	
Fibrinogen, mg/dL, n (%)				**<.001**
>1	340 (51.28)	244 (57.55)	96 (40.17)	
$\leq$1	323 (48.72)	180 (42.45)	143 (59.83)	
D-dimer, mg/dL, n (%)				**<.001**
<3.76	250 (37.71)	185 (43.63)	65 (27.20)	
$\geq$3.76	413 (62.29)	239 (56.37)	174 (72.80)	

(*continued*)

Table 1. (*continued*)

Variables	Total	Non-Bleeding	Bleeding	P
INR, n (%)				0.955
<0.8 or >1.2	568 (85.67)	363 (85.61)	205 (85.77)	
0.8~1.2	95 (14.33)	61 (14.39)	34 (14.23)	
TT, seconds, n (%)				0.145
<20	263 (39.67)	177 (41.75)	86 (35.98)	
≥20	400 (60.33)	247 (58.25)	153 (64.02)	
Total Bilirubin, μmol/L, n (%)				0.449
<21	169 (25.49)	104 (24.53)	65 (27.20)	
≥21	494 (74.51)	320 (75.47)	174 (72.80)	
Direct Bilirubin, μmol/L, n (%)				0.368
<6.7	194 (29.26)	119 (28.07)	75 (31.38)	
≥6.7	469 (70.74)	305 (71.93)	164 (68.62)	
Indirect Bilirubin, μmol/L, n (%)				**0.025**
<6.7	211 (31.83)	122 (28.77)	89 (37.24)	
≥6.7	452 (68.17)	302 (71.23)	150 (62.76)	
AST, U/L, n (%)				0.565
<550	199 (30.02)	124 (29.25)	75 (31.38)	
≥550	464 (69.98)	300 (70.75)	164 (68.62)	
ALT, U/L, n (%)				**<.001**
<500	263 (39.67)	144 (33.96)	119 (49.79)	
≥500	400 (60.33)	280 (66.04)	120 (50.21)	
Absolute neutrophil count, ×10^9/L, n (%)				0.005
>0.5	629 (94.87)	410 (96.70)	219 (91.63)	
≤0.5	34 (5.13)	14 (3.30)	20 (8.37)	
Hemoglobin, g/L, n (%)				**<.001**
>80	508 (76.62)	351 (82.78)	157 (65.69)	
≤80	155 (23.38)	73 (17.22)	82 (34.31)	
Total Protein, g/L, n (%)				**<.001**
<44	88 (13.27)	35 (8.25)	53 (22.18)	
≥44	575 (86.73)	389 (91.75)	186 (77.82)	
Albumin, g/L, n (%)				**<.001**
<30	262 (39.52)	132 (31.13)	130 (54.39)	

(*continued*)

Table 1. (*continued*)

Variables	Total	Non-Bleeding	Bleeding	P
≥30	401 (60.48)	292 (68.87)	109 (45.61)	
Globulin, g/L, n (%)				0.488
<15.3	73 (11.01)	44 (10.38)	29 (12.13)	
≥15.3	590 (88.99)	380 (89.62)	210 (87.87)	
LDH, U/L, n (%)				**<.001**
<1000	326 (49.17)	238 (56.13)	88 (36.82)	
≥1000	337 (50.83)	186 (43.87)	151 (63.18)	
GGT, U/L, n (%)				0.351
<380	622 (93.82)	395 (93.16)	227 (94.98)	
≥380	41 (6.18)	29 (6.84)	12 (5.02)	
ALP, U/L, n (%)				**0.001**
<95	65 (9.80)	32 (7.55)	33 (13.81)	
≥405	154 (23.23)	114 (26.89)	40 (16.74)	
95–405	444 (66.97)	278 (65.57)	166 (69.46)	
Uric Acid, μmol/L, n (%)				**<.001**
>420	201 (30.32)	107 (25.24)	94 (39.33)	
≤420	462 (69.68)	317 (74.76)	145 (60.67)	
Plasma Creatinine, μmol/L, n (%)				**<.001**
<97	549 (82.81)	370 (87.26)	179 (74.90)	
≥97	114 (17.19)	54 (12.74)	60 (25.10)	
CKMB, ug/L, n (%)				0.762
<0.21 or >5	302 (45.55)	195 (45.99)	107 (44.77)	
0.21–5	361 (54.45)	229 (54.01)	132 (55.23)	
CK, U/L, n (%)				**0.007**
<300	406 (61.24)	276 (65.09)	130 (54.39)	
≥300	257 (38.76)	148 (34.91)	109 (45.61)	
Total calcium, mmol/L, n (%)				**< .001**
<2.2 or >3.0	388 (58.52)	217 (51.18)	171 (71.55)	
2.2–3.0	275 (41.48)	207 (48.82)	68 (28.45)	
Ammonia, μmol/L, n(%)				0.213
<9 or >33	446 (67.27)	278 (65.57)	168 (70.29)	
9–33	217 (32.73)	146 (34.43)	71 (29.71)	

(*continued*)

Table 1. (*continued*)

Variables	Total	Non-Bleeding	Bleeding	P
Lactic Acid, mmol/L, n (%)				0.257
<0.7 or >2.1	445 (67.12)	278 (65.57)	167 (69.87)	
0.7–2.1	218 (32.88)	146 (34.43)	72 (30.13)	
CRP, mg/L, n (%)				0.472
<8	48 (7.24)	33 (7.78)	15 (6.28)	
≥8	615 (92.76)	391 (92.22)	224 (93.72)	
Procalcitonin, ng/ml, n (%)				0.354
<0.1	27 (4.07)	15 (3.54)	12 (5.02)	
≥0.1	636 (95.93)	409 (96.46)	227 (94.98)	

may even shift towards a hypercoagulable state [11]. In addition to rebalancing coagulation, there are changes in platelet production due to liver-generated thrombocytopenia, increased von-Willebrand factor due to low-grade endothelial cell activation, and hyperfibrinolysis and fibrinolysis due to synthetic liver dysfunction [14–16]. All these changes contribute to the multifactorial nature of coagulopathy in PALF. The aggressive utilization of plasma or cryoprecipitate for the prophylactic prevention of bleeding in PALF patients may backfire, leading to other complications such as fluid overload, transfusion-related lung injury, and increased risk of thrombosis [6, 17].

Our study also found that infection is an important risk factor for bleeding in PALF children. The reason may be that endotoxins and cytokines produced by infection induce disseminated intravascular coagulation, inhibit platelet function, and enhance the action of nitric oxide. In PALF children, immune dysfunction is usually present, making them more susceptible to bacterial infections and sepsis, and infections in children may be more covert. At the same time, we also found that HRS and MODS in this study are independent risk factors for bleeding in PALF children. We know that in critically ill children, infections often lead to renal injury and multi-organ failure [18]. Therefore, when PALF children show clinical deterioration, there may be covert manifestations of infection, and the active use of antibiotics in PALF children may be more superior to the utilization of plasma or cryoprecipitate in the prevention of bleeding strategies, which requires further confirmation by subsequent large-sample, multi-center prospective studies.

Renal impairment is another important risk factor for bleeding in children with PALF. The kidneys play a crucial role in maintaining fluid, electrolyte balance, and coagulation function. The association between renal impairment and bleeding in PALF is multifactorial. Renal dysfunction can lead to the accumulation of uremic toxins, which may impair platelet function and contribute to coagulopathy [19]. Furthermore, renal impairment is often associated with volume overload and electrolyte disturbances, which can further exacerbate bleeding [20]. Additionally, patients with renal impairment may be more likely to require renal replacement therapy, which can further increase the risk of bleeding due to the use of anticoagulants and the removal of coagulation factors.

Table 2. Multivariate Logistic Regression Analysis of Bleeding Complications in Children with Acute Liver Failure

Variables	β	S.E	Z	P	OR (95%CI)
Infection					
No					1.00 (Reference)
Yes	1.40	0.25	5.56	**<0.001**	4.05 (2.47~6.64)
HRS					
No					1.00 (Reference)
Yes	1.08	0.25	4.41	**<0.001**	2.95 (1.82~4.77)
MODS					
No					1.00 (Reference)
Yes	0.90	0.23	3.93	**<0.001**	2.47 (1.57~3.88)
Utilization of plasma or cryoprecipitate					
No					1.00 (Reference)
Yes	0.29	0.20	1.44	0.149	1.34 (0.90~2.00)
Platelet count, × 10^9/L					
>50					1.00 (Reference)
≤50	0.92	0.24	3.88	**<0.001**	2.51 (1.58~3.99)
APTT, seconds					
<47					1.00 (Reference)
≥47	−0.15	0.23	−0.67	0.503	0.86 (0.55~1.35)
Fibrinogen, mg/dL					
>1					1.00 (Reference)
≤1	0.55	0.22	2.45	**0.014**	1.73 (1.12~2.69)
D−dimer, mg/dL					
<3.76					1.00 (Reference)
≥3.76	−0.11	0.23	−0.48	0.634	0.90 (0.57~1.40)
Indirect Bilirubin, μmol/L					
<6.7					1.00 (Reference)
≥6.7	0.30	0.24	1.25	0.211	1.35 (0.84~2.15)
ALT, U/L					
<500					1.00 (Reference)
≥500	−0.38	0.22	−1.71	0.087	0.69 (0.45~1.06)
Absolute neutrophil count, × 10^9/L					
>0.5					1.00 (Reference)

(continued)

Table 2. (*continued*)

Variables	β	S.E	Z	P	OR (95%CI)
≤0.5	−0.23	0.45	−0.52	0.604	0.79 (0.33~1.91)
Hemoglobin, g/L					
>80					1.00 (Reference)
≤80	0.38	0.24	1.62	0.106	1.47 (0.92~2.34)
Total Protein, g/L					
<44					1.00 (Reference)
≥44	−0.33	0.32	−1.05	0.295	0.72 (0.38~1.34)
Albumin, g/L					
<30					1.00 (Reference)
≥30	−0.03	0.25	−0.11	0.912	0.97 (0.60~1.59)
LDH, U/L					
<1000					1.00 (Reference)
≥1000	−0.08	0.24	−0.34	0.737	0.92 (0.58~1.47)
ALP, U/L					
<95					1.00 (Reference)
≥405	0.03	0.39	0.08	0.938	1.03 (0.48~2.21)
95–405	0.29	0.33	0.89	0.376	1.34 (0.70~2.56)
Uric Acid, μmol/L					
>420					1.00 (Reference)
≤420	−0.08	0.25	−0.32	0.747	0.92 (0.57~1.50)
Plasma Creatinine, μmol/L					
<97					1.00 (Reference)
≥97	−0.24	0.30	−0.79	0.429	0.79 (0.44~1.42)
CK, U/L					
<300					1.00 (Reference)
≥300	−0.02	0.22	−0.11	0.911	0.98 (0.63~1.51)
Total calcium, mmol/L					
<2.2 or >3.0					1.00 (Reference)
2.2–3.0	−0.34	0.23	−1.44	0.150	0.72 (0.45~1.13)

Our study results suggest that MODS may also be an independent risk factor for bleeding in this patient population, consistent with other studies. MODS is a common complication of severe illness, including PALF. Patients with MODS often develop a systemic inflammatory response that can lead to endothelial dysfunction, impaired tissue perfusion, and coagulopathy [21]. The severity of MODS is associated with an increased risk of mortality in patients with PALF. Our findings suggest that MODS may also be an independent risk factor for bleeding in this patient population.

Thrombocytopenia is a well-known risk factor for bleeding. In PALF, thrombocytopenia can occur due to impaired platelet production, increased platelet consumption, or sequestration of platelets in the spleen. [22, 23] Additionally, thrombocytopenia may be exacerbated by the use of medications such as heparin and proton pump inhibitors, which are commonly used in the management of PALF.

Our study also found that routine coagulation indicators such as PT and INR in coagulation function tests are not independent risk factors for bleeding in PALF children, and routine coagulation function tests may not predict the bleeding risk in PALF children well. Routine coagulation tests, including PT and INR, belong to procoagulant factors and ignore the contributions of inhibitors, fibrinolysis, and other cellular components. These tests do not provide information on actual fibrinolysis formation or clot dissolution [24]. In contrast, an increasing number of studies have shown that thromboelastography (TEG) is more comprehensive and complete than routine coagulation tests in assessing coagulation function and truly reflects the low-level "hemostatic rebalancing" state in patients with liver failure [24, 25]. The effectiveness of TEG has been confirmed in studies of adult liver failure [26, 27] and adult trauma critically ill patients [28], providing more accurate assessment of coagulation disorders and helping to reduce the blind utilization of plasma or cryoprecipitate in clinical practice. However, in PALF patients, there is currently a lack of relevant studies on TEG evaluation of coagulation, and large-sample, multi-center prospective studies would be beneficial in providing better clinical decisions for PALF children.

In conclusion, our study has identified key risk factors for bleeding in pediatric patients with PALF, emphasizing the importance of a comprehensive management approach that includes early identification and treatment of infection, renal impairment, and MODS. Active prevention and control of infections, along with maintaining organ function, are crucial in preventing bleeding. Furthermore, close monitoring of platelet counts, and coagulation parameters is essential. While spontaneous bleeding in pediatric acute liver failure is relatively rare, a more comprehensive coagulation evaluation system is needed to better predict bleeding risk and guide clinical decisions in PALF children, as traditional markers like PT and INR are not sufficiently predictive. Further studies are required to evaluate the effectiveness of specific interventions for preventing and treating bleeding in this patient population.

References

1. Ascher Bartlett, J.M., Yanni, G., Kwon, Y., Emamaullee, J.: Pediatric acute liver failure: reexamining key clinical features, current management, and research prospects. Liver Transpl. **28**, 1776–1784 (2022). https://doi.org/10.1002/lt.26500
2. Coagulopathy in acute liver failure. Best Practice & Research Clinical Gastroenterology, 101956 (2024). https://doi.org/10.1016/j.bpg.2024.101956
3. Stravitz, R.T., et al.: Bleeding complications in acute liver failure. Hepatology **67**, 1931 (2018). https://doi.org/10.1002/hep.29694
4. Ow, T.-W., et al.: Prevalence of bleeding and thrombosis in critically Ill patients with chronic liver disease. Thromb. Haemost. **122**, 1006–1016 (2021). https://doi.org/10.1055/a-1667-7293

5. Tujios, S., Stravitz, R.T., Lee, W.M.: Management of acute liver failure: update 2022. Semin. Liver Dis. **42**, 362–378 (2022). https://doi.org/10.1055/s-0042-1755274

6. Bulut, Y., Sapru, A., Roach, G.D.: Hemostatic balance in pediatric acute liver failure: epidemiology of bleeding and thrombosis, physiology, and current strategies. Front. Pediatr. **8**, 618119 (2020). https://doi.org/10.3389/fped.2020.618119

7. Zermatten, M.G., Fraga, M., Calderara, D.B., Aliotta, A., Moradpour, D., Alberio, L.: Biomarkers of liver dysfunction correlate with a prothrombotic and not with a prohaemorrhagic profile in patients with cirrhosis. JHEP Rep. **2**, 100120 (2020). https://doi.org/10.1016/j.jhepr.2020.100120

8. Liver Failure and Artificial Liver Group: Chinese society of infectious diseases: guideline for diagnosis and treatment of liver failure (2024 version). Chinese J. Clin. Infect. Diseases **17**, 1–19 (2024). https://doi.org/10.3760/cma.j.issn.1674-2397.2024.05.001

9. Flamm, S.L., Yang, Y.-X., Singh, S., Falck-Ytter, Y.T.: AGA institute clinical guidelines committee: American gastroenterological association institute guidelines for the diagnosis and management of acute liver failure. Gastroenterology **152**, 644–647 (2017). https://doi.org/10.1053/j.gastro.2016.12.026

10. Samanta, A., Poddar, U.: Pediatric acute liver failure: current perspective in etiology and management. Indian J. Gastroenterol. **43**, 349–360 (2024). https://doi.org/10.1007/s12664-024-01520-6

11. McMurry, H.S., Jou, J., Shatzel, J.: The hemostatic and thrombotic complications of liver disease. Eur. J. Haematol. **107**, 383 (2021). https://doi.org/10.1111/ejh.13688

12. Premkumar, M., Sarin, S.K.: Current concepts in coagulation profile in cirrhosis and acute-on-chronic liver failure. Clin. Liver Disease **16**, 158 (2020). https://doi.org/10.1002/cld.976

13. Jiang, T., et al.: Analysis of etiology and prognosis of 120 children with pediatric acute liver failure. Chinese J. Appl. Clin. Pediatr. 422–425 (2020)

14. Lim, H.I., Cuker, A.: Thrombocytopenia and liver disease: pathophysiology and periprocedural management. Hematology **2022**, 296–302 (2022). https://doi.org/10.1182/hematology.2022000408

15. Groeneveld, D., Poole, L.G., Luyendyk, J.P.: Targeting von Willebrand factor in liver diseases: a novel therapeutic strategy? J. Thrombosis Haemostasis: JTH **19**, 1390 (2021). https://doi.org/10.1111/jth.15312

16. Nightingale, T., Cutler, D.: The secretion of von Willebrand factor from endothelial cells; an increasingly complicated story. J. Thromb. Haemost. **11**, 192 (2013). https://doi.org/10.1111/jth.12225

17. Vlaar, A.P.J., et al.: Transfusion strategies in bleeding critically ill adults: a clinical practice guideline from the European Society of Intensive Care Medicine. Intensive Care Med. **47**, 1368–1392 (2021). https://doi.org/10.1007/s00134-021-06531-x

18. Kozlov, A.V., Grillari, J.: Pathogenesis of multiple organ failure: the impact of systemic damage to plasma membranes. Front. Med. (Lausanne) **9**, 806462 (2022). https://doi.org/10.3389/fmed.2022.806462

19. Qiu, Z., Pang, X., Xiang, Q., Cui, Y.: The crosstalk between nephropathy and coagulation disorder: pathogenesis, treatment, and dilemmas. J. Am. Soc. Nephrol. **34**, 1793 (2023). https://doi.org/10.1681/ASN.0000000000000199

20. Kim, G.-H.: Fluid and electrolyte problems in chronic kidney disease. 收入: Arıcı, M. (编) Management of Chronic Kidney Disease: A Clinician's Guide. 页 327–344. Springer, Cham (2023)

21. Singh, M., Pushpakumar, S., Zheng, Y., Smolenkova, I., Akinterinwa, O.E., Luulay, B., Tyagi, S.C.: Novel mechanism of the COVID-19 associated coagulopathy (CAC) and vascular thromboembolism. NPJ Viruses **1**, 1–9 (2023). https://doi.org/10.1038/s44298-023-00003-3

22. Balaphas, A., et al.: Platelets and platelet-derived extracellular vesicles in liver physiology and disease. Hepatol. Commun. **3**, 855–866 (2019). https://doi.org/10.1002/hep4.1358

23. Stravitz, R.T., et al.: Role of procoagulant microparticles in mediating complications and outcome of acute liver injury/acute liver failure. Hepatology **58**, 304–313 (2013). https://doi.org/10.1002/hep.26307

24. Bannish, B.E., Chernysh, I.N., Keener, J.P., Fogelson, A.L., Weisel, J.W.: Molecular and physical mechanisms of fibrinolysis and thrombolysis from mathematical modeling and experiments. Sci. Rep. **7**, 6914 (2017). https://doi.org/10.1038/s41598-017-06383-w

25. Gv, P., D, P., Gj, W., J, B., E, B., Ak, B.: Infection and hemostasis in decompensated cirrhosis: a prospective study using thrombelastography. Hepatology (Baltimore, Md.). **29** (1999). https://doi.org/10.1002/hep.510290437

26. Goyal, S., et al.: Thromboelastography parameters in patients with acute on chronic liver failure. Ann. Hepatol. **17**, 1042–1051 (2018). https://doi.org/10.5604/01.3001.0012.7205

27. Intrinsic or Nonintrinsic End-stage Liver Disease and Its Association With Thromboelastography-based Coagulation States in Patients Undergoing Liver Transplantation: A Retrospective Cohort Study. J. Cardiothoracic Vasc. Anesthesia **38**, 2368–2376 (2024). https://doi.org/10.1053/j.jvca.2024.07.036

28. Bugaev, N., et al.: Thromboelastography and rotational thromboelastometry in bleeding patients with coagulopathy: practice management guideline from the Eastern Association for the Surgery of Trauma. J. Trauma Acute Care Surg. **89**, 999–1017 (2020). https://doi.org/10.1097/TA.0000000000002944

PMFNet: Pseudo-modal Fusion Network for Obstructive Sleep Apnea Detection Using Single-Lead ECG Signals

Meixin Wang[1], Yanchun Zhang[2]([✉]), Minghao Mo[1], and Yifu Zeng[1]

[1] Guangzhou University, Guangzhou, China
[2] Zhejiang Normal University, Jinghua, China
Yanchun.Zhang@vu.edu.au

Abstract. Obstructive sleep apnea (OSA) is a common sleep-disordered breathing (SDB) characterized by recurrent apnea events during sleep due to partial or complete obstruction of the upper airway, which impairs the patient's quality of sleep and daily life and increases the risk of several chronic diseases. Polysomnography (PSG) is clinically used as the gold standard for detecting OSA, but its expensive, complex and time-consuming procedure limits its widespread use. In this study, we propose a novel pseudo-modal fusion network (PMFNet) using single-lead ECG signals for the task of obstructive sleep apnea. We innovatively propose the concept of "pseudo-modal" in ECG signal analysis, using the QRS wave detection algorithm and the continuous wavelet transform (CWT) to obtain the R-wave data features and time-frequency maps as pseudo-modal data, respectively. Different feature extractors are carefully designed for these two types of pseudo-modal data to complete the time-domain and frequency-domain feature extraction of ECG signals, and a bilinear attention network (BAN) is introduced to effectively integrate our proposed pseudo-modal data. We validate the performance of PMFNet on the publicly available PhysioNet Apnea-ECG dataset and make a fair comparison with previous studies. Extensive experimental results show that PMFNet achieves optimal performance, with specific accuracy, sensitivity, specificity, and F1 scores of 92.79%, 90.90%, 93.95%, and 90.42%, respectively. Our proposed PMFNet is able to determine end-to-end whether an OSA event has occurred for a given ECG signal segment, providing an effective and convenient alternative to current clinical approaches.

Keywords: Obstructive sleep apnea · Deep learning · Electrocardiogram · Classification · Multi-modal

1 Introduction

As economic development continues, fast-paced lifestyles and intense work pressure often lead to disruptions in people's work schedules and a variety of sleep

© The Author(s), under exclusive license to Springer Nature Singapore Pte Ltd. 2025
Y. Zhang et al. (Eds.): CHIP 2024, CCIS 2433, pp. 50–69, 2025.
https://doi.org/10.1007/978-981-96-3752-2_4

problems. On the other hand, economic development has led people to pay attention to and pursue healthy lifestyles, and more and more people are beginning to attach importance to quality sleep. At the same time, the healthcare system in many countries and regions has been improved and medical resources have become more abundant, which can gradually meet people's urgent demand for healthy sleep. Obstructive sleep apnea (OSA) is a common sleep-disordered breathing (SDB) that is closely associated with a variety of sleep problems and manifests as apnea or upper airway obstruction during sleep, leading to sleep rhythm disturbances and sleep fragmentation. People suffering from OSA may experience symptoms such as daytime sleepiness, daily memory loss and poor concentration, which may be complicated by cardiovascular and cerebrovascular pathologies such as hypertension, coronary heart disease, pulmonary heart disease, stroke, etc., and in severe cases psychological, intellectual and behavioural abnormalities may occur [17,24,26]. OSA is diagnosed by an Apnea-Hypopnea Index (AHI) greater than or equal to 5, and the prevalence in the general population ranges from 9% to 38% [29]. Studies have reported that 936 million adults aged 30–69 years worldwide suffer from mild to severe obstructive sleep apnea, with China having the highest number of patients at approximately 176 million [7]. Fortunately, OSA can be effectively improved and treated if it is accurately diagnosed by a doctor in a timely manner and the necessary interventions and adjustments are made as early as possible.

Polysomnography (PSG) is the "gold standard" for diagnosing OSA in clinical settings, recording physiological signals from more than 10 channels, including electrocardiogram (ECG), electroencephalogram(EEG), electrooculogram, oxygen saturation(SaO2), etc., throughout the sleep process. However, during the signal collection process, the subject has to stay in the hospital laboratory all night with a large number of wires and electrodes connected, which makes the subject's experience much less comfortable and interferes with sleep to some extent, which in turn affects the accuracy of the results. At the same time, because PSG is composed of a variety of physiological signals, the huge amount of data requires a lot of time for professionals to collect and analyse it, making the whole process expensive in terms of time and labor. All these difficulties have somewhat limited the use of PSG in daily life. To find alternatives to PSG, few studies have proposed the use of clinically validated features and readily available physiological characteristics to estimate OSA severity using statistical strategies and regression models. For example, Juang et al. [15] proposed an interpretable fuzzy systems using three physiological variables (neck circumference, waist circumference and mean awake blood pressure) with a multi-objective genetic algorithm to rapidly estimate OSA severity. Wu et al. [39] selected changes in blood pressure status at bedtime and early morning and five readily available measurements (age, BMI, etc.) and used stepwise regression to find effective variables. As these methods are highly dependent on domain knowledge, more and more researchers are proposing the possibility of using convenient wearable devices to capture physiological signals (e.g., ECG signals, EEG signals, and SpO2, etc.) for OSA detection. Among these physiological signals, ECG signals are obviously of greater interest. Bacharova et al. [4] showed that patients with OSA have complex morphological changes in the QRS wave complexes, low QRS voltages, and the occurrence of fragmented QRS (fQRS); Salari et al. [28] reported that apnea or hypoventilation reduces the oxygen level in the patient's body, which further leads to a decrease in the heart rate and an increase in R-peak spacing. Various reports continue to demonstrate the strong correlation between OSA and ECG signal transformations, and the use of single-lead ECG signals to detect OSA is a convenient, effective, and cost-effective option.

In this study, we propose a pseudo-modal fusion network, PMFNet, for OSA detection, which fully exploits the time-domain and frequency-domain features of single-lead ECG signals through a well-designed feature extraction and feature fusion mechanism, and validate the model performance on the publicly available PhysioNet Apnea-ECG dataset [25]. Our main contributions are as follows:

* Given a single-lead ECG signal as input, our proposed neural network model PMFNet is able to provide end-to-end information on whether an OSA event is present in the input segment, significantly reducing the error and cost associated with manual feature engineering and offering a promising alternative to PSG. We train and test the model on the publicly available PhysioNet Apnea-ECG dataset, achieving an accuracy of 92.79% on the official withheld set and an average accuracy of 94.0% in a 10-fold cross-validation experiment. Compared to previous studies, the results show that PMFNet has optimal performance.
* Inspired by the idea of multimodal learning, the concept of "pseudo-modality" is innovatively proposed in ECG signal analysis. We use the QRS wave test algorithm and continuous wavelet transform to obtain R-wave feature data and time-frequency maps, which are regarded as two pseudo-modalities of the ECG signal, and design different feature extractors for the two modalities, which can make full use of the time-domain and frequency-domain features of the ECG signal.
* For the task of obstructive sleep apnea detection, our study is the first to introduce a bilinear attention network that effectively fuses our proposed pseudo-modal data using an attention weight capture layer and a bilinear pooling layer.
* Our network model can be openly developed to researchers via Github.

2   Related Work

Several approaches have been proposed to detect OSA using single-lead ECG signals. Some of the studies have been carried out by applying statistical strategies and regression models using basic features obtained from signal analysis. For example, Rajesh et al. [27] obtained discrete features of ECG signals by discrete wavelet transform (DWT) and used correlation-based feature selection (CFS) and particle swarm optimization (PSO) search to obtain the optimal feature vectors to complete the OSA classification. Martin et al. [20] proposed an expert system for OSA detection based on heart rate variability (HRV) features using logistic regression, linear discriminant analysis and quadratic discriminant analysis. Part of the machine learning approach is used to select the appropriate classifier. Fatimah et al. [11] decomposed the ECG signal into multiple Fourier intrinsic band functions (FIBF) with desired cut-off frequencies using Fourier decomposition method (FDM), completed the feature selection and then used multiple classifiers for comparison experiments. The online sleep apnea detection technique proposed by Surrel et al. [35] used the ECG R-wave amplitude and RR intervals to build predictive models by support vector mechanism (SVM), while Song et al. [34] proposed a hidden markov model (HMM)-based OSA detection method by extracting time-domain and frequency-domain features from the ECG and ECG-derived respiration (EDR) signals.

Deep learning, as a branch of machine learning, can extract hidden features from input data and use them to perform highly accurate classification, greatly improving learning efficiency. To minimise the errors caused by automatic feature engineering, Wang et al. [37] proposed a method for OSA classification based on a modified LeNet-5 convolutional neural network, which is capable of effective automatic feature extraction; Sharan et al. [32] used raw HRV data as the input to a one-dimensional CNN model without the need for feature extraction and selection. Wang et al. [38] and Chen et al. [10] both chose to use ECG signal RR intervals and R-wave peaks to represent ECG signal time-domain features; the former proposed a multi-scale neural network URNet integrating ResNet and UNet, which is capable of fusing features collected from both shallow and deep layers by jumping connections to process convolutional blocks at different scales; and the latter proposed a restricted attention mechanism with cascade morphology and temporal attention, which effectively improves the OSA detection performance by adaptively assigning weight importance to suppress redundant features from adjacent segments.

At the same time, deep learning continues to show strong capabilities in the field of computer vision, and image-based research in clinical applications is increasing significantly. In order to make full use of all the information contained in physiological signals, a large number of studies and experiments have begun to attempt to use images to solve the problem of OSA detection. Mashrur et al. [21] trained a lightweight CNN model for OSA detection after converting ECG signals into regular and mixed scale maps using continuous wavelet transform (CWT) and empirical modal decomposition (EMD). Zhou et al. [40] proposed a composite deep neural convolutional network, CCNN, by converting single-lead ECG signals into heart rate variability scalogram images and Gramian Angular Filed (GAF) matrix images. While Nadeem et al. [36] proposed a dual convolutional dual attention network (DCDA-Net) for OSA detection by generating spectrograms and scale maps using short-time Fourier transform (STFT) and CWT for ECG signals respectively.

Existing studies on the task of predicting obstructive sleep apnea using single-lead ECG signals have presented their own brilliant ideas from different perspectives using a variety of different approaches, with surprising results. Unfortunately, these studies have either chosen to use only the 1D ECG data (i.e., the extracted ECG R-wave peaks, RRI intervals, or EDR, etc.) in order to obtain rich time domain features, or they have chosen to convert the 1D ECG signals into a 2D image using other signal processing techniques (e.g., STFT, CWT, etc.) to extract the hidden frequency domain features in the original 1D ECG signals. However, the feature information embedded in these two data representations is complementary, and using only one of them in an isolated manner is bound to miss some important information. Therefore, we propose a novel pseudo-modal fusion network, PMFNet, which fully extracts and fuses the above two data forms of ECG signals by introducing the idea of multimodal learning to deeply mine the data feature information and improve the performance of OSA detection.

3   Method

3.1   Pre-processing

ECG signals are random signals and are susceptible to interference from numerous sources of noise during the nightly acquisition, which may be intrinsic, such as respiration and muscle tremor, or extrinsic, such as poor contact with the equipment or electromagnetic interference present in the environment. In our study a fourth order Butterworth bandpass filter [6] (0.5–48 Hz) was used for filtering to remove high frequency noise interference with and signals affected by baseline drift (Fig. 1).

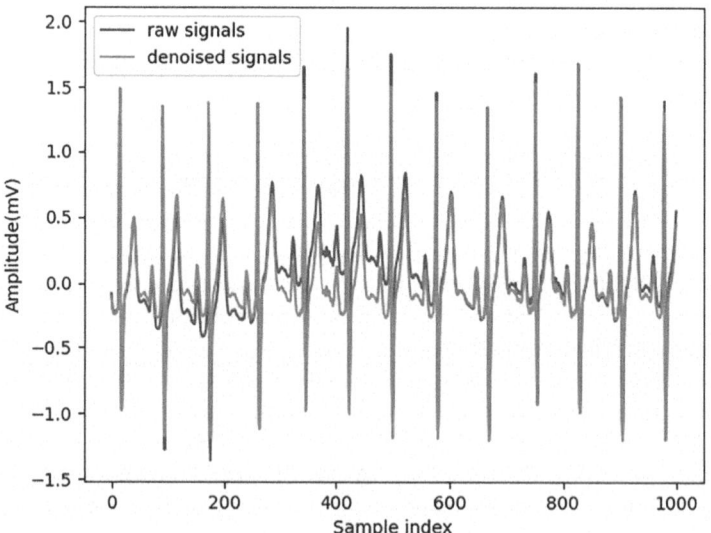

Fig. 1. Raw signal vs. denoised signal

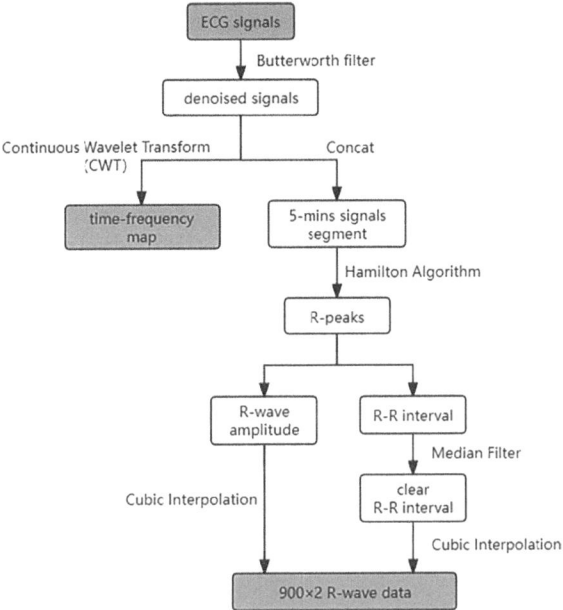

Fig. 2. Pre-processing flow chart

Based on the filtered signals, we obtained two types of data using different ways of transformations. On the one hand, we used CWT to obtain time-frequency maps of the ECG signals. ECG signals are non-smooth signals whose frequency varies with time, and the time-frequency representation of the signals helps to extract complex and high-dimensional signal features. SFTF aims to extract frequency information from the signal at the cost of losing temporal information, and CWT takes the idea of STFT localisation and develops it further, overcoming the disadvantage that the window size does not vary with frequency [27]. And it works exceptionally well when evaluating non-smooth signals [1]. In this study we use the generalized Morse wavelet for CWT with the following Eq. 1:

$$C\left(a, b; X(t), \psi(t)\right) = a^{-\frac{1}{2}} \int_{-\infty}^{+\infty} X(t)\bar{\psi}\left(\frac{t - b}{a}\right) dt \qquad (1)$$

where $a > 0$, a is the scale parameter, b is the position parameter, t and ψ denote the time value and the mother wavelet respectively, the mother wavelet chosen here is the Generalized Morse Wavelet, which is one of the good choices for time-frequency analysis using CWT.

On the other hand, several previous studies [8,10,14] have shown that RR interval (RRI) and R-wave amplitude in ECG signals are effective in sleep apnea detection tasks, both of which are closely related to respiratory airflow, which is one of the most important bases for physicians to determine whether a subject has OSA in clinical applications. In addition, adjacent ECG signals have been shown to help improve OSA detection performance [32,37]. We followed these findings in our study. We used the ECG central marker segment (target segment, one minute in length) and its surrounding ±2 segments (two minutes before and two minutes after) merged into a whole, and used Hamilton's algorithm [13] to locate the R-peaks of the filtered ECG signal, extract the R-peak amplitudes, and calculate the corresponding RRI. To eliminate the possibility of some physiologically unexplained points in the RRI, the median filter [9] was used to provide a robust estimate of the RRI. Finally, to satisfy the model inputs, we finally used a cubic spline interpolation technique to fix the input length at 900, and hereafter refer to the RRI and R-wave amplitude inputs (900 × 2) as simply the R-wave features. The entire pre-processing procedure can be summarised in Fig. 2.

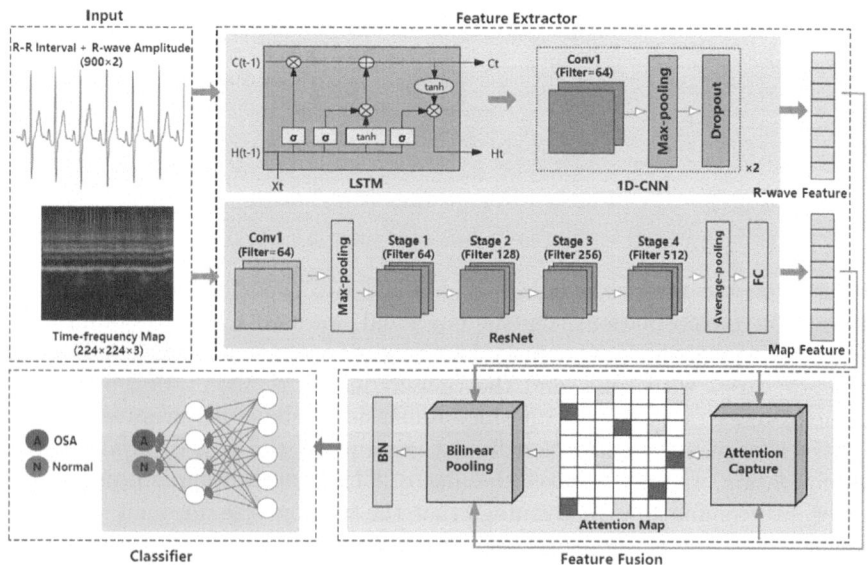

Fig. 3. The architecture of our proposed PMFNet

3.2   Proposed PMFNet

The overall architecture of our proposed deep learning model for predicting a given ECG signal segment as OSA or normal is as follows (Fig. 3). Specifically, our proposed PMFNet consists of three main modules: a feature extraction module, a feature fusion module and a classification module. In the final classification module we use two successive fully connected layers to predict whether an OSA event occurs in the target segment. In the next two subsections, the feature extraction module and the feature fusion module are described in detail.

Feature Extractor. As described in Sect. 3.1, we performed a series of pre-processing operations on the ECG signal to obtain two data forms, R-wave data and time-frequency maps. Therefore, in the feature extraction stage, we designed different feature extraction networks for these two data forms.

For R-wave data, we use a combination of Long Short-Term Memory (LSTM) and One-Dimensional Convolutional Neural Network (1D-CNN) for feature extraction. LSTM is able to effectively capture and record long-term dependent information through its unique gating mechanism, and is highly sensitive to processing time series data, while ECG signals happen to be inextricably linked to time series. In recent years' research, LSTM and its variants have shown good performance in processing ECG signals to complete classification, abnormality detection and disease diagnosis [5,31]. In this study we first use LSTM with 256 cells to generate a high-dimensional feature map that can well reflect the time series features. Then we use to two repeated 1D-CNN blocks, specifically composed of convolutional layer, max pooling layer and dropout layer, through which this structure makes the high dimensional feature map dimensions descend to the specified embedding dimensions to obtain the embedding representation $S_R = \{s_R^1, s_R^2, s_R^3, \ldots, s_R^N\}$, $S_R \in \mathbb{R}^{D_R \times N}$, where D_R is the embedded feature dimension of the R-wave data, N is the embedded feature length, and S_R can be specifically calculated by the following Eq. 2:

$$S_R^{(l+1)} = CNN\left(W_c^{(l)}, b_c^{(l)}, S_R^{(l)}\right) \tag{2}$$

where $W_c^{(l)}$ and $b_c^{(l)}$ represent the learnable matrix and bias vector of the l-th CNN block, respectively, and $S_R^{(1)} = \{H_1, H_2, \ldots H_n\}$ represents the R-wave feature representation after passing through the LSTM, and the specific H_t can be obtained from the Eq. 3 to Eq. 8:

$$f_t = \sigma\left(W_f\left[H_{t-1}, x_t\right] + b_f\right) \tag{3}$$

$$i_t = \sigma\left(W_i\left[H_{t-1}, x_t\right] + b_i\right) \tag{4}$$

$$C_t' = \tanh\left(W_C\left[H_{t-1}, x_t\right] + b_C\right) \tag{5}$$

$$C_t = f_t * C_{t-1} + i_t * C_t' \tag{6}$$

$$o_t = \sigma\left(W_o\left[H_{t-1}, x_t\right] + b_o\right) \tag{7}$$

$$H_t = o_t * \tanh\left(C_t\right) \tag{8}$$

where x_t is the current input, f_t, i_t, and o_t are the value of the forgetting gate, the memory gate value, and the output gate value, respectively, C_t' is the temporary cell state, C_t is the current cell state, and W and b represent the learning parameter and the bias vector of the corresponding gate, respectively.

For the time-frequency maps, we chose to use the pre-trained ResNet-50 for feature extraction. Since it was first proposed in 2015, ResNet has made a great impact in various application areas of deep learning, especially in many visual recognition tasks, and its innovative "residual learning" mechanism captures and integrates multiscale features well, effectively solving the problem of gradient disappearance or gradient explosion. Ma et al. [19] and Guan et al. [12] converted ECG signals into 2D images and used ResNet to classify arrhythmias. Wang et al. [38] and Li et al. [18] accomplished the tasks of sleep staging and obstructive sleep apnea detection, respectively, by extending ResNet. The ResNet architecture used in this study consists of five main stages. The first stage, which we call the image preprocessing stage, starts with 64 convolutional filters ($7{\times}7$), followed by a batch normalization, a nonlinear rectification function ReLU, and a max pooling layer. In the next four stages two similar residual blocks are used (Fig. 4), the right branch of the residual block is usually called Identity, which can transform the shape of the input X to the same shape as the output of the convolutional part, and after completing the jump connections the whole output is activated by the ReLU activation function. The number of filters in the four stages is incremented (64, 128, 256, 512).

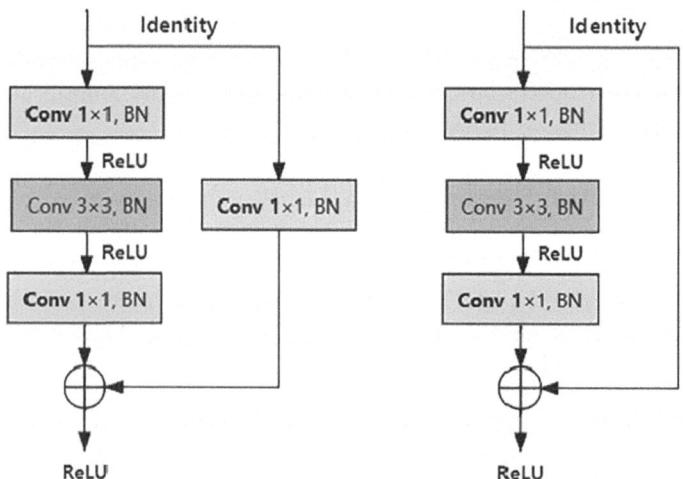

Fig. 4. Residual block of ResNet

Finally the embedded feature $S_P = \{s_P^1, s_P^2, s_P^3, \ldots, s_P^M\}$, $S_P \in \mathbb{R}^{D_P \times M}$, where D_p is the dimension of the embedded feature of the time-frequency map and M is the length of the embedded feature, is obtained after passing through the average pooling layer and the full connectivity layer in turn.

Feature Fusion. Bilinear Attention Networks (BAN) is an attention-based multimodal learning model proposed by Kim et al. [16] and originally used in the field of computer vision to solve Visual Question Answering (VQA) problems. In the context of this task, BAN uses a low-rank bilinear pool to extract a joint representation of the multimodal multichannel inputs, seamlessly exploiting the given visual-textual information and providing satisfactory text-image matching answers. Compared to previous studies, BAN extends the single attention network to provide a richer joint representation of the multimodal multichannel.

In this study, in order to make full use of the multidimensional information of the ECG signal, we use both one-dimensional ECG signal change data and time-frequency domain maps. Considering that these two types of data contain the time-domain and frequency-domain information of the ECG signal, respectively, and their data structures are spatially different, we can naturally associate these two types of data with multimodal data. Therefore, inspired by multimodal learning, we propose the concept of "pseudo-modality". We consider R-wave data and time-frequency maps as two kinds of pseudo-modalities, and apply BAN to design an ECG pseudo-modal fusion representation extraction module. Specifically it can be divided into two layers: the (1) attentional weight capture layer and the (2) bilinear pooling layer.

Given two pseudo-modal representations S_R and S_P from Subsect. 3.2.1, The attentional weight capture layer aims to obtain a bilinear attentional mapping $\mathcal{A} \in \mathbb{R}^{N \times M}$ between modalities, specifically the element $\mathcal{A}_{i,j}$ in $\mathcal{A}$ can be represented as:

$$\mathcal{A}_{i,j} = q^T \left(U^T s_R^i \right) \circ \left(V^T s_P^j \right) \tag{9}$$

where $U \in \mathbb{R}^{D_R \times K}$ and $V \in \mathbb{R}^{D_P \times K}$ are the learnable weights of the R-wave representation and the time-frequency map representation, respectively, $q \in \mathbb{R}^K$ is a learnable weight vector, and $\circ$ represents the Hadamard product. The attention weight capture layer maps the R-wave representation and the time-frequency map representation to the same feature space through the weight matrices U and V. The bilinear attention mapping graph is obtained by learning the Hadamard product and the weight vector q. To obtain the final cross-modal fusion representation $f \in \mathbb{R}^K$, we introduce a bilinear pooling layer and a summing pool on the bilinear attention mapping graph.

$$\begin{aligned} f'_k &= \left(S_R \right)^T U \Big)_k^T \mathcal{A} \left(S_P \right)^T V \Big)_k \\ &= \sum_{i=1}^{N} \sum_{j=1}^{M} \mathcal{A}_{i,j} \left(s_R^i \right)^T \left(U_k V_k^T \right) s_P^j \end{aligned} \tag{10}$$

where the subscript k is the index of the column in the matrix, and the weight matrices U and V are shared with the previous layer, in the form of shared parameters to reduce the number of parameters while mitigating the overfitting problem.

$$f = Sumpool \left(f', s \right) \tag{11}$$

The sum pool reduces the dimension of the fusion representation decrease from K to K/s by the step s, resulting in a more compact fusion representation. Furthermore, by adding a new weight vector q, the entire fusion representation extraction process can be easily extended to a multi-head form (Fig. 5), and the final pseudo-modal fusion representation can be represented as the sum of the computed sums of multiple heads, two of which are used in our proposed architecture.

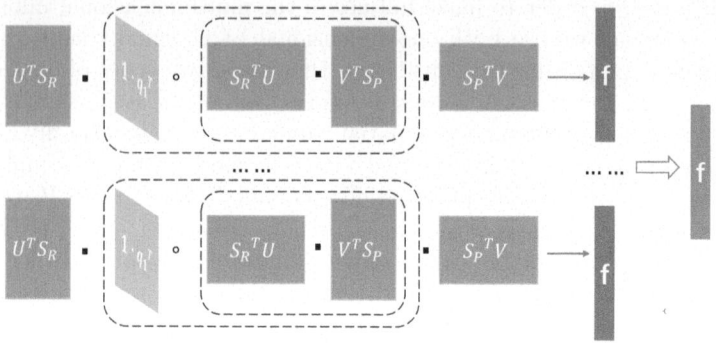

Fig. 5. Bilinear Attention Networks with Multiple Heads

4 Experiment and Results

4.1 Database

In the present study we used a well-known and widely used public dataset: the PhysioNet Apnea-ECG dataset. This dataset was provided by the Phillips University of Marburg, Germany, in 2000 and contains 70 single-lead ECG signal recordings sampled at 100 Hz, divided into an open release set of 35 recordings (a01 to a20, b01 to b05, and c01 to c10) and a retained set of 35 recordings (x01 to x35), with experts marking the occurrence of apnea events in one minute units. Subjects in the dataset were aged 27–63 years, weighed 53–135 kg, and each recording was between 401 and 578 min in length, and the details of the data distribution are shown in Fig. 6.

In order to make a fair comparison of our model performance with previous studies, two different segmentation strategies are applied to the dataset in this study. One segmentation strategy comes from the way the dataset is officially divided, using the public release set as the training set and the withheld set as the test, and our processed dataset segments include 16840 training samples and 17041 test samples, as shown in Table 1.

Since the Apnea-ECG dataset is a medium size publicly available dataset, the use of 10-fold cross-validation can provide more training samples for the training process of the deep learning model and it can ensure that the model is robust under different test datasets. There are many studies that have used 10-fold cross-validation to evaluate the performance of the proposed model [2,3,23,40]. In this study, the total data is divided into 10 subsets, one subset is selected as the test set each time and the remaining nine subsets are used as the training set and the process is repeated 10 times. Finally, the mean value of each evaluation metric was taken as the model performance estimate.

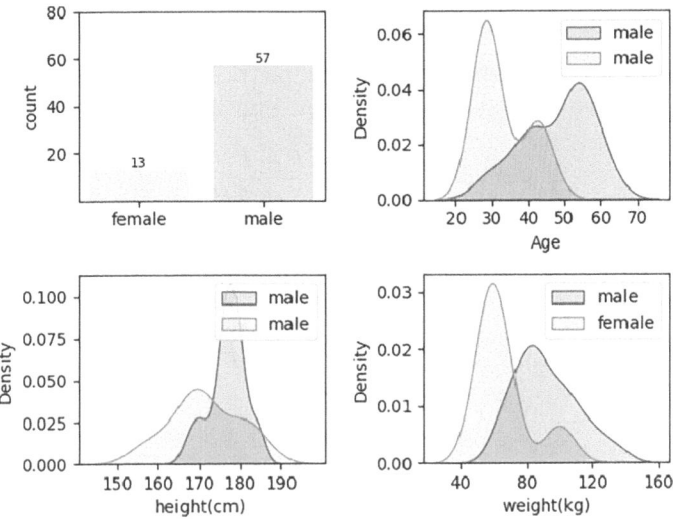

Fig. 6. Kernel density plot of the data distribution for the dataset

Table 1. PhysioNet Apnea-ECG database description after preprocessing

Database	OSA	Normal	The total
Released set	6484	10356	16840
Withheld set	6506	10535	17041
The total	12990	20891	33881

4.2   Experiment Setup

The architecture proposed in this paper has been trained and tested on a single NVIDIA GeForce GTX 3090 GPU. The architecture is implemented on PyCharm 2023.2.3 based on Python 3.8 using the Pytorch and Scikit-learn libraries, and the data pre-processing part is done by calling MATLAB R2022a. In our experiments we use a grid search algorithm to find the best hyperparameters. In the end we set the batch size to 64, used the binary cross-entropy loss as the loss function, and used Adam optimisation with a learning rate of 3e−4. We let the model to run for up to 50 epochs on the chosen dataset and at the end of each epoch we evaluated the test set, saving the test results with the file of the more optimal model. Finally the model with the best performance on the test set is selected as the basis for our comparison with other previous studies.

4.3   Evaluation Metrics

The model is estimated using the following metrics: accuracy, sensitivity, specificity and F1 score. These metrics are defined in the Eqs. (12)–(15).

$$Accuracy = \frac{TP + TN}{TP + TN + FP + FN} \tag{12}$$

$$Sensitivity = \frac{TP}{TP + FN} \tag{13}$$

$$Specificity = \frac{TN}{TN + FP} \tag{14}$$

$$F1 = \frac{2 * TP}{2 * TP + FP + FN} \tag{15}$$

4.4   Result

Table 2 shows the performance metrics of our proposed model PMFNet and various previous studies under the official splitting strategy of the Apnea-ECG dataset, while the evaluation results of other studies are taken from their literature records. To maintain consistency in data presentation, all results in the table are rounded to only one decimal place. Our proposed PMFNet obtained an accuracy of 92.8%, a sensitivity of 91.0%, a specificity of 94.0% and an F1 value of 90.4% on the task of detecting OSA in each 1-minute segment. Compared to studies using the same statistical strategy and machine learning approach [20,34], the accuracy, sensitivity and specificity of PMFNet improved on average by 7.3 %, 8.95%, and 6.35%, respectively. The significant improvement in each metric indicates that our proposed deep learning model is able to better capture and learn the complex and abstract features in ECG signals. Compared to other studies in the table [10,22,33,37,38], our model additionally uses time-frequency maps based on 1D ECG signal variation data, which proves the effectiveness of the graph data in feature representation. Wang et al. [38] obtained better specificity, which we believe may be due to the fact that the Apnea-ECG dataset is not a balanced dataset, and its data distribution may affect the specificity of our method. The F1 score is taken from the reconciled mean of precision and recall, which is unaffected by unbalanced data distributions and is often considered a better performance metric, where we still achieve optimal performance.

Table 3 records the performance comparison between our proposed model PMFNet and previously studied models under 10-fold cross-validation. Figure 7 records the distribution of PMFNet's performance metrics during the 10-fold cross-validation process, where the middle point of each violin represents the average performance of the ten experiments. Obviously, the 10-fold average of PMFNet's accuracy, sensitivity, specificity, and F1 values on the OSA detection task for each one-minute segment are 93.90%, 93.53%, 96.71%, 91.84%, respectively. Among these existing studies listed, both Wang et al. [40] and Niroshana et al. [23] chose to obtain images through data transformation as

Table 2. Performance results of our proposed model and previous models on Apnea-ECG database

Method	Accuracy (%)	Sensitivity (%)	Specificity (%)	F1 (%)	
An Expert System	84.8	81.5	86.6	-	
Song et al. [34]	HMM + SVM 86.2	82.6	88.4	-
LeNet-5	87.6	83.1	90.3	-	
MSDA-1DCNN	89.4	89.8	89.1	-	
URNet	90.4	83.3	**94.8**	89.6	
SE-ResNext50	91.1	88.7	92.6	-	
RAFNet	91.4	88.7	93.0	88.7	
PMFNet	**92.8**	**91.0**	94.0	**90.4**	

Table 3. Results of 10-fold cross-validation of our proposed model and previous models on the Apnea-ECG database

Reference	Method	Accuracy (%)	Sensitivity (%)	Specificity (%)
Rajesh et al. [27]	DWT+RF	90.3	86.6	92.59
Wang et al. [40]	OSA-CCNN	90.93	83.68	95.29
Almutairi et al. [2]	CNN + LSTM	90.92	91.24	90.36
Niroshana et al. [23]	2D-CNN	92.4	92.3	92.6
Fatimah et al. [11]	FFT+SVM	92.59	89.7	94.67
Proposed model	PMFNet	**93.90**	**93.53**	**96.71**

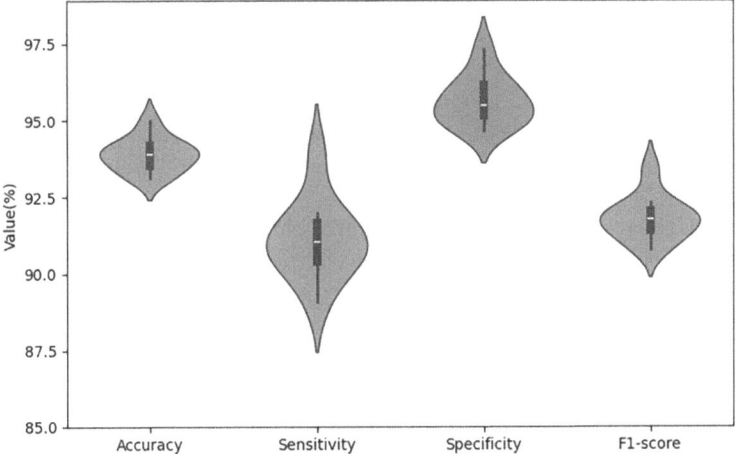

Fig. 7. Ten-fold cross-validation results for the PMFNet

model inputs, while Almutairi et al. [2] used one-dimensional ECG signal variation data as inputs, which is the most common form of input, and Rajessh et
al. [27] and Fatimah et al. [11] obtained a large number of discrete features of
the ECG signals via DWT and FDM, which is also a form of representation of
one-dimensional data. Compared to these studies, PMFNet shows a significant
improvement in all metrics, which not only proves that PMFNet has a surprising predictive performance, but also demonstrates that the use of multimodal
data is complementary rather than independent for the characterisation of ECG
signals.

5   Discussion

5.1   Ablation Study

To verify the validity of the adjacent segments as well as the individual components of our proposed model, we performed a large number of ablation experiments on the Apnea-ECG dataset. In the following we refer to our proposed
PMFNet model as the control group. To ensure the accuracy of the results, the
environment, hyperparameters and evaluation metrics used in all the experiments were the same as those used in the control group, and each experiment
was conducted five times. The specific experimental settings were as follows:

(A) Target segment only: R-wave feature data were constructed using the ECG
centre marker segment (one minute target segment).
(B) Target segment + adjacent segments: R-wave feature data were constructed
by combining the ECG central marker segment and ±1 segment around it
(i.e. one minute before and one minute after, for a total of three minutes)
as a whole.
(C) R-wave data only: Using only the extracted R-wave data as input data, a
CNN and LSTM model is constructed to complete OSA detection.
(D) Resnet only: Using only the time-frequency maps obtained from the transformation as input data, OSA detection was performed using the ResNet-50
model.
(E) Modal Concat: The R-wave data features obtained in the feature extraction
stage are concatenated with the time-frequency map features and passed
directly to the fully connected layer for classification, replacing the BAN
module in PMFNet.

We comparing model (A) and model (B) with the control group, we used different strategies for introducing the adjacent segments. The experimental results
(Fig. 8) showed that the accuracy of model (A) using only the target fragment
was 89.82%, and that of model (B) based on the three minutes combined fragment was 90.15%, and all the evaluated metrics were lower than that of the
control in both cases, further illustrating that the use of adjacent fragments can
effectively provide the detection performance of OSA.

In addition we designed groups C, D and E to be compared with the control
group. From the experimental results (Fig. 9), we can see that compared with

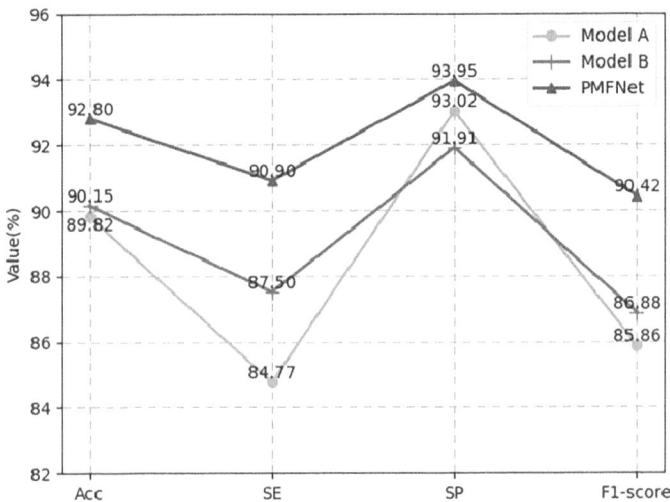

Fig. 8. Performance Comparison of different inputs in ablation experiments

models C and D, which use only R-wave data and only graph data as inputs, both model E and the control group, which use both pseudo-modal data as inputs, achieve better performance, which not only proves the validity of the concept of pseudo-modality, but also shows that the strategy of using multiple modal data as inputs can contribute additional effective information based on the use of single data information. If we further compare the effects of model E and the control group, we can see that the control group outperforms model E in all the metrics, further proving that the bilinear attention network used by PMFNet is more conducive to cross-modal feature fusion than the simple concatenation operation.

5.2 Future Work

The PMFNet proposed in this paper is based on single-lead ECG signals, and transforms to obtain two types of pseudo-modal data, namely the R-wave data features extracted from a group of five minutes ECG segments, and the ECG time-frequency maps obtained by transforming from a one minute central target segment. Previous studies and a large number of ablation experiments have demonstrated the effectiveness of introducing adjacent segments to improve OSA detection, so in the subsequent work, we will consider using five minutes (or other time lengths) as a window, and use the sliding window mechanism to transform to obtain time-frequency maps that cover the five minutes ECG time-frequency domain change information. In addition, considering that the introduction of adjacent segments brings redundant information to a certain extent, we try a series of ideas and experiments to consider how to effectively control the effect of redundant features on the central target segment, so that our network can

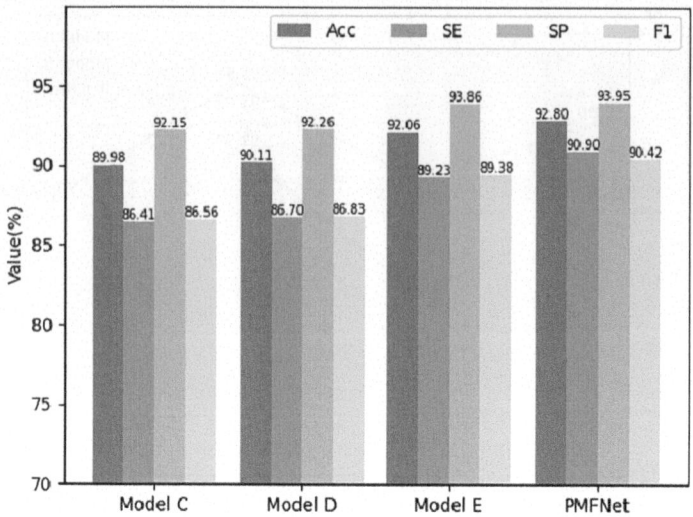

Fig. 9. Performance comparison of different models in ablation experiments

learn the central target segment more intensively while combining the features of adjacent segments effectively.

Furthermore, based on the survey [30] we learnt that there are limitations in the data labelling of the PhysioNet Apnea-ECG dataset. In particular, the labelled value for each minute (A for OSA event, N for normal) are labelled according to whether an OSA event occurred in the first data point sampled in that minute or not, and this labeling method will label the segments in which an OSA event occurs after the first sampling point as negative, i.e., false negative labeling, thus bringing some impact on the model training results. According to Table 1, the number of positive samples in the pre-processed training dataset is 6484, accounting for 38.5 % of the total samples in the training set, which shows that there is some imbalance in the sample distribution of this dataset. To address some of the labelling deficiencies in the publicly available dataset, and also to validate and improve the generalisation ability of PMFNet in real clinical applications, we are in the process of establishing a multi-centre sleep apnea detection dataset with relevant healthcare organisations.

6   Conclusion

In this paper, we propose a pseudo-modal fusion network, PMFNet, which is influenced by multimodal learning, to complete the detection of obstructive sleep apnea using single-lead ECG signals, providing an effective alternative to the use of PSG to complete OSA detection. We have innovatively proposed the concept of "pseudo-modality" in the use of ECG signals, carefully designed different feature extractors for different modalities and effectively fused cross-modal features.

Overall, given a one-minute sleep ECG segment of a subject, PMFNet is able to automatically extract effective features without relying on the experience or domain knowledge of professional researchers for feature processing, enabling an end-to-end OSA classification task. Extensive experimental results on the publicly available PhysioNet Apnea-ECG dataset show that our proposed PMFNet has very competitive experimental results, with a specific test set accuracy of 92.79%, sensitivity of 90.90%, specificity of 93.95% and F1 score of 90.42%, and a tenfold cross-validation strategy is used to demonstrate the robustness of PMFNet. At the same time, we also used a 10-fold cross-validation strategy to demonstrate the robustness of PMFNet, with an average test set accuracy of 93.9%, verifying that our proposed pseudo-modal data are complementary rather than isolated in characterising ECG signals. Our study is a successful application case of multimodal learning ideas in the field of ECG signal analysis.

References

1. Addison, P.S.: Wavelet transforms and the ECG: a review. Physiol. Meas. **26**(5), R155 (2005)
2. Almutairi, H., Hassan, G.M., Datta, A.: Classification of obstructive sleep Apnoea from single-lead ECG signals using convolutional neural and long short term memory networks. Biomed. Sig. Process. Control **69** (2021)
3. Almutairi, H., Hassan, G.M., Datta, A.: Detection of obstructive sleep Apnoea by ECG signals using deep learning architectures. In: 2020 28th European Signal Processing Conference (EUSIPCO), pp. 1382–1386 (2021)
4. Bacharova, L., Triantafyllou, E., Vazaios, C., Tomeckova, I., Paranicova, I., Tkacova, R.: The effect of obstructive sleep apnea on QRS complex morphology. J. Electrocardiol. **48**(2), 164–170 (2015)
5. Bahrami, M., Forouzanfar, M.: Detection of sleep apnea from single-lead ECG: comparison of deep learning algorithms. In: 2021 IEEE International Symposium on Medical Measurements and Applications (MeMeA), pp. 1–5 (2021)
6. Basu, S., Mamud, S.: Comparative study on the effect of order and cut off frequency of butterworth low pass filter for removal of noise in ECG signal. In: 2020 IEEE 1st International Conference for Convergence in Engineering (ICCE), pp. 156–160 (2020)
7. Benjafield, A.V., et al.: Estimation of the global prevalence and burden of obstructive sleep Apnoea: a literature-based analysis. Lancet Respir. Med. **7**(8), 687–698 (2019)
8. de Chazal, P., Heneghan, C., Sheridan, E., Reilly, R., Nolan, P., O'Malley, M.: Automatic classification of sleep apnea epochs using the electrocardiogram. In: Computers in Cardiology 2000(Cat. 00CH37163), vol. 27 , pp. 745–748 (2000)
9. Chen, L., Zhang, X., Song, C.: An automatic screening approach for obstructive sleep apnea diagnosis based on single-lead electrocardiogram. IEEE Trans. Autom. Sci. Eng. **12**(1), 106–115 (2015)
10. Chen, Y., Yue, H., Zou, R., Lei, W., Ma, W., Fan, X.: RafNnet: restricted attention fusion network for sleep apnea detection. Neural Netw. **162**, 571–580 (2023)
11. Fatimah, B., Singh, P., Singhal, A., Pachori, R.B.: Detection of apnea events from ECG segments using Fourier decomposition method. Biomed. Sig. Process. Control **61**, 102005 (2020)

12. Guan, Y., An, Y., Xu, J., Liu, N., Wang, J.: Ha-resnet: residual neural network with hidden attention for ECG arrhythmia detection using two-dimensional signal. IEEE/ACM Trans. Comput. Biol. Bioinf. **20**(6), 3389–3398 (2023)

13. Hamilton, P.: Open source ECG analysis. In: Computers in Cardiology, pp. 101–104 (2002)

14. Huang, G., Ma, F.: Concad: contrastive learning-based cross attention for sleep apnea detection (2021)

15. Juang, C.F., Pan, G.R., Huang, W.C., Wen, C.Y., Wu, M.F.: Multiobjective optimization of interpretable fuzzy systems and applicable subjects for fast estimation of obstructive sleep apnea-hypopnea severity. IEEE Trans. Fuzzy Syst. **31**(7), 2225–2237 (2023)

16. Kim, J.H., Jun, J., Zhang, B.T.: Bilinear attention networks. In: Bengio, S., Wallach, H., Larochelle, H., Grauman, K., CesaBianchi, N., Garnett, R. (eds.) Advances in Neural Information Processing Systems 31 (NIPS 2018). Advances in Neural Information Processing Systems, vol. 31 (2018), 32nd Conference on Neural Information Processing Systems (NIPS), Montreal, Canada, 02–08 December 2018

17. Labarca, G., Sanchez-de-la Torre, M., Jorquera, J.: Systemic involvement in obstructive sleep apnea: personalized medicine to improve health outcomes. Front. Med. **9** (2022)

18. Li, W., Gao, J.: Automatic sleep staging by a hybrid model based on deep 1d-resnet-se and LSTM with single-channel raw EEG signals. PeerJ Comput. Sci. **9** (SEP 26 2023)

19. Ma, K., Zhan, C.A., Yang, F.: Multi-classification of arrhythmias using resnet with CBAM on CWGAN-GP augmented ECG Gramian angular summation field. Biomed. Sig. Process. Control **77**, 103684 (2022)

20. Martín-González, S., Navarro-Mesa, J.L., Juliá-Serdá, G., Kraemer, J.F., Wessel, N., Ravelo-García, A.G.: Heart rate variability feature selection in the presence of sleep apnea: An expert system for the characterization and detection of the disorder. Comput. Biol. Med. **91**, 47–58 (2017)

21. Mashrur, F.R., Islam, M.S., Saha, D.K., Islam, S.R., Moni, M.A.: SCNN: scalogram-based convolutional neural network to detect obstructive sleep apnea using single-lead electrocardiogram signals. Comput. Biol. Med. **134**, 104532 (2021)

22. Nguyen, A.T., Nguyen, T., Le, H.K., Pham, H.H., Do, C.: A novel deep learning-based approach for sleep apnea detection using single-lead ECG signals. In: 2022 Asia-Pacific Signal and Information Processing Association Annual Summit and Conference (APSIPA ASC), pp. 2046–2052 (2022)

23. Niroshana, S.M.I., Zhu, X., Nakamura, K., Chen, W.: A fused-image-based approach to detect obstructive sleep apnea using a single-lead ECG and a 2D convolutional neural network. PLOS ONE **16**(4) (2021)

24. Peker, Y., et al.: Obstructive sleep apnea and cardiovascular disease: where do we stand? Anatolian J. Cardiol. **27**(7), 375–389 (2023)

25. Penzel, T., Moody, G., Mark, R., Goldberger, A., Peter, J.: The apnea-ECG database. In: Computers in Cardiology 2000 (Cat. 00CH37163), vol. 27, pp. 255–258 (2000)

26. Piccirillo, F., Crispino, S.P., Buzzelli, L., Segreti, A., Incalzi, R.A., Grigioni, F.: A state-of-the-art review on sleep apnea syndrome and heart failure. Am. J. Cardiol. **195**, 57–69 (2023)

27. Rajesh, K., Dhuli, R., Kumar, T.S.: Obstructive sleep apnea detection using discrete wavelet transform-based statistical features. Comput. Biol. Med. **130**, 104199 (2021)

28. Salari, N., et al.: Detection of sleep apnea using machine learning algorithms based on ECG signals: a comprehensive systematic review. Expert Syst. Appl. **187**, 115950 (2022)
29. Senaratna, C.V., et al.: Prevalence of obstructive sleep apnea in the general population: a systematic review. Sleep Med. Rev. **34**, 70–81 (2017)
30. Seo, D.W., Kim, J., Lee, H.W., Suh, Y.K.: A deep neural network based wake-after-sleep-onset time aware sleep apnea severity estimation scheme using single-lead ECG data. IEEE Access **11**, 43720–43732 (2023)
31. Shao, S., Han, G., Wang, T., Song, C., Yao, C., Hou, J.: Obstructive sleep apnea detection scheme based on manually generated features and parallel heterogeneous deep learning model under IOMT. IEEE J. Biomed. Health Inform. **26**(12), 5841–5850 (2022)
32. Sharan, R.V., Berkovsky, S., Xiong, H., Coiera, E.: ECG-derived heart rate variability interpolation and 1-D convolutional neural networks for detecting sleep apnea. In: 2020 42nd Annual International Conference of the IEEE Engineering in Medicine and Biology Society (EMBC), pp. 637–640 (2020)
33. Shen, Q., Qin, H., Wei, K., Liu, G.: Multiscale deep neural network for obstructive sleep apnea detection using RR interval from single-lead ECG signal. IEEE Trans. Instrum. Meas. **70**, 1–13 (2021)
34. Song, C., Liu, K., Zhang, X., Chen, L., Xian, X.: An obstructive sleep apnea detection approach using a discriminative hidden Markov model from ECG signals. IEEE Trans. Biomed. Eng. **63**(7), 1532–1542 (2016)
35. Surrel, G., Aminifar, A., Rincón, F., Murali, S., Atienza, D.: Online obstructive sleep apnea detection on medical wearable sensors. IEEE Trans. Biomed. Circuits Syst. **12**(4), 762–773 (2018)
36. Ullah, N., Mahmood, T., Kim, S.G., Nam, S.H., Sultan, H., Park, K.R.: DCDA-net: dual-convolutional dual-attention network for obstructive sleep apnea diagnosis from single-lead electrocardiograms. Eng. Appl. Artif. Intell. **123**, 106451 (2023)
37. Wang, T., Lu, C., Shen, G., Hong, F.: Sleep apnea detection from a single-lead ECG signal with automatic feature-extraction through a modified Lenet-5 convolutional neural network. PEERJ **7** (2019)
38. Wang, Z., et al.: Single-lead ECG based multiscale neural network for obstructive sleep apnea detection. Internet Things **20** (2022)
39. Wu, M.F., et al.: A new method for self-estimation of the severity of obstructive sleep apnea using easily available measurements and neural fuzzy evaluation system. IEEE J. Biomed. Health Inform. **21**(6), 1524–1532 (2017)
40. Zhou, Y., He, Y., Kang, K.: OSA-CCNN: obstructive sleep apnea detection based on a composite deep convolution neural network model using single-lead ECG signal. In: 2022 IEEE International Conference on Bioinformatics and Biomedicine (BIBM), pp. 1840–1845 (2022)

VisionLLM-Based Multimodal Fusion Network for Glottic Carcinoma Early Detection

Zhaohui Jin[1], Yi Shuai[2], Yongcheng Li[1], Lingcong Cai[1], Yun Li[2], Huifen Liu[1(✉)], and Xiaomao Fan[1(✉)]

[1] Shenzhen Technology University, Shenzhen, China
liuhuifen@sztu.edu.cn, astrofan2008@gmail.com
[2] First Affiliated Hospital of Sun Yat-sen University, Guangzhou, China

Abstract. The early detection of glottic carcinoma is critical for improving patient outcomes, as it enables timely intervention, preserves vocal function, and significantly reduces the risk of tumor progression and metastasis. However, the similarity in morphology between glottic carcinoma and vocal cord dysplasia results in suboptimal detection accuracy. To address this issue, we propose a vision large language model-based (VisionLLM-based) multimodal fusion network for glottic carcinoma detection, known as MMGC-Net. By integrating image and text modalities, multimodal models can capture complementary information, leading to more accurate and robust predictions. In this paper, we collect a private real glottic carcinoma dataset named SYSU1H from the First Affiliated Hospital of Sun Yat-sen University, with 5,799 image-text pairs. We leverage an image encoder and additional Q-Former to extract vision embeddings and the Large Language Model Meta AI (Llama3) to obtain text embeddings. These modalities are then integrated through a laryngeal feature fusion block, enabling a comprehensive integration of image and text features, thereby improving the glottic carcinoma identification performance. Extensive experiments on the SYSU1H dataset demonstrate that MMGC-Net can achieve state-of-the-art performance, which is superior to previous multimodal models.

Keywords: Multimodal machine learning · Large-scale foundation model · Llama3 · Glottic carcinoma early detection

1 Introduction

Glottic carcinoma is a common malignant tumor of the head and neck that can severely affect the patient's voice, swallowing, breathing function, and even overall health [8]. The early detection of glottic carcinoma heavily relies on the manual interpretation of laryngoscopic results. However, vocal cord dysplasia, a

---

Z. Jin and Y. Shuai—Contribute equally.

© The Author(s), under exclusive license to Springer Nature Singapore Pte Ltd. 2025
Y. Zhang et al. (Eds.): CHIP 2024, CCIS 2433, pp. 70–77, 2025.
https://doi.org/10.1007/978-981-96-3752-2_5

kind of precancerosis is hard to distinguish from glottic carcinoma under laryngoscopy [16]. Moreover, the small size of lesions, coupled with the limitations of specialist expertise may lead to a high misdiagnosis rate [2,5,15]. Therefore, the development of an automated approach to assist laryngologists in the early detection of glottic carcinoma is of paramount importance.

Recently, significant progress has been made in deep learning techniques for tackling real-world classification tasks in computer vision and natural language processing. Many researchers have sought to apply these models to the detection of laryngeal cancer, yielding promising outcomes. However, most existing methods only utilize laryngoscopic images as input, including UC-DenseNet [12], MTANet [19], DLGNet [17], RedFormer [3], and SAM-FNet [18]. Although these methods have demonstrated improved performance in laryngeal cancer detection, they mainly neglected the potential benefits of incorporating text modality to further enhance classification accuracy. Therefore, we have curated the SYSU1H dataset from the First Affiliated Hospital of Sun Yat-sen University, which includes both laryngoscopic images and corresponding clinical reports. This comprehensive dataset enables the integration of multimodal information, offering a significant advantage in improving the performance and robustness of classification models.

In this paper, we propose a simple yet effective multimodal fusion framework, termed MMGC-Net, for early detection of glottic carcinoma. Specifically, we introduce a laryngoscopic image encoder [10] to extract image embeddings from laryngoscopic images and Llama3 [4] to derive text embeddings from clinical reports. Additionally, we design a laryngeal feature fusion block that integrates these two modalities, enabling the model to capture joint features from both the visual data and the corresponding clinical reports. The combination of these modalities allows the model to better exploit the complementary information provided by the images and texts, enhancing its classification capability. Extensive experiments on our collected SYSU1H dataset demonstrate that our proposed MMGC-Net can achieve state-of-the-art results with a significant margin. Overall, our main contributions can be summarized as follows:

- We present the SYSU1H dataset, collected from the First Affiliated Hospital of Sun Yat-sen University, which includes both laryngoscopic images and clinical reports, providing a unique resource for laryngeal cancer detection.
- We employ the pre-trained image encoder and Q-Former to extract well-aligned features from laryngoscopic images, and introduce Llama3, leveraging its advanced natural language processing capabilities, to extract text embeddings from clinical reports.
- We propose MMGC-Net, a novel VisionLLM-based multimodal fusion network for the early detection of glottic carcinoma, which is the first application of multimodal learning to this specific task.
- Extensive experiment results conducted on our collected SYSU1H dataset demonstrate that our proposed MMGC-Net can achieve state-of-the-art results with a significant margin.

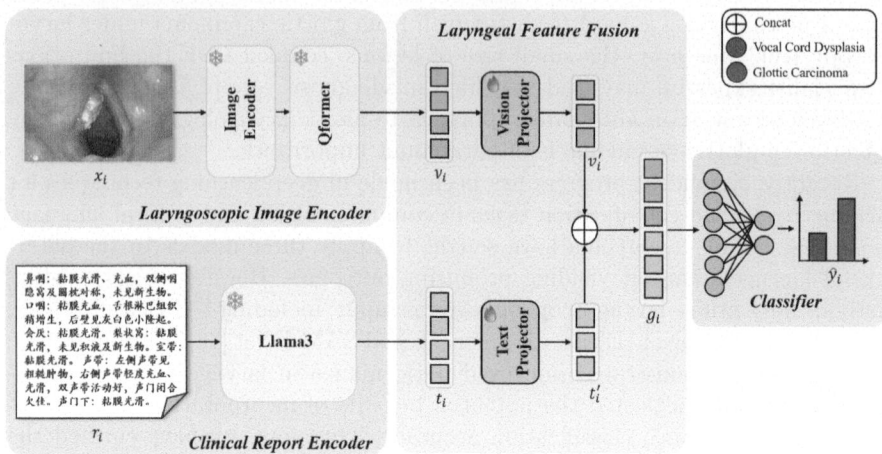

Fig. 1. The overall architecture of our proposed MMGC-Net.

2   Methodology

Figure 1 illustrates the overall architecture of our proposed MMGC-Net, which consists of three main components: laryngoscopic image encoder, clinical report encoder, and laryngeal feature fusion block. The laryngoscopic image encoder extracts embeddings from laryngoscopic images, while the text encoder processes clinical reports to obtain text embeddings. These embeddings are then integrated via the laryngeal feature fusion block. Finally, a fully connected layer is utilized for classification. The detailed information is outlined as follows:

2.1   Laryngoscopic Image Encoder

Solely utilizing an image encoder (i.e. ViT [1]) to extract image features may result in significant discrepancies between image and text features, potentially resulting in a decline in classification performance. To address this issue, we leverage an additional Q-Former [10] in our laryngoscopic image encoder to extract the image feature most relevant to the text. Formally, let $f_{enc}(\cdot)$ and $f_q(\cdot)$ represent the image encoder and Q-Former respectively. Given a image x_i, the image feature v_i can be obtained by:

$$v_i = f_q(f_{enc}(x_i; \theta_{enc}); \theta_q), \tag{1}$$

where θ_{enc}, θ_q are the parameter of image encoder and Q-Former. It is noteworthy that we use the pre-trained weight of BLIP-2 as the parameters for our laryngoscopic image encoder, since a great number of studies have demonstrated the effectiveness of BLIP2 in downstream tasks [9,13,20]. It ensures that the extracted image features are well-aligned with the text features, which can mitigate the catastrophic consequences that could arise from modality discrepancies.

2.2   Clinical Report Encoder

For the text modality, we employ Llama3, a sophisticated large language model renowned for its robust multilingual and long-text processing capabilities. Compared to other large language models, Llama3 excels in handling Chinese clinical reports, making it particularly well-suited for our application. Formally, let $f_{Llama3}(\cdot)$ denote the clinical report encoder. Given a clinical report r_i, the encoder can be expressed as:

$$t_i = f_{Llama3}(r_i, \theta_l), \tag{2}$$

where t_i represents the text embedding generated by the clinical report encoder, and θ_l denotes the encoder's parameters.

2.3   Laryngeal Feature Fusion

To fuse the image and text modalities, we introduce a laryngeal feature fusion block. Specifically, we first leverage the vision projector $f_{vp}(\cdot)$ and text projector $f_{tp}(\cdot)$, which map the image and text embeddings v_i and t_i into a unified representation space, formulated as:

$$v_i' = f_{vp}(v_i; \theta_{vp}), \tag{3}$$
$$t_i' = f_{tp}(t_i; \theta_{tp}), \tag{4}$$

where v_i' and t_i' represent the transformed image and text features, and θ_{vp}, θ_{tp} denote the respective parameters of $f_{vp}(\cdot)$ and $f_{tp}(\cdot)$. Additionally, we apply L2-normalization to both features, yielding $v_i'' = \frac{v_i'}{\|v_i'\|_2}$ and $t_i'' = \frac{t_i'}{\|t_i'\|_2}$. Finally, the normalized features v_i'' and t_i'' are concatenated to form the vision-language joint feature, denoted as $g_i = Concat(v_i'', t_i'')$. The vision-language joint feature g_i is then passed through a classifier f_{fc}, which can be defined as follows:

$$\hat{y}_i = f_{fc}(g_i, \theta_{fc}) \tag{5}$$

where θ_{fc} represents the parameters of the classifier and $\hat{y}$ is the predicted probability distribution by the model. To optimize the MMGC-Net, this study utilizes the cross-entropy loss function, denoted as $\mathcal{L}_{ce}$, which can be expressed as follows:

$$\mathcal{L}_{CE} = -\sum_{i=1}^{C} y_i \log(\hat{y}_i) \tag{6}$$

where C is the number of classes and y represents the one-hot encoded ground truth labels.

3   Experiment

3.1   Dataset

SYSU1H: The dataset, collected from the First Affiliated Hospital of Sun Yat-sen University, comprises 5,799 image-text pairs classified into two categories:

vocal cord dysplasia and glottic carcinoma. Each image-text pair contains a laryngoscopic image and a corresponding laryngoscopy report (written by a professional doctor). This dataset is collected and organized for the first time, and it has unique clinical value, which can effectively support the early detection research of glottic carcinoma. The dataset has been split into training, validation, and test sets following an 8:1:1 ratio, providing sufficient data support for this study and ensuring the reliability and representativeness of the experimental results.

3.2   Implementation Details

All experiments are carried out on a dedicated server featuring eight NVIDIA A6000 GPUs with a total of 196 GB of video memory. The system runs on Ubuntu 20.04.5 LTS, utilizing Pytorch 1.9.1 and Scikit-learn 1.3.1 for the implementation. In this study, we employ the AdamW to optimize MMGC-Net with an initial learning rate of 0.00001, with a warm-up and cosine learning schedules to dynamically control the learning rate. MMGC-Net is trained for 80 epochs.

Table 1. Comparison with the state-of-the-art multimodal machine learning models. The best performance is in **bold** and the second best is indicated with underline.

Methods	Overall results				Recall for different classes	
	Accuracy (%)	Precision (%)	Recall (%)	F_1 score (%)	VCD (%)	GC (%)
CLIP [14]	67.24 ± 2.7	67.49 ± 2.6	66.26 ± 2.7	67.57 ± 3.6	63.76 ± 7.0	70.75 ± 3.8
BLIP [11]	58.95 ± 1.9	59.30 ± 1.7	59.02 ± 1.9	59.13 ± 1.1	49.31 ± 7.5	68.70 ± 4.2
VILT [7]	59.10 ± 0.1	59.07 ± 0.1	59.08 ± 0.1	59.07 ± 0.1	49.13 ± 4.9	69.01 ± 4.4
ALIGN [6]	62.31 ± 2.0	62.51 ± 0.9	56.81 ± 3.3	61.80 ± 1.9	33.13 ± 7.9	$\underline{80.48 \pm 8.3}$
MMGC-Net (Ours)	$\mathbf{76.10 \pm 0.2}$	$\mathbf{76.70 \pm 0.2}$	$\mathbf{76.16 \pm 0.2}$	$\mathbf{74.41 \pm 0.5}$	$\mathbf{68.83 \pm 1.4}$	$\mathbf{83.48 \pm 1.1}$

3.3   Experimental Results

To demonstrate the effectiveness of our proposed MMGC-Net, we compare our method with four state-of-the-art methods, including CLIP [14], BLIP [11], VILT [7], and ALIGN [6]. The average results from five trials of various benchmark models, along with our proposed model, are presented in Table 1. MMGC-Net demonstrates promising performance, achieving accuracy, precision, recall, and F_1 score of 76.10%, 76.70%, 76.16%, and 74.41%, respectively. Notably, our model surpasses the second-best model by 8.86% and 9.90% in accuracy and recall, respectively. Regarding the single-class recall, MMGC-Net achieves 68.83% for vocal cord dysplasia and 83.48% for glottic carcinoma. Compared to other state-of-the-art models, MMGC-Net demonstrates significant enhancements in both accuracy and recall, indicating its superior capability in identifying glottic carcinoma.

Table 2. Ablation study of MMGC-Net.

Variants	Image	Report	Accuracy (%)	Precision (%)	Recall (%)	F_1 score (%)
M1	✓		66.72 ± 2.6	67.82 ± 2.5	67.44 ± 3.0	67.63 ± 2.7
M2		✓	65.36 ± 0.8	71.51 ± 2.4	64.56 ± 1.6	61.59 ± 1.3
M3	✓	✓	76.10 ± 0.2	76.70 ± 0.2	76.16 ± 0.2	74.41 ± 0.5

3.4   Ablation Studies

To verify the effectiveness of our method for early detection of glottic laryngeal cancer, we compare variants of our method by using only the image modality or text modality: (1) M1 represents using only the image modality; (2) M2 represents using only the text modality; (3) M3 represents using both image and text multimodal data.

As shown in Table 2, The model variant M3, which integrates both image and text modality, demonstrates the best overall performance across all metrics. Specifically, M3 achieves an accuracy of 76.10%, precision of 76.70%, recall of 76.16%, and an F_1 score of 74.41%, which outperforms M1 and M2 with a significant margin. These results clearly indicate that using both image and report data significantly enhances the model's performance compared to using either modality alone.

4   Conclusion

In this paper, we propose MMGC-Net, a novel model for the early detection of glottic carcinoma. MMGC-Net integrates a laryngoscopic image encoder, a clinical report encoder, and a laryngeal feature fusion block. These two modules efficiently extract embeddings from laryngoscopic images and clinical reports, respectively. Leveraging the laryngeal feature fusion block, MMGC-Net captures intrinsic patterns from these multimodal embeddings. Extensive experiments on our SYSU1H dataset demonstrate that MMGC-Net achieves a new state-of-the-art baseline with a substantial performance improvement.

Acknowledgment. This work is partially supported by the National Natural Science Foundation of China (62473267), the Basic and Applied Basic Research Project of Guangdong Province (2022B1515130009), the Special subject on Agriculture and Social Development, Key Research and Development Plan in Guangzhou (2023B03J0172), and the Natural Science Foundation of Top Talent of SZTU (GDRC202318).

References

1. Alexey, D.: An image is worth 16x16 words: transformers for image recognition at scale. arXiv preprint arXiv:2010.11929 (2020)
2. Azam, M.A., et al.: Deep learning applied to white light and narrow band imaging videolaryngoscopy: toward real-time laryngeal cancer detection. Laryngoscope **132**(9), 1798–1806 (2022)
3. Cui, C., Ma, Y., Lu, J., Wang, Z.: Redformer: radar enlightens the darkness of camera perception with transformers. IEEE Trans. Intell. Veh. (2023)
4. Dubey, A., et al.: The llama 3 herd of models. arXiv preprint arXiv:2407.21783 (2024)
5. Irjala, H., Matar, N., Remacle, M., Georges, L.: Pharyngo-laryngeal examination with the narrow band imaging technology: early experience. Eur. Arch. Otorhinolaryngol. **268**, 801–806 (2011)
6. Jia, C., et al.: Scaling up visual and vision-language representation learning with noisy text supervision. In: International Conference on Machine Learning, pp. 4904–4916. PMLR (2021)
7. Kim, W., Son, B., Kim, I.: VILT: vision-and-language transformer without convolution or region supervision. In: International Conference on Machine Learning, pp. 5583–5594. PMLR (2021)
8. Kwon, I., et al.: Diagnosis of early glottic cancer using laryngeal image and voice based on ensemble learning of convolutional neural network classifiers. J. Voice (2022)
9. Lee, C., Jang, J., Lee, J.: Personalizing text-to-image generation with visual prompts using blip-2 (2023)
10. Li, J., Li, D., Savarese, S., Hoi, S.: Blip-2: bootstrapping language-image pre-training with frozen image encoders and large language models. In: International Conference on Machine Learning, pp. 19730–19742. PMLR (2023)
11. Li, J., Li, D., Xiong, C., Hoi, S.: Blip: bootstrapping language-image pre-training for unified vision-language understanding and generation. In: International Conference on Machine Learning, pp. 12888–12900. PMLR (2022)
12. Luo, X., Zhang, J., Li, Z., Yang, R.: Diagnosis of ulcerative colitis from endoscopic images based on deep learning. Biomed. Sig. Process. Control **73**, 103443 (2022)
13. Nguyen, T., Gadre, S.Y., Ilharco, G., Oh, S., Schmidt, L.: Improving multimodal datasets with image captioning. In: Advances in Neural Information Processing Systems, vol. 36 (2024)
14. Radford, A., et al.: Learning transferable visual models from natural language supervision. In: International Conference on Machine Learning, pp. 8748–8763. PMLR (2021)
15. Tamagawa, S., et al.: Primary laryngeal cryptococcosis resembling laryngeal carcinoma. Auris Nasus Larynx **42**(4), 337–340 (2015)
16. Unger, J., Lohscheller, J., Reiter, M., Eder, K., Betz, C.S., Schuster, M.: A non-invasive procedure for early-stage discrimination of malignant and precancerous vocal fold lesions based on laryngeal dynamics analysis. Cancer Res. **75**(1), 31–39 (2015)
17. Wang, K.-N., et al.: DLGnet: a dual-branch lesion-aware network with the supervised gaussian mixture model for colon lesions classification in colonoscopy images. Med. Image Anal. **87**, 102832 (2023)
18. Wei, J., Li, Y., Qiu, M., Chen, H., Fan, X., Lei, W.: Sam-FNET: Sam-guided fusion network for laryngo-pharyngeal tumor detection. arXiv preprint arXiv:2408.05426 (2024)

19. Zhou, W., Dong, S., Lei, J., Lu, Yu.: MTAnet: multitask-aware network with hierarchical multimodal fusion for RGB-T urban scene understanding. IEEE Trans. Intell. Veh. **8**(1), 48–58 (2022)
20. Zhu, D., Chen, J., Haydarov, K., Shen, X., Zhang, W., Elhoseiny, M.: ChatGPT asks, blip-2 answers: automatic questioning towards enriched visual descriptions. arXiv preprint arXiv:2303.06594 (2023)

RAG Combined with Instruction Tuning for Traditional Chinese Medicine Syndrome Differentiation Thinking

Chunliang Chen, Ming Guan, Wenjing Yue, Xinyu Wang, Yuanbin Wu, and Xiaoling Wang[✉]

East China Normal University, Shanghai, China
{clchen,mguan}@stu.ecnu.edu.cn, xlwang@cs.ecnu.edu.cn

Abstract. The rapid advancements of large language models (LLMs) have opened new avenues for data processing and knowledge extraction, particularly in the medical domain. This paper investigates the application of LLMs in Traditional Chinese Medicine (TCM), with a focus on enhancing the models' capabilities in syndrome differentiation thinking tasks. We propose a method that delineates the syndrome differentiation process in TCM into four critical steps: clinical information extraction, pathogenesis inference, syndrome inference, and explanatory summarization, with tailored prompting strategies designed for each step. By integrating Retrieval-Augmented Generation (RAG) with instruction tuning, we generated 800 instruction data entries rich in localized knowledge and instruction tuning of a pre-trained model. Experimental results indicate that our approach significantly improves the models' performance in TCM syndrome differentiation thinking, achieving top rankings in both the A and B leaderboards, with scores of 45.12 and 44.37, respectively.

Keywords: Instruction Tuning · RAG · TCM LLM

1 Introduction

In recent years, large language models (LLMs) have exhibited significant advancements in data processing [2], knowledge extraction [10], and information integration [4,5], creating new opportunities for applications in the medical domain [6,16,27]. These models hold considerable promise in areas such as improving diagnostic precision, facilitating personalized treatment approaches, and supporting clinical decision-making processes.

As an essential component of modern healthcare systems, Traditional Chinese Medicine (TCM) has also benefited from advancements in LLMs [8,18], enabling more precise and intelligent approaches to disease prevention and treatment. These advancements substantively facilitate the modernization and internationalization of TCM, which is defined by its unique and intricate knowledge framework, deeply informed by extensive clinical insights captured in medical case records and syndrome differentiation is fundamental to TCM diagnostics [3,23,26], guiding both clinical diagnosis and treatment approaches.

© The Author(s), under exclusive license to Springer Nature Singapore Pte Ltd. 2025
Y. Zhang et al. (Eds.): CHIP 2024, CCIS 2433, pp. 78–89, 2025.
https://doi.org/10.1007/978-981-96-3752-2_6

CHIP2024-Chinese Medicine Syndrome Differentiation Thinking task has collected and refined high-quality medical case data, structuring syndrome differentiation thinking into a model based on TCM principles. This task categorizes syndrome differentiation thinking into four key steps: clinical information recognition and extraction, pathogenesis inference, syndrome inference, and interpretative summary. The objective is to provide language models with a standardized, highly reliable, and quantifiable benchmark for evaluating reasoning in complex scenarios.

In this competition, we employed the internlm2-chat-20b-sft [1] as the base model for the evaluation tasks. To align with the characteristics of TCM reasoning, we designed specific prompts and generated 800 instruction data entries based on the four key steps from the training data to fine-tune the model. Additionally, we integrated Retrieval-Augmented Generation (RAG) with instruction tuning techniques to enhance the model's comprehension and improve the accuracy of results. Our method scored 45.12 points on the A scale and 44.37 points on the B scale. Both of these scores are among the highest, demonstrating the effectiveness of our method.

Specifically, the main contributions of this paper are as follows:

1. We treated the four key steps as independent reasoning tasks and used a staged output strategy to generate results sequentially, effectively reducing the model's performance demand in a single reasoning pass.
2. We proposed a strategy that combined RAG with instruction tuning. Using a text embedding model, we retrieved the most relevant TCM knowledge from a local knowledge base and incorporated it into the instruction data. This approach enhanced the model's understanding of TCM knowledge and improved its capability across the four reasoning tasks.
3. We conducted experimental validation on the dataset for this evaluation task, including the design of ablation studies, which further demonstrated the importance of the RAG strategy in the instruction data and its positive impact on model performance.

2   Related Work

In this section, we present the work related to our proposed methodology, including Retrieval-Augmented Generation and TCM LLM.

2.1   Retrieval-Augmented Generation

RAG addresses the limitations faced by LLMs in domain-specific and knowledge-intensive tasks, particularly the generation of hallucinations [11,14] and reliance on outdated information [13]. By retrieving relevant content from external databases, RAG enhances LLM performance through continuous knowledge updates and the incorporation of domain-specific information.

Several studies demonstrate the effectiveness of RAG in various contexts. MedGraphRAG [20] establishes connections between entities and foundational medical knowledge derived from medical journals and dictionaries, thereby providing the model with empirical citations and precise definitions of medical terminology. i-MedRAG [21] employs an iterative feedback mechanism in which insights from previous iterations inform query generation for subsequent rounds, thereby enhancing performance in multi-turn information retrieval tasks. Retcare [19] integrates authoritative medical literature to improve the interpretability of predictive results, contextualizing this information within the healthcare domain to offer detailed reasoning that supports clinical decision-making.

2.2 TCM LLM

Due to the constraints in pre-trained models' knowledge within the realm of TCM, the majority of large models pertinent to TCM have been fine-tuned using publicly accessible datasets, including classical texts, TCM literature, and educational materials [8,17,22]. Some models have incorporated proprietary data, such as clinical case records and TCM patents, to enhance their specificity and expertise. Notably, certain large models have undertaken in-depth research focused on specific disease domains, driven by the characteristics of this proprietary data. For example, The BianCang-TCM-LLM [15] integrated clinical data from cardiology, whereas the CMLM-ZhongJing [9] concentrated on gynecological prescriptions within TCM.

Furthermore, evaluation datasets specific to the TCM domain have begun to emerge. TCMBench [24] has proposed a comprehensive benchmark designed to assess the performance of LLMs in TCM, compiling 5,473 questions from the Traditional Chinese Medicine Licensing Examination. This dataset encompasses a wide range of competencies in TCM, including foundational knowledge and clinical practice. The Qibo-benchmark [25] has introduced an evaluative tool that assesses LLM performance in TCM from multiple perspectives, including subjective and objective evaluations, as well as three distinct TCM NLP tasks. While both benchmarks effectively evaluate foundational TCM knowledge, they do not specifically address the syndrome differentiation reasoning capabilities of LLMs, thus limiting the potential for advancements and optimizations in language models tailored to the TCM domain.

3   Method

The CHIP2024 competition dissects the syndrome differentiation thinking inherent in TCM into a distinct natural language processing tasks. A key challenge lies in the interdependence of the tasks; inaccuracies in earlier outputs can lead to cumulative errors and a decline in overall accuracy. Given that the competition does not impose restrictions on model types or open-source resources, we adopted instruction fine-tuning methods to enhance the performance of LLMs in TCM reasoning tasks. To improve LLM capabilities, we employed RAG, starting with the design of prompt templates that emphasize causal relationships for each task. We then enriched the instruction data with locally relevant knowledge using text embedding models and organized the output to extract pertinent information that aligns with our requirements. Through these strategies, we aim to significantly boost the accuracy and effectiveness of TCM reasoning tasks within the competition.

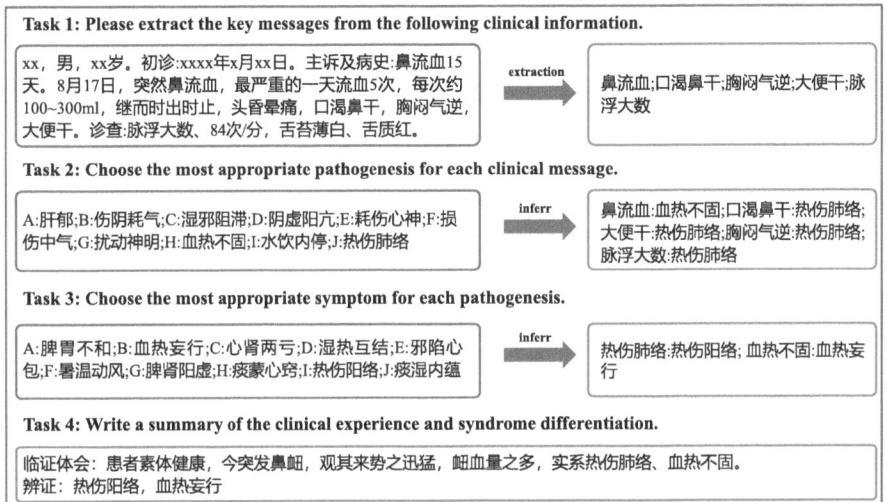

Fig. 1. A figure outlines the sequential processes of Information Extraction, Pathogeny Inference, and Dialectical Reasoning, illustrating their interconnections in analyzing clinical data.

3.1 Task Decomposition

We outline the generation of instruction data for the four distinct tasks, as illustrated in the Fig. 1. The initial task, Information Extraction, is designed to identify and extract pertinent clinical information from the textual case data. This includes general symptoms and signs, tongue and pulse diagnoses, etiological factors, and examination findings.

The subsequent task, Pathogeny Inference, involves correlating the extracted clinical key information with predefined options based on the data gathered in the first step. By utilizing the pathogeny identified in this stage, we synthesize it with the clinical information to deduce the dialectical outcomes, which encompass the syndrome information.

Finally, we integrate the aforementioned steps to articulate and summarize the syndrome differentiation thinking process. This comprehensive summary comprises two essential components: clinical insights derived from practice and the resultant syndrome differentiation conclusions.

3.2 Incorporation Based RAG

In the instruction data for Tasks 2,3,4, we integrated local knowledge based on the principle of RAG. We conceptualize the reasoning tasks in TCM as akin to an open-book exam; directly inputting relevant knowledge into publicly available models like gpt4o is comparable to taking an exam without prior study. However, by equipping the model with relevant knowledge during the fine-tuning phase, we can effectively guide it on how to extract desired outcomes from reference materials, ultimately enhancing its reasoning capabilities.

As illustrated in Fig. 2, the local knowledge base was partitioned into distinct segments, referred to as chunks, and vector models were employed to generate embeddings. Specifically, let Q denote the question to be addressed. The knowledge base is represented as $D = \{d_1, d_2, \ldots, d_n\}$, where each d_i corresponds to a chunk of the document. Embeddings for each chunk are generated using a vector model, denoted as $E = \{e_1, e_2, \ldots, e_n\}$. Each embedding is defined as $e_i = f(d_i)$, with f representing the embedding generation function. The similarity matching is established through cosine similarity, defined as follows:

$$\text{sim}(e_i, Q) = \frac{e_i \cdot Q}{\|e_i\|\|Q\|} \tag{1}$$

where $\| \cdot \|$ represents the vector norm, and chunks exhibiting the highest similarity are selected to form the matched document set D':

$$D' = \{d_j \in D \mid \text{sim}(e_j, Q) \geq \theta\} \tag{2}$$

In this expression, θ represents a predefined similarity threshold. Finally, the reference knowledge is integrated into the instructional data I, thereby enhancing reasoning capabilities across three tasks during practical evaluations.

3.3 Formatting Processing

In light of the inconsistency between the model's output format and the desired answer structure, we implement a processing step following each result generation. We systematically extract clinical information, infer the pathogenesis, deduce the symptom, and summarize clinical experiences from the output of each task. Subsequently, we integrate these components in accordance with the specified structural requirements, ensuring a coherent and academically rigorous presentation of the findings.

4 Experiments

4.1 Experimental Setup

In this experiment, all tests were conducted on a single A6000 GPU equipped with 48GB of memory. The base model we selected is internlm2-chat2-20b-sft.

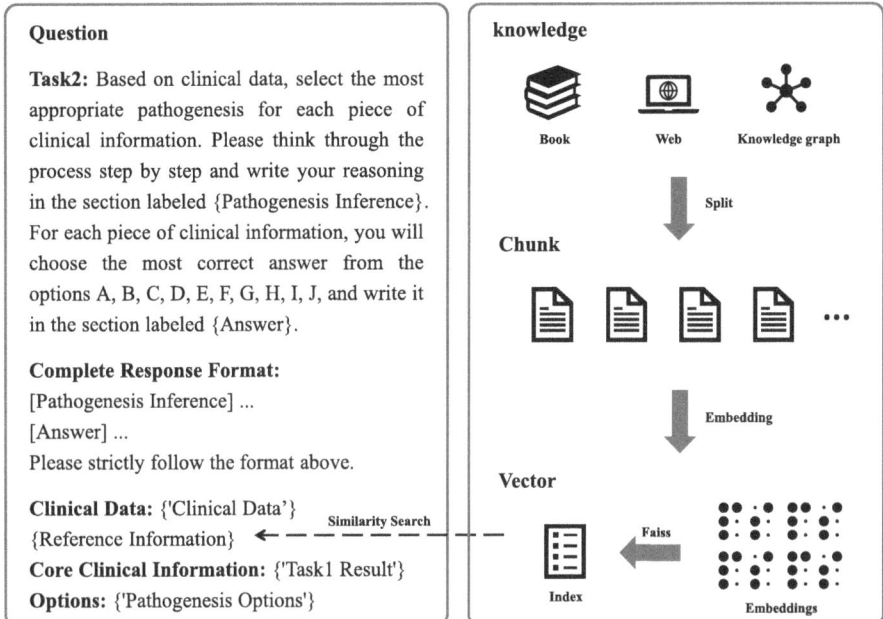

Fig. 2. A schematic representation of the methodology for integrating local information using RAG in the TCM syndrome differentiation thinking task, exemplifying Task 2.

This model not only supports the processing of complex scenarios but also integrates extensive knowledge of TCM during its training, providing a strong foundation for applications in related fields. Notably, the model is capable of effectively handling simple TCM QA tasks without any fine-tuning, establishing a solid basis for subsequent fine-tuning efforts. We use gte-Qwen2-7B-instruct [12] as text embedding model, both embedding and pre-training models can be downloaded from the Hugging Face Hub[1].

To further enhance the model's performance, we generated 800 instruction data points based on task decomposition from the training dataset. We employed Llama Factory with LoRA [7] for instruction tuning, setting the learning rate to 2e-4 and the number of training epochs to 5.0. After the fine-tuning was completed, we only needed to merge the fine-tuned parameters for application. This approach not only improved the model's accuracy but also accelerated the training process, enabling it to quickly adapt to new task requirements in practical applications.

4.2   Evaluation Metrics and Dataset

In this study, the task organization collected and processed a dataset comprising 300 clinical cases to establish a proprietary database. This database was

---

[1] https://huggingface.co/.

constructed using high-impact public platforms such as the "Journal of Traditional Chinese Medicine" and the "Clinical Case Database of Traditional Chinese Medicine," thereby ensuring the quality and representativeness of the data. The 300 case samples were meticulously organized and annotated by the research team, categorizing them into various dimensions, including clinical data and experiential insights.

As shown in Table 1, the task organization has established five evaluation metrics-extracted information, pathogen inference, symptom inference, overall quality, and final score-based on the inherent key steps in the process of TCM syndrome differentiation. These metrics are designed to assess the reasoning process and logical framework of the model when dealing with general clinical cases. A scoring system will be employed to comprehensively evaluate the model's overall capability in handling these cases. In this context, GroundTruth represents the core information extracted manually, score represents the score of the question, Correct represents the number of correct answers selected by the model, while Total represents the sum of both the correct and incorrect answers. All scores are restricted to the interval of 0 to 1.

Table 1. Evaluation Metrics

Task	Index	Method
Task1	Extracted Information	$P_1 = Extracted/GroundTruth$
Task2	Pathogen Inference	$P_2 = Score \times Correct/Total$
Task3	Symptom Inference	$P_3 = Score \times Correct/Total$
Task4	Overall Quality	$P_4 = \text{Rouge-L}$
Total Score	Final Score	$P = 0.2 \times P_1 + 0.3 \times P_2 + 0.4 \times P_3 + 0.1 \times P_4$

4.3 Main Results

In the CHIP2024 Evaluation Task 1, we submitted results for both the A and B leaderboards, which are based on entirely distinct sets of 50 test data. For both submissions, we employed the same methodology and model, requiring only a single fine-tuning of the model to fulfill the evaluation criteria. Our results yielded a score of 45.12 on the A leaderboard and 44.37 on the B leaderboard, positioning us at the forefront among 239 competing teams. Table 2 shows the specific results of the two leaderboards on the five metrics. The experimental findings suggest that our trained model exhibits a robust capacity for dialectical reasoning when provided with accurate local knowledge.

4.4 Case Study

Since we used a combination of RAG and directive tuning, we categorised the processes and used an example to thoroughly evaluate the impact of each com-

Table 2. For the five metrics scores of Leaderboard A and Leaderboard B, both Leaderboard A and B have a total score of 50 points, accurate to two decimal places.

Leaderboard	Task1	Task2	Task3	Task4	Total Score
A	8.68	13.05	19.37	4.02	45.12
B	8.39	13.59	18.10	4.29	44.37

ponent on the performance of the framework. Specific case information, disease mechanism options, evidence candidates, and references are shown in Fig. 3.

- *Only RAG:* In this configuration, the results of local knowledge are incorporated into the question context at the same position and subsequently input into the currently superior GPT-4o[2] to derive outcomes.
- *Only SFT:* This setting indicates that the model is fine-tuned exclusively using instruction data, with no integration of local knowledge within the instruction data itself.

Clinical Information

王某，男，45岁。主诉及病史：2个月前于外出路上，突然下肢无力，跌倒在地，当时未予注意，但自觉数天来腰背酸软，下肢乏力，多走数步则肢体下沉，容易跌倒，以后又连续跌倒两次，乃去某医学院附属医院神经科检查，脊髓腔造影显示：4、5腰椎管狭窄，脊髓神经及下行纤维受到压迫，诊断为"椎管狭窄症"，治疗1个月未见好转，乃转求中医治疗。诊查：患者脉沉细，舌暗淡，苔薄黄。腰椎部有酸胀感及压痛，下肢表面无异常，触觉亦正常，但不敢久站，久站则欲倾倒，饮食睡眠尚好。

Pathogenesis Options

A:少阳证;B:脾阳虚久;C:久郁致瘀;D:血虚;E:肾气不足;F:清窍受蒙;G:痰浊;H:气滞血瘀;I:内热;J:血虚生风

Syndrome Options

A:肝肾阴亏;B:心包肝胆热迫;C:肝风夹痰;D:肝亢风动;E:湿热下注;F:肝风内动;G:痰饮化热;H:胃热;I:血虚生风;J:阳虚

Reference Information

风痱为肢体不用之症，系因下元虚衰，虚阳上浮，痰浊随之上泛，堵塞窍道，以致下厥上冒，肢体不用，历代医家多有论述，如《金匮要略》说："....中风痱，身体不能自收持，口不能言，冒昧不知痛处，或拘急不能转侧。"尤在泾说："痱者厥也，精神不持，筋骨不用，非特邪气之扰，亦真气之衰也。"《黄帝素问宣明论方》云"地黄饮子治暗痱，肾虚厥逆，语声不出，足废不用。"根据上述论述，可以看出古人对于风痱已确立了一定的理论基础和治疗方法。通过对本例治疗，说明脊髓病变按风痱治疗是会取得效果的。

Fig. 3. Relevant information regarding the case.

Figure 4 presents the results and corresponding prompts under three different settings, with Ground Truth representing the answers in the dataset. The results show that for Task 1, the outputs across all three settings are relatively close to the Ground Truth, indicating that the model performs reasonably well on this task. However, for Task 2 and Task 3, which involve more complex inferences related to pathogenesis and syndrome differentiation, the outputs are still suboptimal, even with the advanced GPT-4o model and additional local knowledge. This suggests that GPT-4o has limitations in handling the nuanced reasoning required for TCM syndrome differentiation. Task 2 and Task 3 uses a multiple-to-multiple question format, increasing the complexity of reasoning and negatively

---

[2] https://chatgpt.com/.

Task1 Prompt: 任务一：请你从下面的临床资料中抽取出关键的信息\n请你一步一步思考并将关键信息写在【核心临床信息】和<eoe>之间。\n完整的回答的格式如下：\n【核心临床信息】... <eoe>\n请你严格按照上述格式作答。\n病例资料如下：\n临床资料：{'临床资料'}

Only SFT: 腰背酸软;下肢乏力;脉象沉细;舌暗淡;苔薄黄;腰椎部有酸胀感及压痛;下肢表面无异常;触觉正常;但不能久站

Only RAG: 腰背酸软;下肢乏力;肢体下沉;脉沉细;舌暗淡;苔薄黄;腰椎部位酸胀及压痛;下肢触觉正常但不敢久站;久站则有倾倒感

Our: 腰背酸软;下肢乏力;行走不稳;脉沉细;舌暗淡;苔薄黄;腰椎部有酸胀感及压痛;下肢表面无异常触觉亦正常;但不敢久站;久站则欲倾倒

Ground Truth: 腰背酸软;下肢乏力;肢体下沉;脉沉细;舌暗淡;苔薄黄;不敢久站;久站则欲倾倒

Task2 Prompt: 任务二：根据临床资料给每一个临床信息选择最合适的病机，请你一步一步思考并将思考结果写在【病机推断】和<eoe>之间。你将从A，B，C，D，E，F，G，H，I，J中给每一个临床信息选择最正确的答案，并写在【答案】和<eoa>之间。\n完整的回答的格式如下：\n【病机推断】... <eoe>\n【答案】... <eoa>\n请你严格按照上述格式作答。\n题目如下：\n临床资料：{'临床资料'}\n{'参考资料'}\n核心临床信息：{task1 result}\n选项：{'病机选项'}

Only SFT: 腰背酸软:肾气不足;下肢乏力:肾气不足;脉象沉细:肾气不足;舌暗淡:肾气不足;苔薄黄:内热;腰椎部有酸胀感及压痛:肾气不足;但不能久站:肾气不足

Only RAG: 腰背酸软:肾气不足; 下肢乏力:肾气不足; 肢体下沉:气滞血瘀; 脉沉细:血虚; 舌暗淡:血虚; 苔薄黄:内热; 腰椎部位酸胀及压痛:气滞血瘀; 下肢触觉正常但不敢久站:肾气不足; 久站则有倾倒感:肾气不足

Our: 腰背酸软:肾气不足;下肢乏力:肾气不足;脉象沉细:肾气不足;舌暗淡:肾气不足;苔薄黄:肾气不足;腰椎部有酸胀感及压痛:肾气不足;但不能久站:血虚生风;久站则欲倾倒:血虚生风

Ground Truth: 腰背酸软:肾气不足;下肢乏力:肾气不足;肢体下沉:肾气不足;脉沉细:肾气不足;舌暗淡:肾气不足;苔薄黄:肾气不足;不敢久站:血虚生风;久站则欲倾倒:血虚生风

Task3 Prompt: 任务三：根据临床资料给每一个病机选择最合适的症候，请你一步一步思考并将思考结果写为【症候推断】和<eoe>之间。你将从A，B，C，D，E，F，G，H，I，J中给每一个病机选择最正确的答案，并写在【答案】和<eoa>之间。\n完整的回答的格式如下：\n【症候推断】... <eoe>\n【答案】... <eoa>\n请你严格按照上述格式作答。\n题目如下：\n临床资料：{'临床资料'}\n{'参考资料'}\n核心病机：{task2 result}\n选项：{'证候选项'}

Only SFT: 肾气不足:肝肾阴亏;内热:肝肾阴亏

Only RAG: 肾气不足:肝肾阴亏;气滞血瘀:肝阴夹痰;血虚:血虚生风;内热:痰饮化热

Our: 肾气不足:血虚生风;血虚生风:血虚生风

Ground Truth: 肾气不足:血虚生风;血虚生风:血虚生风

Task4 Prompt: 任务四：根据临床资料、核心病机、核心症候为该病历写总结以及辨证分析，\n完整的回答的格式如下：\n【病例总结】... <eoe>\n【辨证】... <eoa>请你严格按照上述格式作答。\n资料如下：\n临床资料：{'临床资料'}\n{'参考资料'}\n核心病机：{task2 result}\n核心证候：{task3 result}

Only SFT: 患者主要病机为肾气不足，内热。肾气不足则腰府失养，故见腰背酸软；气虚则肢体无力，故下肢乏力、久站欲倾倒；内热则舌苔薄黄。其核心证候为肝肾阴亏，肝肾阴虚则筋脉失养，进一步加重了肢体的酸软无力。因此，本病治疗应以滋补肝肾、清泄内热为主，辅以益气养血、通络止痛，以期达到缓解症状、改善体质的目的。

Only RAG: 本病例核心病机为肾气不足，气滞血瘀，血虚内热。患者肝肾阴亏，肾虚致下元无力，故下肢乏力，伴腰背酸软；气滞血瘀导致经络不通，气血运行不畅，故下肢沉重易倾倒。脉沉细，舌暗淡，苔薄黄，提示肝肾亏虚及血虚生风之证。根据肾气不足、肝肾夹痰之核心病机，痰浊阻络，气血不畅，致下厥上冒，引发风痹症候。本病辨证应以补肾益气、活血化瘀、祛风化痰为主，选用相应治疗以改善症状。

Our: 根据中医理论，风痱是一种因下元虚衰，虚阳上浮，痰浊堵塞窍道所致的疾病，表现为肢体不用，精神不持等症状。本例患者主诉及临床表现与风痱的描述相符，结合其脉舌象，可辨证为肾气不足，血虚生风。治疗方法应以补肾益气，养血息风为主，兼以化痰通窍，以达到恢复肢体功能的目的。

Ground Truth: 临证体会：本病为肾亏所致。腰为肾之府，脊椎为督脉所在，督脉属肾，肾气不足则督脉亦亏；下肢为少阴通络，督脉统辖下肢，督脉空虚，下肢无主，则易跌倒。古称"风痱"，盖血虚生风，痱者废也，故下肢废软无力。

Fig. 4. Prompts for Tasks 1–4, along with the results for 'only RAG,' 'only SFT,' and our solution, based on the cases presented in Fig. 3.

impacting model performance. For fine-tuned models, the existing knowledge base is insufficient to support accurate answers to all questions, leading to lower accuracy. Furthermore, as Tasks 1 to 4 form a continuous reasoning process, error accumulation may contribute to the incorrect responses observed in the other two settings.

5   Conclusion

The application of large language models across various fields has revealed substantial development opportunities and research implications. However, their capability in syndrome differentiation for TCM remains limited, posing a significant barrier to research progress. To address this limitation, we propose a novel approach that combines RAG with instruction tuning. By integrating local knowledge with the training set, our method forms instruction data designed to improve the model's comprehension of retrieved information. Additionally, we decompose the dialectical reasoning process into four consecutive tasks, thereby reducing the instability commonly seen in single-instance reasoning. Extensive offline experiments and online submissions have demonstrated our method's strong performance. Nonetheless, our approach depends considerably on the accuracy of information retrieved by RAG, which remains relatively straightforward. In future research, we aim to enhance retrieval capabilities to further improve the model's effectiveness.

References

1. Cai, Z., et al.: Internlm2 technical report. arXiv preprint arXiv:2403.17297 (2024)
2. Chen, D., et al.: Data-juicer: a one-stop data processing system for large language models. In: Companion of the 2024 International Conference on Management of Data, pp. 120–134 (2024)
3. Chen, Z., Zhang, D., Liu, C., Wang, H., Jin, X., Yang, F., Zhang, J.: Traditional Chinese medicine diagnostic prediction model for holistic syndrome differentiation based on deep learning. Integrative Med. Res. **13**(1), 101019 (2024)
4. Dai, S., Xu, C., Xu, S., Pang, L., Dong, Z., Xu, J.: Bias and unfairness in information retrieval systems: new challenges in the llm era. In: Proceedings of the 30th ACM SIGKDD Conference on Knowledge Discovery and Data Mining, pp. 6437–6447 (2024)
5. Ghosh, A., Acharya, A., Jain, R., Saha, S., Chadha, A., Sinha, S.: Clipsyntel: clip and llm synergy for multimodal question summarization in healthcare. In: Proceedings of the AAAI Conference on Artificial Intelligence, vol. 38, pp. 22031–22039 (2024)
6. Hager, P., Jungmann, F., Holland, R., Bhagat, K., Hubrecht, I., Knauer, M., Vielhauer, J., Makowski, M., Braren, R., Kaissis, G., et al.: Evaluation and mitigation of the limitations of large language models in clinical decision-making. Nat. Med. **30**(9), 2613–2622 (2024)
7. Hu, E.J., et al.: Lora: low-rank adaptation of large language models. arXiv preprint arXiv:2106.09685 (2021)

8. Hua, R., Dong, X., Wei, Y., Shu, Z., Yang, P., Hu, Y., Zhou, S., Sun, H., Yan, K., Yan, X., et al.: Lingdan: enhancing encoding of traditional chinese medicine knowledge for clinical reasoning tasks with large language models. J. Am. Med. Inform. Assoc. **31**(9), 2019–2029 (2024)

9. Kang, Y., Chang, Y., Fu, J., Wang, Y., Wang, H., Zhang, W.: Cmlm-zhongjing: Large language model is good story listener (2023). https://github.com/pariskang/CMLM-ZhongJing

10. Kirk, J.R., Wray, R.E., Lindes, P., Laird, J.E.: Improving knowledge extraction from llms for task learning through agent analysis. In: Proceedings of the AAAI Conference on Artificial Intelligence, vol. 38, pp. 18390–18398 (2024)

11. Li, A., Shrestha, R., Jegatheeswaran, T., Chan, H.O., Hong, C., Joshi, R.: Mitigating hallucinations in large language models: a comparative study of rag-enhanced vs. human-generated medical templates. medRxiv, pp. 2024–09 (2024)

12. Li, Z., Zhang, X., Zhang, Y., Long, D., Xie, P., Zhang, M.: Towards general text embeddings with multi-stage contrastive learning. arXiv preprint arXiv:2308.03281 (2023)

13. Mousavi, S.M., Alghisi, S., Riccardi, G.: Is your llm outdated? benchmarking llms & alignment algorithms for time-sensitive knowledge. arXiv preprint arXiv:2404.08700 (2024)

14. Shuster, K., Poff, S., Chen, M., Kiela, D., Weston, J.: Retrieval augmentation reduces hallucination in conversation. In: Findings of the Association for Computational Linguistics: EMNLP 2021, pp. 3784–3803 (2021)

15. Sibo Wei, Wenpeng Lu*, J.W.Y.F.W.W.Z.S.L.H.G.L.Z.: Biancang: A traditional chinese medicine large language model. https://github.com/QLU-NLP/BianCang-TCM-LLM (2024)

16. Singhal, K., et al.: Large language models encode clinical knowledge. Nature **620**(7972), 172–180 (2023)

17. Tan, Y., Zhang, Z., Li, M., Pan, F., Duan, H., Huang, Z., Deng, H., Yu, Z., Yang, C., Shen, G., et al.: Medchatzh: a tuning llm for traditional Chinese medicine consultations. Comput. Biol. Med. **172**, 108290 (2024)

18. Wang, Z., Li, K., Ren, Q., Yao, K., Zhu, Y.: Traditional Chinese medicine formula classification using large language models. In: 2023 IEEE International Conference on Bioinformatics and Biomedicine (BIBM), pp. 4647–4654. IEEE (2023)

19. Wang, Z., et al.: Retcare: Towards interpretable clinical decision making through LLM-driven medical knowledge retrieving. In: Artificial Intelligence and Data Science for Healthcare: Bridging Data-Centric AI and People-Centric Healthcare (2024). https://openreview.net/forum?id=jqo1vk63qE

20. Wu, J., Zhu, J., Qi, Y.: Medical graph rag: towards safe medical large language model via graph retrieval-augmented generation. arXiv preprint arXiv:2408.04187 (2024)

21. Xiong, G., Jin, Q., Wang, X., Zhang, M., Lu, Z., Zhang, A.: Improving retrieval-augmented generation in medicine with iterative follow-up questions. arXiv preprint arXiv:2408.00727 (2024)

22. Yang, Q., Wang, R., Chen, J., Su, R., Tan, T.: Fine-tuning medical language models for enhanced long-contextual understanding and domain expertise. arXiv preprint arXiv:2407.11536 (2024)

23. Yu, J., Zhang, L., Xu, N., Fa, L., Yang, K.: Application of constraint-based frequent closed itemsets mining in tcm clinical data analysis. In: 2023 IEEE International Conference on Bioinformatics and Biomedicine (BIBM), pp. 4689–4696. IEEE (2023)

24. Yue, W., Wang, X., Zhu, W., Guan, M., Zheng, H., Wang, P., Sun, C., Ma, X.: Tcmbench: A comprehensive benchmark for evaluating large language models in traditional chinese medicine. arXiv preprint arXiv:2406.01126 (2024)
25. Zhang, H., Wang, X., Meng, Z., Jia, Y., Xu, D.: Qibo: a large language model for traditional Chinese medicine. arXiv preprint arXiv:2403.16056 (2024)
26. Zhang, Y., et al.: Study on the rule of diagnosis and treatment of primary epilepsy in ancient medical cases. In: 2023 IEEE International Conference on Bioinformatics and Biomedicine (BIBM), pp. 4726–4732. IEEE (2023)
27. Zijia, C., Wenxi, P., Dezheng, Z., Xin, L., Zhifei, W.: The application, challenges, and prospects of large language models in the field of traditional Chinese medicine. Medical Journal of Peking Union Medical College Hospital (2024)

Drug Prediction and Knowledge Map

MBF-DTI: A Fused Multi-dimensional Biochemical Feature-Based Drug Target Prediction Method Based on Heterogeneous Graph Attention Networks

Haixue Zhao[1] ⓘ, Kui Yao[1] ⓘ, Yunjiong Liu[1] ⓘ, Chao Che[2] ⓘ, and Lin Tang[2(✉)] ⓘ

[1] Key Laboratory of Advanced Design and Intelligent Computing, Ministry of Education, Dalian University, Dalian 116622, China
[2] School of Software Engineering, Dalian University, Dalian 116622, China
tanglin@dlu.edu.cn

Abstract. Drug-target interaction prediction help reduce the cost and time of drug development. However, existing research often overlooks the complexity of biological interactions. To address this issue, this paper proposes a DTI prediction model that integrates multi-dimensional biochemical features. Specifically, the model utilizes a heterogeneous graph attention network to capture the topological relationships among biological entities from diverse data, providing a deep understanding of the interactions among drugs, proteins, diseases, and side effects. A molecular attention Transformer network and a CBiNet module are used to extract the key structural features of drugs and targets. By automatically optimizing the weight distribution between drugs and targets, the model enhances the information transfer during network training, significantly improving model performance. Experimental results on real-world datasets demonstrate that the proposed model outperforms the current state-of-the-art methods in the field. Among the top 50 novel COVID-19 therapeutic drugs predicted by our model, 30 have been supported by clinical trials or scientific literature, further demonstrating the effectiveness of our proposed method in drug repurposing. Experimental data and supplementary materials are available online at: https://github.com/Eadog/MBF-DTI.

Keywords: Drug-target interaction · Drug repurposing · Heterogeneous network · Graph neural network · Data mining

1 Introduction

Drugs exert significant therapeutic effects on specific diseases by interacting with multiple targets and regulating their functions. Accurate prediction of drug-target interactions (DTI) is crucial for understanding the mechanisms of drug action, discovering new targets, and drug repurposing [1]. However, traditional drug repurposing methods

---

H. Zhao and K. Yao—Contribute equally to this work.

© The Author(s), under exclusive license to Springer Nature Singapore Pte Ltd. 2025
Y. Zhang et al. (Eds.): CHIP 2024, CCIS 2433, pp. 93–110, 2025.
https://doi.org/10.1007/978-981-96-3752-2_7

are often time-consuming, expensive, and high-risk. Computational methods can effectively improve the success rate of drug discovery and reduce research costs. With the rapid development of internet technology, the accumulation of data related to drug compounds, targets, and interactions has accelerated, further promoting the advancement of drug repurposing.

Currently, DTI prediction methods are mainly categorized into: structure-based methods [2], ligand similarity-based methods [3, 4], and network-based methods [5, 6]. Structure-based methods typically require knowledge of the three-dimensional structure of target proteins and drugs [7], and they often perform poorly for proteins with unknown structures. Ligand similarity-based methods utilize the structural similarity of drugs to predict DTI. These methods are computationally efficient, but they do not account for complex biochemical properties or molecular physicochemical properties, which may lead to inaccurate DTI predictions [8].

Network-based methods have now become a mainstream technique for DTI prediction [9, 10], which employ heterogeneous networks or knowledge graphs to express potential relationships between drugs and target proteins, mining the topological relationships between entities to predict potential correlations between drugs and targets [11]. As the most used method in network-based DTI prediction research, Graph Neural Network (GNN) [12–14] can effectively capture the complex relationships and structural features of the drug and target protein through networks [15], thereby improving model prediction accuracy. However, current DTI prediction methods based on GNN usually do not explore biological knowledge fully, such as drug chemical structures, protein sequences, and thus cannot adequately represent potential features of the network entities. Moreover, external knowledge such as drug side effects and protein interactions, which are equally important for DTI prediction, is also not considered. Therefore, effectively integrating knowledge from different domains into GNN models is an urgent problem that needs to be solved. In addition, node representations in graphs are usually high-dimensional and sparse, which increases the computational complexity and resource requirements, as well as the risk of overfitting. Therefore, accurately characterizing the node feature is another problem that needs to be addressed in the network-based DTI prediction methods.

To address the abovementioned issues, this paper proposes a method for drug-target interaction prediction based on multi-dimensional biochemical features fusion (MBF-DTI). MBF-DTI employs a molecular attention transformer to extract the structural features of drugs. For protein biological feature extraction, it utilizes the CBiNet network, which is composed of convolutional neural networks (CNN) and bidirectional long short-term memory networks (BiLSTM). The extracted features are then integrated into the message-passing process of a heterogeneous graph attention network. MBF-DTI optimizes edge weight distribution during the message passing process to better learn the associative features between drugs and targets by considering network topology and biological knowledge. Ultimately, MBF-DTI obtains node-level feature embeddings from heterogeneous graph to predict new DTIs. In comprehensive performance comparisons, MBF-DTI outperforms many state-of-the-art methods. Furthermore, we evaluated the COVID-19 repurposed drugs predicted by MBF-DTI through extensive literature research. The results show that out of the 50 innovative COVID-19 treatments predicted by MBF-DTI, the top 30 have been proven to be therapeutic, further confirming the effectiveness of MBF-DTI in drug repurposing.

The main contributions of this paper are as follows:

1. A heterogeneous graph attention network technique is introduced to construct a known network with multiple entities and edges by collecting and incorporating biochemical knowledge of proteins and drugs. This technique dynamically adjusts the information aggregation process between nodes, flexibly capturing the importance and relevance between them.

2. We utilize a molecular attention Transformer network to extract the structural information of drugs from molecular graphs and integrate it into heterogeneous networks. The rich physicochemical information is utilized to efficiently represent drug node features and extract unscaled features.

3. A CBiNet network is proposed to capture key local features of protein sequences at different scales using CNN. Additionally, BiLSTM is utilized to capture long-distance dependencies and global context information in protein sequences.

4. We develop a fused multi-dimensional biochemical feature-based DTI prediction method. Extensive experiments show that the proposed method outperforms state-of-the-art methods, and the repurposed drugs prediction experiment demonstrates the method's ability to discover therapeutic drugs.

2 Related Work

The prediction of drug-target relationships is increasingly linked to drug repurposing and has become a popular research topic in this field. Computational methods for DTI prediction are gaining increasing attention. Currently, the DTI prediction methods fall into four categories [16]: feature-based methods, matrix decomposition-based methods, and network-based methods.

2.1 Feature-Based DTI Prediction Method

Feature-based methods predict DTI by combining multiple features of the drugs and targets. Such methods usually represent each drug-target combination as a feature vector pair of specific length. They often use binary labels to mark whether there is an interaction between the drug and target. Aman Sharma et al. [17] used the Repi package and the PROFEAT web server to obtain the features of drug and target, which improves the performance of the model. Wail Ba-alawi et al. [18] proposed DASPfind model, which uses a graph-based feature extraction method to characterize the DTI. Song et al. [19] proposed a multi-scale feature fusion method (DeepFusion) based on deep learning. DeepFusion uses CNN to extract global structural features of drugs and protein molecules and employs Transformer network to extract semantic features of the local chemical substructures, which captures the complex relationships between drugs and proteins.

2.2 Matrix Factorization-Based DTI Prediction Method

Matrix decomposition-based methods [20] utilize existing drug-target interaction data and employ mathematical techniques to decompose these data into simpler forms to predict new or unknown interaction relationships. Bence Bolgár et al. [21] proposed the Variational Bayesian Multiple Kernel Logistic Matrix Factorization (VB-MK-LMF) method. VB-MK-LMF combines techniques, such as multiple kernel learning, weighted observations, graph Laplacian regularization, and probabilistic modeling, to enhance DTI prediction accuracy. While this method has been demonstrated to outperform other machine learning approaches, the rapid growth in both the volume and diversity of drug and target data far exceeds the analytical capabilities of matrix-based data representation and current algorithms.

2.3 Network- Based DTI Prediction Method

Network-based methods employ graph algorithms to perform DTI prediction tasks. They predict potential relationships between drugs and targets by utilizing the topological relationships of entities in drug-target networks. This approach is among the simplest and most effective inference methods. Additionally, several methods integrate drug similarity networks, protein similarity networks, and known DTI networks into heterogeneous networks (HN), such as DTINet [5], MSCMF [22], and HNM [23], to further enhance DTI prediction accuracy. However, these methods still have some limitations to address. For instance, MSCMF uses similarity matrices of relevant drugs and proteins to normalize matrix decomposition operations of specific DTI networks. These similarity matrices are created by combining multiple data sources using weighted averaging methods, which may lead to significant information loss.

DTINet was the first method to extract low-dimensional feature representations of drugs and targets from HN using unsupervised methods. It applies inductive matrix completion to predict new DTIs using learned features [24]. In such frameworks, separate feature learning is impractical because the learned features through unsupervised learning may not be the optimal final representations of drugs or targets. Therefore, the information obtained from model data may not yield the best solutions.

To address the above issues, information transmission and aggregation techniques extend GNNs to large-scale graph data and integrate attention mechanisms, resulting in significant performance improvements [25, 26] in relevant prediction tasks. This has led us to combine more effective deep learning models to extract more complex information from HN and discover new DTIs.

Currently, GNNs have been widely applied to heterogeneous graphs. For example, heterogeneous graph attention network (HAN) [27, 28] learns the importance of various meta-paths [29] and the importance of nodes based on a hierarchical attention mechanism. Then, the information of the surrounding neighbors is hierarchically aggregated based on the meta-paths. Meta-path aggregated graph neural Network (MAGNN) [30] consists of a node content transformation component for capturing node attributes, an intra-metapath component for aggregating node features within a meta-path, and a component for aggregating information from various meta-paths. Graph Transformer Networks(GTN) [31] creates new graph structures by discovering beneficial information between nodes in the original network and extracts valuable node embeddings on the new graph.

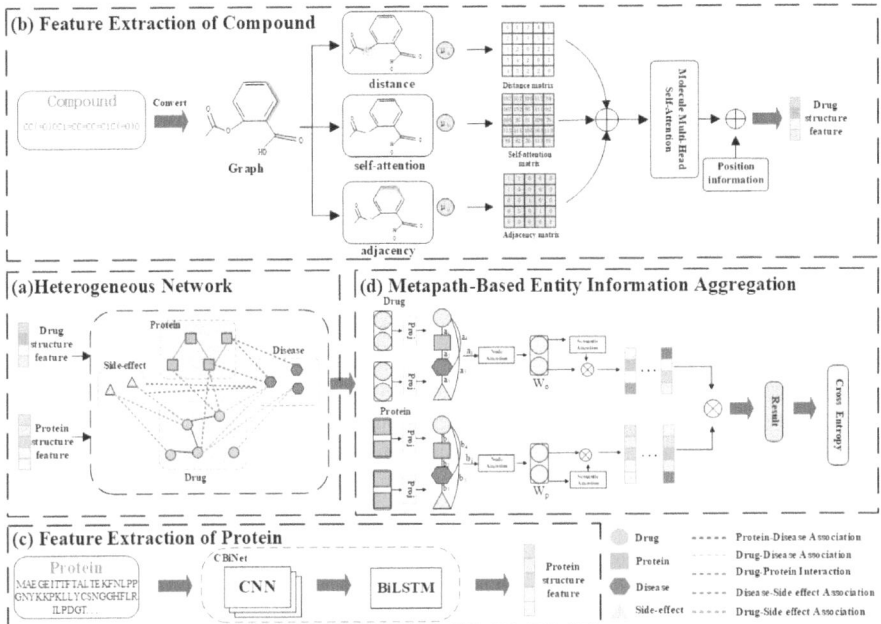

Fig. 1. MBF-DTI Model Architecture: (a) Construction of the HN; (b) Extracting structural features of drugs from their SMILES sequences and updating these features in the HN. (c) Using the CBiNet network, composed of CNN and BiLSTM, to extract structural features from protein sequences and updating these features in the HN. (d) Using HAN and the message-passing phase to extract network topological features and predict DTI.

3   Method

MBF-DTI integrates multi-dimensional biochemical information from heterogeneous data. It embeds representations of drug molecular structures and protein sequence data, which directly participate in the message passing process of the heterogeneous GNN, optimizing information weights during transmission. As shown in Fig 1(a)-(d), the MBF-DTI process is divided into four steps. First, MBF-DTI constructs an HN containing drugs, proteins, diseases, and drug side effects. Second, it uses a molecular attention Transformer network [32] to extract 3D structural features from the molecular graph of drugs, which are converted from their SMILES [33]. These features are used to represent the drug nodes in the HN. Moreover, a CBiNet network is proposed to extract biological features from protein sequences, which are used to represent target nodes in the HN. MBF-DTI employs a heterogeneous attention network (HAN) to capture topological information in the HN, projecting all types of nodes into a unified feature space. Node-level attention learns the weights of node pairs based on meta-paths, and semantic-level attention is used to fuse the semantic-specific node embeddings by combining the weights of each meta-path. Finally, MBF-DTI applies a cross-entropy loss (CEL) function to optimize the entire model and predict potential DTIs.

3.1 Heterogeneous Network

The HN is described as an undirected graph G = (V, E), where V = $\{v_1, v_2, \ldots, v_n\}$ represents the set of nodes, and E = {E(1), E(2), ..., E(k) }, E(i) = $\{e_{i1}, e_{i2}, \ldots, e_{im}\}$ represents the set of k types of edges.

In this paper, a complete heterogeneous information network is constructed, which includes information about drug-drug interactions, drug-protein interactions, drug-disease associations, drug-side effect associations, protein-protein interactions, and protein-disease association networks, as shown in Fig. 1(a). The network represents objects such as drugs, targets, diseases, and side effects as nodes, while associations and interactions between nodes are represented as edges. In the framework proposed in this paper, each node belongs to only one type of entity and all edges are undirected and non-negative weighted. A node's message is first sent to its first-order neighbors and then propagated to its higher-order neighbors through the network edges, which is a process known as message passing. The message-passing formula in a heterogeneous graph is as follows:

$$h_v^{l+1} = \sigma(\sum_{t \in T} \sum_{u \in N_t(v)} W_t^{(l)} h_u^{(l)}) \tag{1}$$

where h_v^{l+1} represents the feature vector of node v at layer $l + 1$; T represents the set of edge types; σ is the activation function, such as ReLU, used to introduce non-linearity; $N_t(v)$ represents the set of neighbors of node v of type t; $W_t^{(l)}$ is the weight matrix at layer l, controlling the weighting of node features.

3.2 Feature Extraction of Compound Structure

The MBF-DTI model uses the SMILES sequences of drug molecules as input to learn the characteristic representations of drug molecular structures. Since the structure of SMILES sequences is very similar to that of natural language sentences, we can use the contextual and structural information of atoms to understand molecular features. SMILES sequences are symbols that encode the molecular structure of chemical substances. Specifically, each atom has interactions with other atoms, and the SMILES sequence contains both nearby atoms and atoms that are far away. However, many methods fail to associate long-distance atoms when representing molecules; we use an improved version of the Transformer model to overcome this problem. We first process SMILES sequences into a graph structure using the RDKit toolkit [34]. Since SMILES sequences all have different lengths, we chose SMILES sequences with a maximum length of 100 characters to create an efficient representation able to cover at least 90% of the compounds in the dataset. Sequences longer than the maximum length are truncated, while shorter sequences are padded with zeros. Afterward, we use the molecule attention Transformer (MAT) [32] to encode the data. We replace all self-attention layers in the original Transformer [35] encoder with molecular multi-head self-attention layers. MBF-DTI interprets the self-attention as a soft adjacency matrix between the elements of the input sequence. It enhances the self-attention mechanism by incorporating inter-atomic distances and molecular graph structures. This results in a feature representation of the drug structure S_{drug}, which includes information about the bonds and distances between atoms in the molecule. The molecular polytope self-attention equation is as follows:

$$A^{(i)} = \left(\mu_b \rho \left(\frac{Q_i K_i^T}{\sqrt{d_k}} \right) + \mu_a g(D) + \mu_c A \right) V_i \tag{2}$$

where $A \in \{0,1\}^{N_{atoms} \times N_{atoms}}$ denotes the adjacency matrix of the molecular graph and $D \in R^{N_{atoms} \times N_{atoms}}$ denotes the distance between atoms. $Q_i = XW_i^q$, $K_i = XW_i^k$, $V_i = XW_i^v$ are the query vector matrices, the key vector matrices, and the value vector matrices, respectively, in which W is a learnable parameter. $i \in (1, ..., c)$, c is the number of heads of the multi-head attention. μ_α, μ_b and μ_c are the weights assigned to each part of the attention module, μ_α is the scalar parameter of the weighted distance matrix, which measures the importance of distance in attention; μ_b is the scalar parameter of the self-attention matrix, which measures the importance of the self-attention in the overall attention mechanism; μ_c is the scalar parameter of the neighbor matrix, which measures the importance of the neighbor relationship in attention.

3.3 Feature Extraction of Protein Structure

The MBF-DTI model uses Fasta-format sequences [36] of proteins to restore structural features. Since protein sequences all have different lengths, we choose sequences with a maximum of 1000 characters to create a valid representation that will cover at least 90% of the data in the dataset. Sequences larger than the maximum length are truncated, while shorter sequences are padded with preset characters.

The sequences are passed through the CNN layer of CBiNet for feature extraction. As shown in Fig. 1(c), we use three consecutive 1D convolutional layers for each CNN block. The number of convolutional kernels increases with the number of layers, with the second layer using double the number of convolutional kernels and the third layer using three times the number of convolutional kernels of the first layer. The CNN efficiently extracts localized features from the protein sequence. Next, CBiNet employ a BiLSTM layer to receive the features from the convolutional layers, which utilize positional information to capture the long-range dependencies and global contextual information in the protein sequence. The final output is the structural feature $S_{protein}$ of the protein, which is computed as shown below:

$$x_t = max \left(\sum_{a=1}^{n} \sum_{b=0}^{m-1} \omega_{\alpha,b} x_{a,t+b} \right) \tag{3}$$

$$S_{protein} = \left(LSTM_F \left(\overrightarrow{h}_{t-1}, x_t \right), LSTM_B \left(\overleftarrow{h}_{t+1}, x_t \right) \right) \tag{4}$$

where $\omega_{\alpha,b}$ and m denote the weight matrix and convolution window size, respectively; h is the BiLSTM hidden layer state and x is the feature representation of the protein sequence.

3.4 Metapath-Based Entity Information Aggregation

The purpose of learning heterogeneous graph representation is to seek an appropriate vector representation for each node in an HN for convenience. However, this task is difficult because it needs to consider both the heterogeneous characteristics and heterogeneous contents associated with each node in addition to integrating the information of the nodes and edges that make up the heterogeneous structure. To address this problem, we extract the topological features of heterogeneous information network using HAN [27]. As shown in Fig. 1(d). the HAN employs a hierarchical attention strategy. It uses node-level attention to learn the neighborhood weights based on meta-paths, aggregates them to generate semantically specific node embeddings, and distinguishes between different meta-paths through semantics-level attention to obtain the optimal weighted combination of node embeddings for a specific task.

The message passing is operated after obtaining the appropriate feature representation. To summarize the message passing process, we consider an HN with the embedding formula of the initialized nodes as $f^0: V \rightarrow R^d$, where $f^0(v)$ represents the d-dimensional mapping of each node v. The information aggregation of neighbor node v is defined as:

$$f_v = \sigma \left(\frac{1}{K} \sum_{k=1}^{K} \sum_{u \in N_v} \alpha_{uv} W f^0(u) \right) \tag{5}$$

$$\alpha_{uv} = \frac{exp(AconC(\alpha^T [W f^0(u) || W f^o(v)]))}{\sum_{k \in N_u} exp(AconC(\alpha^T [W f^0(u) || W f^0(k)]))} \tag{6}$$

where σ denotes the nonlinear activation function during neural network propagation, K indicates the number of attention layers, N_v represents all neighboring nodes of node v, W is the shared weight parameter, and a_{uv} denotes the weight vector of the attention mechanism. In particular, $AconC(*)$ [37] is a novel activation function for adaptive learning.

In addition, after obtaining the drug structural feature S_{drug} and protein structural feature $S_{protein}$, we update the node embedding in Eq. (5), which is calculated as follows:

$$f'_{drug} = \sigma \left(concat \left(f_{drug}, S_{drug} \right) \right) \tag{7}$$

$$f'_{protein} = \sigma \left(concat \left(f_{protein}, S_{protein} \right) \right) \tag{8}$$

3.5 DTI Prediction

After acquiring the drug and protein representations, we use the inner product to determine the probability of interaction [37] between them as shown in Fig. 1(d). Given a drug node u and a protein node v, f_u and f_v denote their feature representations, respectively. The probability that there is an interaction between u and v is calculated as follows:

$$p^{uv} = \sigma \left((f_u)^T f_v \right) \tag{9}$$

where σ is the sigmoid function and p^{uv} denotes the interaction prediction score between u and v.

We use the CEL to train the model. CEL is a loss function often used in classification problems. Since the error of the output affects the learning rate, using CEL as the loss function avoid the problem of learning rate degradation that occurs in gradient descent with the sigmoid function. The formula of the CEL loss function is defined as:

$$\pounds = \sum\nolimits_{r \in R} -y_r log(p_r) - (1 - y_r)log(1 - p_r) \qquad (10)$$

where R denotes the set of relationship types; y_r is the label of sample r, with positive instances labeled 1 and negative instances labeled 0; p_r denotes the likelihood that sample r will be predicted as a positive instance. We want the model to assign the highest possible edge probability for positive samples and the lowest possible edge probability for negative samples by using CEL.

4 Experiment

4.1 Dataset

In this study, we conducted DTI prediction experiments on Luo dataset [5]. To capture the biological features, we added the SMILES sequences of all drug molecules and the structural sequence data of proteins to the dataset. The statistical information of nodes and edges in the dataset is shown in Tables 1 and 2. The dataset contained six independent drug-protein association networks. All data had binary edge weights.

Table 1. Statistics of node information in the dataset.

Node Type	Count
Drug	708
Protein	1512
Disease	5603
Side effect	4192

Table 2. Statistics of association information between nodes in the dataset.

Edge Type	Count	Source
Drug–protein interaction	1,923	DrugBank version 3.0 [39]
Drug–drug interaction	10,036	DrugBank version 3.0 [39]
Protein–protein interaction	7,363	HPRD Release 9 [40]
Drug–disease association	199,214	Comparative Toxicogenomics Database [41]
Protein–disease association	1,596,745	Comparative Toxicogenomics Database [41]
Drug-side-effect association	80,164	SIDER Release 2 [42]

4.2   Experimental Settings

DTI prediction can be regarded as a binary classification task. We first constructed an HN using 90% of the positive and negative samples in the dataset, and then used these samples to train the MBF-DTI model. The remaining 10% were used as a test set. We tested the model's performance using 10-fold cross-validation and evaluated the effectiveness of the method using the area under the receiver operating characteristic (AUROC) and the area under the precision-recall curve (AUPR) metrics.

The model proposed in this paper consists of three main modules: the CBiNet module, the MAT module and the HAN module. The parameter settings used in the model are shown in Table 3. In addition, we use the Adam optimizer to update the weights of the neural network.

Table 3. Parameter settings in the experiment.

Parameter	Value
Epoch	1,000
Batch size	128
Learning rate	0.001
Dropout rate	0.1
CNN input size	64/128/192
CNN kernel size	128
BiLSTM input size	192
HAN input size	1,024
MAT multi-head attention number	16
MAT stack number	8

4.3   Comparison with Other DTI Prediction Methods

In this study, we randomly sampled negative samples, extracted all positive samples, and set the ratio of negative to positive samples to 10:1 to simulate real-world scenarios. The comparative methods we used are briefly described as follows:

MSCMF [22]: MSCMF utilizes collaborative matrix factorization to discover low-dimensional feature representations of drugs and targets.

HNM [23]: HNM uses an iterative algorithm to calculate similarity scores between diseases and drugs to infer new treatments for diseases.

DTINet [5]: DTINet is an integrated HN method that considers both the local and global topology of each network.

NeoDTI [43]: NeoDTI uses multiple HNs to predict DTIs and employs a multi-objective optimization approach to reconstruct the topology of the input data.

EEG-DTI [44]: EEG-DTI is a heterogeneous graph convolutional network used to learn low-dimensional feature representations of different types of edges in a HN for DTI prediction.

SHGCL-DTI [45]: SHGCL-DTI is a novel semi-supervised heterogeneous graph contrastive learning framework that generates node representations through neighbor views and meta-path views and reconstructs the original heterogeneous network to predict potential DTIs.

We compared the performance of MBF-DTI with the state-of-the-art methods in the field, and the experimental results are shown in Fig. 2. MBF-DTI achieves the optimal results in all evaluation metrics, with a significant improvement in performance compared to other DTI methods. Its AUPR is 0.892, representing a 3.7% improvement compared to the suboptimal method, NeoDTI. Additionally, its AUROC is 0.965, a 2.2% improvement over NeoDTI. Among these methods, MSCMF used network inference and the topology of the data to improve the prediction results through matrix transformation. However, compared with the deep learning methods that have performed well in recent years, MSCMF cannot sufficiently explore the hidden information or neighboring nodes in the embedding of the data matrix, and this leading to the poorer performance. HNM did not adopt the mainstream heterogeneous data embedding methods, which limit the HNM's feature expression ability, generalization ability and prediction accuracy. As a result, the prediction performance of the final model was relatively poor. DTINet, NeoDTI, and EEG-DTI further mined the hidden information through matrix-transformed neural networks, and were able to fit the node features more accurately than MSCNF and HNM. SHGCL-DTI employed a graph comparison learning method to capture the structural information in heterogeneous graphs. This was achieved by maximizing the similarity of positive sample pairs and minimizing the similarity of negative sample pairs. However, SHGCL-DTI cannot fully utilize the rich semantic information and complex interactions in heterogeneous graphs, which limits its performance in processing complex biological data.

However, none of these methods fully use the drug molecular structure and protein sequence information, and ignore the information (e.g., NeoDTI constructs HNs only by calculating the similarity between drugs and proteins). Existing methods also ignore the information loss problem caused by node information embedding. Unlike the above methods, MBF-DTI extracted the compound structure information through the molecular attention Transformer network containing all types of neighboring nodes, which is added to the HAN, thus fully exploiting the hidden information between different types of nodes. In addition, features extracted from sequences were dynamically added to the drug and protein node networks to update the node embeddings. In this process, the weights of drug and protein node information were gradually amplified, allowing the final node embedding reasonably utilized the information from different types of nodes, optimized the weights of node information, and ultimately improved the predictive ability of the model.

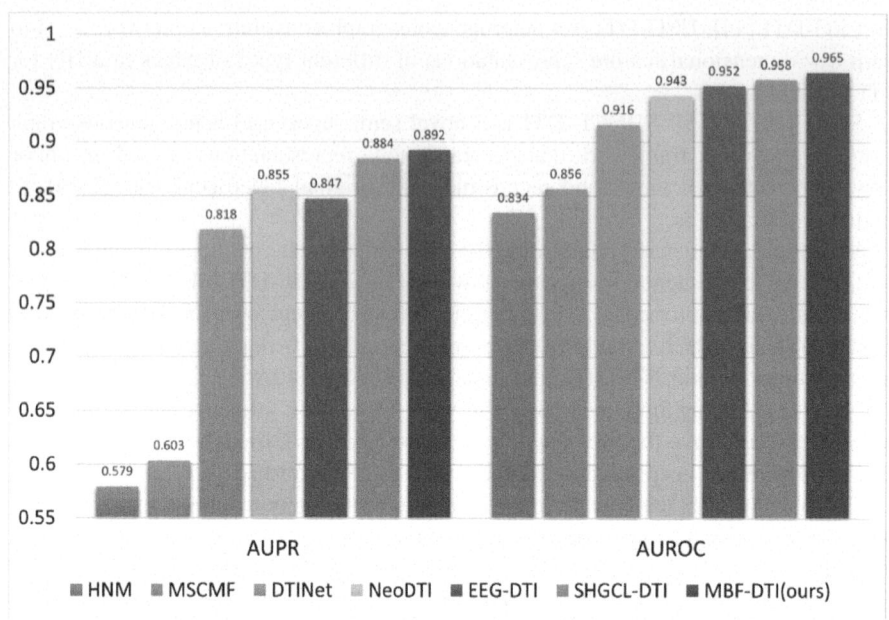

Fig. 2. AUPR and AUROC performance of each model.

Table 4. Number of drugs, targets and DTIs included in the redundant data.

Redundant data	Drug number	Target number	DTI number
DTI of similar drugs or targets	146	78	955
DTI of drugs with similar drug interactions	101	0	366
DTI of drugs with similar side effects	17	0	51

4.4 Robustness Experiment

To further evaluate the reliability of MBF-DTI, we conducted robustness experiments to further validate the model's predictive performance considering the possible presence of redundant drug and target data in the dataset. First, we removed some redundant data from the dataset: (1) DTIs of similar drugs or targets; (2) DTIs of drugs with similar interactions; (3) DTIs of drugs with similar side effects. Table 4 lists the removed data.

As shown in Fig 3(a), after removing similar drugs and targets, the performance of MBF-DTI is 3.1% higher than that of the suboptimal method NeoDTI. In Fig 3(b), after removing DTIs of drugs with similar drug interactions, the performance of the MBF-DTI model significantly surpasses the suboptimal method, with the AUPR metric improving by 2.4%. In Fig. 3(c), under the condition of removing drugs with similar side effects, the performance of MBF-DTI improves by 2.5% compared to NeoDTI.

The results of this test scheme indicate that the model's performance weakened after removing a large amount of specific DTI data, but MBF-DTI remains the optimal model in terms of AUPR, demonstrating that the performance of MBF-DTI is stable and robust. Additionally, we treated the drug-protein interactions as a special case in the experiments. To verify the impact of such treatment on the experimental results, we separately handled special drug-target relationships and conventional drug-target relationships to more objectively evaluate the predictive performance of MBF-DTI. Specifically, the model was first trained on a dataset where the interactions between drugs and proteins were not unique, and then tested on a unique dataset. As shown in Fig 3(d), MBF-DTI significantly outperforms the suboptimal method, with an AUPR improvement of 3.5%. This indicates that MBF-DTI has a stronger generalization ability than baseline methods in predicting whether drugs will interact with a target.

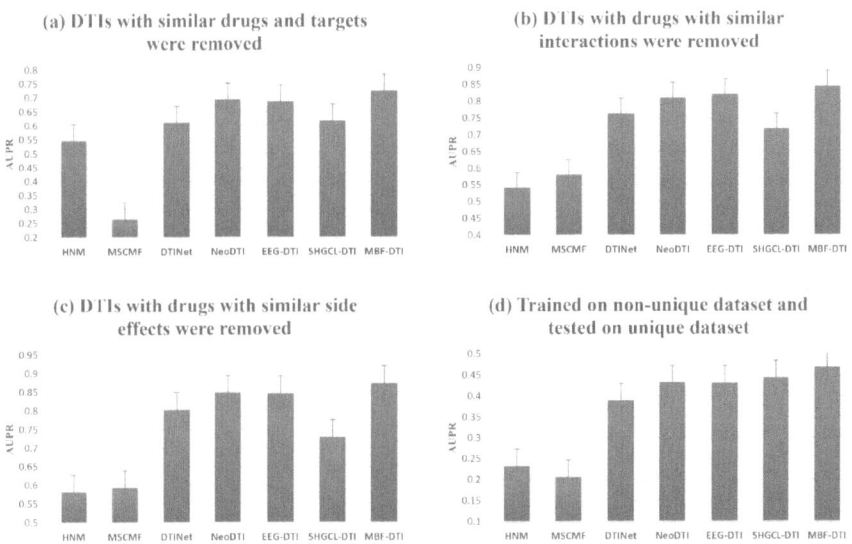

Fig. 3. AUPR performance of each model after adjustment of the dataset.

4.5 Ablation Experiment

We also performed ablation experiments to verify the effect of each MBF-DTI module. The experimental results are shown in Table 5. ProSFE denotes the protein structure feature extraction module and DruSFE denotes the drug compound structure feature extraction module.

The Effectiveness of the Protein Structure Feature Extraction Module. As shown in Table 5, the presence of the ProSFE module improved the model's performance by 0.8% in terms of AUROC and by 2% in terms of AUPR. ProSFE effectively retained the biological structure information of proteins and optimized the message passing weight of protein nodes in the GNN, thereby improving the DTI prediction performance.

The Effectiveness of the Drug Compound Structure Feature Extraction Module. As shown in Table 5, the presence of the DruSFE module significantly

Table 5. Evaluation of the impact of MBF-DTI modules on performance.

Method	AUROC	AUPR
w/o ProSFE	0.957	0.872
w/o DruSFE	0.954	0.867
w/o ProSFE and DruSFE	0.952	0.860
MBF-DTI	**0.965**	**0.892**

w/o denotes corresponding module was removed; Bolded numbers are the best performance.

improved the model's performance, with AUROC and AUPR increasing by 1.1% and 2.5%, respectively. DruSFE fully extracted the structural features of the drugs, enhancing their weights in the message passing process and improving the model's prediction performance.

The results indicate that MBF-DTI effectively extracts the biological structural features of drugs and proteins. By deeply exploring the chemical structures, physical properties, and biological functions of drugs and proteins, MBF-DTI can capture the complex interactions between them, further enhancing the predictive ability of drug-protein interactions. Additionally, we found that the structural information of drug molecules appears to be more useful than that of proteins. We believe this is because the molecular attention module used for extracting drug features can fully capture their structural characteristics, better representing their physicochemical information. Furthermore, drugs with similar chemical structures often exhibit the same biological activity [47], thus requiring further attention to the correlations between drug molecules.

5   Case Study

In this section, we apply the MBF-DTI method to predict interactions [46] between existing drugs and COVID-19 targets to identify potential treatments for COVID-19. We extracted targets closely related to COVID-19 from the Comparative Toxicogenomic Database and DrugBank database. Among these, 146 targets appeared in the heterogeneous dataset used in this study. We used the trained model to predict interactions between these targets and 708 drugs, and visualized the results. As shown in Fig. 4, the orange squares represent targets, the blue circles represent candidate drugs, and larger circles indicate higher confidence in the drug's therapeutic effect. We conducted literature searches for drugs with high confidence in their therapeutic effects.

Imatinib [48] and Dasatinib [49] are both tyrosine kinase inhibitors with antitumor activity that show in vitro antiviral activity against the replication and spread of the COVID-19 virus. Studies have shown that tyrosine kinase inhibitors can interfere with the process of viral entry into host cells, thereby inhibiting viral infection [48]. Sorafenib [50] inhibits the serine protein kinase pathway, which plays a critical role in the replication of various viruses. By targeting this pathway, Sorafenib reduces the replication of severe acute respiratory syndrome coronavirus 2. Currently, several clinical trials are investigating the safety of Sorafenib in treating COVID-19. Minocycline [51] has

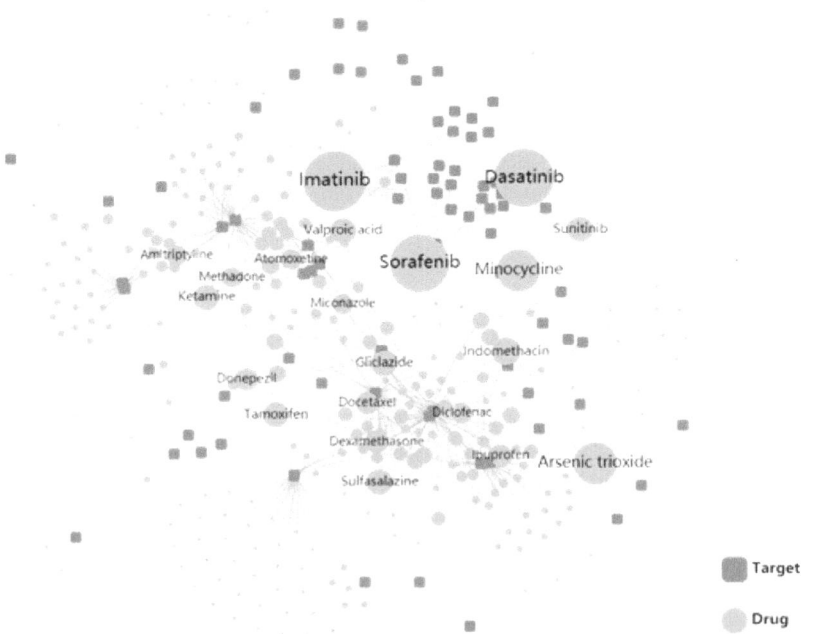

Fig. 4. Visualization result of DTI prediction for COVID-19. In the figure, larger circles indicate higher confidence in the possibility of a therapeutic effect of the drug.

significant anti-cytokine and anti-inflammatory effects. when used in combination with hydroxychloroquine, which has anti-cytokine and anti-COVID-19 effects, it shows good efficacy in treating moderate to severe COVID-19 infections. This combination may also help prevent morbidity and complications.

6 Conclusion

In this study, we propose a novel DTI prediction method that extracts biological features from protein sequences and the molecular graphs of drug compounds, incorporating them into a heterogeneous network for message passing. The model can acquire more biological information with each iteration, optimizing the weights of drug and target information, ultimately achieving excellent experimental results. In several challenging and realistic DTI prediction scenarios, the MBF-DTI model significantly outperforms other state-of-the-art methods. The strong performance of MBF-DTI indicates that leveraging rich heterogeneous information and biological knowledge can enhance the model's ability to identify new drug indications. Additionally, we used the trained MBF-DTI model to evaluate drugs that may have therapeutic effects against COVID-19. Among the 50 drugs predicted by the model, 30 have already appeared in clinical studies, further demonstrating the effectiveness of the MBF-DTI model. In the future, we aim to further enhance the model's generalizability by integrating more drug-target information and to predict potential therapeutic drugs for a wider range of diseases, such as coronary heart disease. This approach aims to improve the drug development process and reduce its cost.

Acknowledgments. This work was supported by the National Natural Science Foundation of China (Grants No. 62076045), the Basic Project for Universities from the Educational Department of Liaoning Province (Grants No. LJKFZ20220290), the 111 Project (Grants No. D23006) and the Interdisciplinary Project of Dalian University (Grants No. DLUXK-2023-YB-003 andDLUXK-2023-YB-009).

Disclosure of Interests. We have no conflicts of interests to disclose.

References

1. Chu, Y., Shan, X., Chen, T., et al.: DTI-MLCD: predicting drug-target interactions using multi-label learning with community detection method. Brief Bioinform. **22**(3) (2021)
2. Morris, G.M., Huey, R., Lindstrom, W., et al.: AutoDock4 and AutoDockTools4: automated docking with selective receptor flexibility. J. Comput. Chem. **30**(16), 2785–2791 (2009)
3. Mathai, N., Kirchmair, J.: Similarity-based methods and machine learning approaches for target prediction in early drug discovery: performance and scope. Int. J. Mol. Sci. **21**(10) (2020)
4. Lian, M., Wang, X., Du, W.: Integrated multi-similarity fusion and heterogeneous graph inference for drug-target interaction prediction. Neurocomputing **500**, 1–12 (2022)
5. Luo, Y., Zhao, X., Zhou, J., et al.: A network integration approach for drug-target interaction prediction and computational drug repositioning from heterogeneous information. Nat. Commun. **8**(1), 573 (2017)
6. Yuan, Q., Gao, J., Wu, D., et al.: DrugE-Rank: improving drug-target interaction prediction of new candidate drugs or targets by ensemble learning to rank. Bioinformatics **32**(12), i18–i27 (2016)
7. Singh, S., Malik, B.K., Sharma, D.K.: Molecular drug targets and structure based drug design A holistic approach. Bioinformation (2006)
8. Ozturk, H., Ozkirimli, E., Ozgur, A.: A comparative study of SMILES-based compound similarity functions for drug-target interaction prediction. BMC Bioinformatics **17**, 128 (2016)
9. Zeng, X., Zhu, S., Lu, W., et al.: Target identification among known drugs by deep learning from heterogeneous networks. Chem. Sci. **11**(7), 1775–1797 (2020)
10. Wang, J., Wang, H., Wang, X., Chang, H.: Predicting Drug-target Interactions via FM-DNN Learning. Current Bioinform. **15**(1), 68–76 (2020)
11. Bingjie, H., Ling, N., Abbas, S.J.: Research on drug-target interactions prediction: network similarity-based approaches. In: Proceedings of the 2020 IEEE 10th International Conference on Electronics Information and Emergency Communication (ICEIEC), pp. 168–173 (2020)
12. Jiao, Q., Qiu, Z., Wang, Y., et al.: Edge-gated graph neural network for predicting protein-ligand binding affinities. In: 2021 IEEE International Conference on Bioinformatics and Biomedicine (BIBM), pp. 334–339 (2021)
13. Zhang, X., Chen, C., Meng, Z., et al.: CoAtGIN: Marrying convolution and attention for graph-based molecule property prediction. In: 2022 IEEE International Conference on Bioinformatics and Biomedicine (BIBM), pp. 374–379 (2022)
14. Xia, L.Y., Yang, Z.Y., Zhang, H., Liang, Y.: Improved prediction of drug-target interactions using self-paced learning with collaborative matrix factorization. J. Chem. Inf. Model. **59**(7), 3340–3351 (2019)

15. Langley, G.R., Adcock, I.M., Busquet, F., et al.: Towards a 21st-century roadmap for biomedical research and drug discovery: consensus report and recommendations. Drug Discov. Today **22**(2), 327–339 (2017)

16. Yansen Su, Z.H., etal.: AMGDTI: drug–target interaction prediction based on adaptive metagraph learning in heterogeneous network. Briefings in Bioinformatics **25**(1) (2024)

17. Sharma, A., Rani, R.: BE-DTI': ensemble framework for drug target interaction prediction using dimensionality reduction and active learning. Comput. Methods Programs Biomed. **165**, 151–162 (2018)

18. Ba-Alawi, W., Soufan, O., Essack, M., et al.: DASPfind: new efficient method to predict drug-target interactions. J. Cheminform. **8**, 15 (2016)

19. Song, T., Zhang, X., Ding, M., et al.: DeepFusion: a deep learning based multi-scale feature fusion method for predicting drug-target interactions. Methods **204**, 269–277 (2022)

20. Huang, Y.A., You, Z.H., Chen, X.: A systematic prediction of drug-target interactions using molecular fingerprints and protein sequences. Curr. Protein Pept. Sci. **19**(5), 468–478 (2018)

21. Bolgar, B., Antal, P.: VB-MK-LMF: fusion of drugs, targets and interactions using variational Bayesian multiple kernel logistic matrix factorization. BMC Bioinform. **18**(1), 440 (2017)

22. Zheng, X., Ding, H., Mamitsuka, H., Zhu, S.: Collaborative matrix factorization with multiple similarities for predicting drug-target interactions. In: Proceedings of the 19th ACM SIGKDD International Conference on Knowledge Discovery and Data Mining, pp. 1025–1033 (2013)

23. Wang, W., Yang, S., Zhang, X., Li, J.: Drug repositioning by integrating target information through a heterogeneous network model. Bioinformatics **30**(20), 2923–2930 (2014)

24. Natarajan, N., Dhillon, I.S.: Inductive matrix completion for predicting gene-disease associations. Bioinformatics **30**(12), i60-68 (2014)

25. Gilmer, J., Schoenholz, S.S., Riley, P.F., et al.: Neural message passing for quantum chemistry. In: Proceedings of the International Conference on Machine Learning, pp. 1263–1272 (2017)

26. Hamilton, W., Ying, Z., Leskovec, J.: Inductive representation learning on large graphs. Advances in neural information processing systems, 30 (2017)

27. Wang, X., Ji, H., Shi, C., et al.: Heterogeneous graph attention network. In: Proceedings of the the World Wide Web Conference, pp. 2022–2032 (2019)

28. Sun, Y., Han, J., Yan, X., et al.: Pathsim: Meta path-based top-k similarity search in heterogeneous information networks. Proc. VLDB Endowment **4**(11), 992–1003 (2011)

29. Yu, D., Liu, H., Yao, S.: Drug–target interaction prediction based on improved heterogeneous graph representation learning and feature projection classification. Expert Syst. Appl. **252**, 124289 (2024)

30. Fu, X., Zhang, J., Meng, Z., King, I.: MAGNN: metapath aggregated graph neural network for heterogeneous graph embedding. Proceedings of The Web Conference **2020**, 2331–2341 (2020)

31. Yun, S., Jeong, M., Kim, R., et al.: Graph transformer networks. Advances in neural information processing systems, 32 (2019)

32. Maziarka, Ł., Danel, T., Mucha, S., et al.: Molecule attention transformer. arXiv preprint arXiv:200208264 (2020)

33. Toropov, A.A., Toropova, A.P., Mukhamedzhanoval, D.V., Gutman, I.: Simplified molecular input line entry system (SMILES) as an alternative for constructing quantitative structure-property relationships (QSPR) (2005)

34. GL a others. Rdkit: open-source cheminformatics software (2016)

35. Vaswani, A.: Attention is all you need. arXiv preprint arXiv:170603762 (2017)

36. Villesen, P.: FaBox: an online toolbox for fasta sequences. Mol. Ecol. Notes **7**(6), 965–968 (2007)

37. Ma, N., Zhang, X., Liu, M., Sun, J.: Activate or not: Learning customized activation. In: Proceedings of the IEEE/CVF Conference on Computer Vision and Pattern Recognition, pp. 8032–8042 (2021)

38. Long, Q., Jin, Y., Song, G., et al.: Graph structural-topic neural network. In: Proceedings of the 26th ACM SIGKDD International Conference on Knowledge Discovery & Data Mining, pp. 1065–1073 (2020)
39. Knox, C., Law, V., Jewison, T., et al.: DrugBank 3.0: a comprehensive resource for 'omics' research on drugs. Nucleic Acids Res, 2011, 39(Database issue): D1035-1041
40. Zeyuan Wang, Q.Z., Shuang-Wei HU, Haoran Yu, Xurui Jin, Zhichen Gong, Huajun Chen. Multi-level protein structure pre-training via prompt learning. In: The Eleventh International Conference on Learning Representation (2023)
41. Davis, A.P., Murphy, C.G., Johnson, R., et al.: The Comparative Toxicogenomics Database: update 2013. Nucleic Acids Res. 41(Database issue), D1104–1114 (2013)
42. Kuhn, M., Campillos, M., Letunic, I., et al.: A side effect resource to capture phenotypic effects of drugs. Mol. Syst. Biol. 6, 343 (2010)
43. Wan, F., Hong, L., Xiao, A., et al.: NeoDTI: neural integration of neighbor information from a heterogeneous network for discovering new drug-target interactions. Bioinformatics 35(1), 104–111 (2019)
44. Peng, J., Wang, Y., Guan, J., et al.: An end-to-end heterogeneous graph representation learning-based framework for drug-target interaction prediction. Brief Bioinform 22(5) (2021)
45. Yao, K., Wang, X., Li, W., et al.: Semi-supervised heterogeneous graph contrastive learning for drug-target interaction prediction. Comput. Biol. Med. 163, 107199 (2023)
46. Huang, L., Luo, H., Li, S., et al.: Drug-drug similarity measure and its applications. Brief Bioinform. 22(4) (2021)
47. T P V a C G Meyer. The COVID-19 epidemic. Tropical medicine & international health 25(3), 278 (2020)
48. B-B D Morales-Ortega, A., et al.: Imatinib for COVID-19: A case report. Clinical Immunology 218, 108518 (2020)
49. Weisberg, E., Parent, A., Yang, P.L., et al.: Repurposing of Kinase Inhibitors for Treatment of COVID-19. Pharmaceutical Res. 37, 167 (2020)
50. Jacobs, C.F., Eldering, Eric, Kater, Arnon P. Kinase inhibitors developed for treatment of hematologic malignancies: implications for immune modulation in COVID-19. Blood Advances 5(3), 913–925 (2021)
51. Gautam, S.S., et al.: Combining hydroxychloroquine and minocycline: potential role in moderate to severe COVID-19 infection. Expert Rev. Clin. Pharmacology 13(11), 1183–1190 (2020)

Structure and Pseudo-Ligand Based Drug Discovery for Disease Targets

Weixin Xie[1,2], Youjun Xu[3], Weilin Zhang[3], Luhua Lai[1,4(✉)],
and Jianfeng Pei[1(✉)]

[1] Center for Quantitative Biology, Academy for Advanced Interdisciplinary Studies,
Peking University, 100871 Beijing, China
{lhlai,jfpei}@pku.edu.cn
[2] Interdisciplinary Institute for Medical Engineering, Fuzhou University,
350108 Fuzhou, China
[3] Infinite Intelligence Pharma, 100083 Beijing, China
[4] BNLMS, Peking-Tsinghua Center for Life Sciences at the College of Chemistry
and Molecular Engineering, Peking University, 100871 Beijing, China

Abstract. Structure-based drug design (SBDD) accelerates drug discovery but traditionally relies on labor-intensive, simulation-based methods. Deep generative models offer a data-driven alternative, but the currently prevalent ligand-based models are often constrained by the availability of active compounds. Here, we present a new SO(3)-equivariant generative model for SBDD, using a pseudo-ligand point-cloud representations of protein cavities to optimize ligands and generate stable 3D molecules. Our model accurately models the chemical space of the protein-binding compounds. We evaluated our model on three therapeutic targets: Janus kinase 2 (JAK2), peptidylprolyl isomerase (hPin1), and Mycobacterium tuberculosis malate synthase. Our model successfully rediscovered moieties involved in key interaction with the proteins and proposed alternative moieties with bioactivity supported by the literature among the highly ranked generated samples. This work approach offers a new way to ligand optimization and drug discovery, advancing the field of public health science by enhancing the precision and efficiency of molecular design in therapeutic development.

Keywords: Drug discovery · Disease targets · Pseudo-ligand
representation · 3D generative model

1 Introduction

Identifying drug candidates that bind to specific targets, such as disease-related proteins, is a fundamental step in drug discovery. Given the vastness of chemical space, this search is often likened to finding a needle in a haystack. High-throughput screening (HTS) against specific targets in bioassays is one method, but its high cost and low success rate have spurred the development of computational alternatives. Virtual screening, using molecular docking or ligand-based

© The Author(s), under exclusive license to Springer Nature Singapore Pte Ltd. 2025
Y. Zhang et al. (Eds.): CHIP 2024, CCIS 2433, pp. 111–129, 2025.
https://doi.org/10.1007/978-981-96-3752-2_8

similarity methods, enables large-scale compound library searches for potential hits. While effective in identifying novel active compounds [22,27], virtual screening is still limited by the scope of available chemical libraries.

Deep generative technologies offer an innovative approach to molecular design, covering broad areas of chemical space and generating molecules in a rule-free fashion [33]. Advances in this area have led to the exploration of diverse model architectures and optimization strategies. Conditional molecular generative models, which generate specialized compound libraries based on user-defined conditions such as molecular properties [4,8,15,19], scaffolds [3,17,20], or pharmacophores [11,32], are particularly promising. Generative models conditioned on receptor structures are of special interest in structure-based drug discovery. The increasing availability of structural data from sources like the Protein Data Bank (PDB) [5] and advancements in protein structure prediction methods such as AlphaFold [12] enable the development of receptor structure-based generative models.

For instance, Xu et al. [31] developed a structure-based generative model that integrates the 3D structural information of protein binding sites, represented by the eigenvalues of the Coulomb matrix of coarse-grained virtual atoms, into a recurrent neural network (RNN) to generate drug-like molecules. Although their model utilizes 3D structures, the eigenvalue decomposition and generation of SMILES outputs limit its ability to identify ligand-protein interactions. While docking programs are often used to predict ligand binding poses, understanding how the model builds ligands within the protein pocket remains challenging when it outputs 2D molecules. More recently, efforts have focused on structure-based models that generate 3D molecules. Ragoza and colleges developed liGAN, a conditional variational autoencoder with 3D convolutional blocks, to directly generate 3D molecules within protein pockets [24]. A notable feature of liGAN is its ability to capture receptor structural variations, making it suitable for structure-based drug design. However, liGAN generates molecules as atomic density grids, requiring rule-based inference for atom coordinates and bond types. Li and colleges proposed L-Net, a model that integrates an internal coordinate system and a graph convolutional neural network to generate 3D molecules with high validity and conformational stability [18]. When combined with Monte Carlo tree search, L-Net can perform structure-based molecular generation tasks. However, their approach relies on a predefined scoring function to guide the search process, and inaccuracies in the scoring function may bias the output distribution of generated compounds.

Most structure-based generative models represent receptor structures either as atomic density grids, capturing the types and shapes of protein atoms, or as graphs that describe spatial proximity between atoms or residues. These representations, however, often lack roto-translational equivariance. Alternative computational methods, such as the pseudo-ligand representation, offer potential solutions by enabling direct comparison between receptor binding sites and their cognate ligands [25]. Katigbak et al. [13] introduced AlphaSpace 2.0, a tessellation-based pseudo-ligand representation that mimics the shape and molecular properties of potential binders, building on their previous work [26]. In addition to characterizing binding pockets and guiding pocket-based docking, they demonstrated AlphaSpace's potential in guiding ligand optimization through retrospective analysis.

In this study, we introduce a novel 3D molecular generative model conditioned on receptor structures. Our model uses a pseudo-ligand representation as an input condition to generate 3D molecules within specific binding cavities. This representation, which incorporates both shape and pharmacophoric information, serves as a negative imprint of the binding pocket, capturing the likely positions and atoms of potential binders. Our model directly generates 3D molecules at target binding sites while simultaneously extracting pocket information. Using the PDBBind v2019 dataset, we developed this conditional generative model in an autoregressive fashion, predicting atoms, bonds, and distances sequentially. Our model accurately captures the chemical space of protein-binding ligands, producing molecules in stable conformation that dock well within the protein pockets. Our model was further evaluated on ligand optimization tasks against three important therapeutic targets: Janus kinase 2 (JAK2), peptidylprolyl isomerase (hPin1), and Mycobacterium tuberculosis malate synthase. It successfully rediscovered fragments involved in key interactions within protein-ligand complexes and proposed other bioactive structures among the top-ranked generated samples. Our method demonstrates practical utility for efficient ligand optimization and drug development for public health.

2   Materials and Methods

2.1   Model Overview

To replicate structure-based molecular design, we employ a pocket-aware approach to generate 3D molecules, directly facilitating the growth of molecules within protein binding pockets. Our model learns both the chemical principles governing molecular structures and the specific characteristics of protein binding sites, such as shape and pharmacophoric features. The model architecture is shown in Fig. 1. We construct the generative model using a factorization scheme as follows:

$$p(L|S) = p(\mathbf{A}_1, \mathbf{A}_2, \ldots, \mathbf{A}_n|S)$$
$$= p(\mathbf{A}_1|S) \prod_{t=2}^{n} p(\mathbf{A}_t|L_{t-1}, S) \tag{1}$$

where L represents the ligand structures, L_t denotes the existing structures at step t, and S refers to the binding sites. The sequence $\mathbf{A}_1, \mathbf{A}_2, \ldots, \mathbf{A}_N$ comprises multi-actions that sequentially construct the ligand L through a deterministic process. A multi-action involves three components: selecting the next atom type e, determining the bond types $\boldsymbol{b}$ with all existing atoms, and assigning the next atom's position in Cartesian coordinates $\boldsymbol{r}$. As there is no canonical ordering

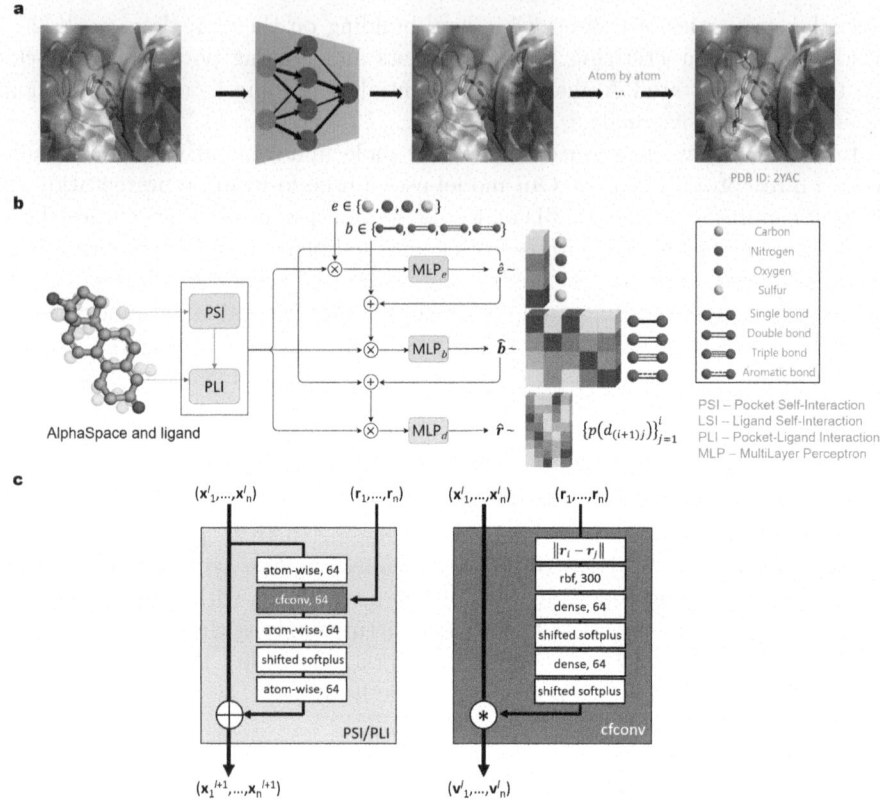

Fig. 1. Overview. (a) Schematic diagram of generating a ligand inside the protein pocket in a auto-regressive fashion. (b,c) The model architecture and interaction modules inspired by SchNet

for atom placement, we generated multiple structural assembly trajectories and used them as a data augmentation strategy, which is explained in Sect. 2.2.

A key distinction from most previous models is that our approach predicts bond types between the newly added atom and all existing atoms, eliminating the need for further connectivity inference, which remains an open challenge [30]. For atoms not connected by a chemical bond, we introduced two virtual bond types to account for the relative position of atoms separated by a topological path of length two or greater. Predicting bond types also facilitates automatic closure of ring structures, which is critical for generating these structures. Additionally, the joint distribution can be rewritten using Bayes' theorem as:

$$p(\mathbf{A}_t|L_{t-1}, S) = p(e_t|L_{t-1}, S) \cdot p(\boldsymbol{b}_t|e_t, L_{t-1}, S) \cdot p(\boldsymbol{r}_t|e_t, \boldsymbol{b}_t, L_{t-1}, S) \quad (2)$$

A crucial aspect is modeling the interaction between the partial ligands L_t and protein pockets S. Proper representation of protein pockets is essential for enabling the generative model to capture these interactions effectively. We represent pocket surfaces using β-clusters, a tessellation-based pseudo-ligand representation provided by AlphaSpace 2.0 [13]. The process of extracting β-clusters is detailed in Sect. 2.2. Briefly, β-clusters and their constituent β-atoms mimic the shape and molecular properties of potential binders, guiding the ligand design process.

Inspired by G-SchNet [9], which employed auxiliary tokens to interact with 3D molecules and direct their growth, we utilize the β-clusters of protein pockets to interact with ligands during their growth. The interaction between ligands and pockets is modeled using SchNet [28], a continuous-filter convolutional neural network originally designed to model quantum interactions within molecules. We specify distinct neighbor relationships for different atom types to regulate the information flow and ensure a stable learning process. Ligand atoms consider both β-atoms and other ligand atoms as neighbors, while β-atoms only interact with other β-atoms. This approach maintains a "static" representation of the pocket environment throughout ligand generation, while the ligand representation evolves as new atoms are added. The state representation of ligands and β-clusters is given as:

$$\tilde{L}_t = \text{PLI}(L_t, \tilde{S}), \tilde{S} = \text{PSI}(S) \tag{3}$$

2.2   Dataset and Data Augmentation

To generate 3D molecules that fit and interact with protein pockets, we trained our model using structures of existing protein-ligand complexes. Data for this training set was sourced from the PDBBind database (v2019) [21], a comprehensive collection of biomolecular complexes with experimentally determined binding affinity data. Both the general set and the refined set were utilized.

To ensure the model learns meaningful protein-ligand interactions, we applied a multi-step filtering pipeline, removing complexes with low binding affinity and poor X-ray resolution (see Fig. 2a). The inclusion of the general set aimed to increase the usable data, retrieving entries without exact K_i/K_d values that were removed from the refined set intended for docking or scoring studies. For instance, PDB entry 3UYT, originally excluded from the refined set, contains a highly bioactive and drug-like ligand and is now included in our dataset (Fig. 2b). Furthermore, we followed the guidelines for compiling the refined set to remove undesired complexes from the general set (Fig. 2a). The final dataset comprised 7,612 complex structures, which we randomly split into training and test sets of 7,550 and 62 complexes, respectively.

We then extracted the ligands from these complexes, representing their corresponding binding sites using a pseudo-ligand approach. Specifically, we used the AlphaSpace2 program with default parameters to extract β-clusters of protein binding sites, along with attributes for each β-atom in the clusters. These attributes included overall and non-polar α-space, as well as docking scores for probe atoms corresponding to one of nine Vina atom types (C, N, O, F, P, S, Cl, Br, and I) placed at each β-atoms location. All attributes were concatenated into

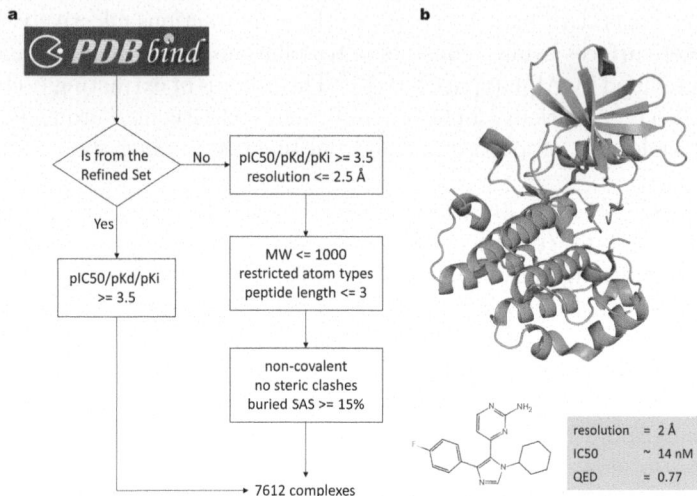

Fig. 2. Dataset curation workflow. (a) Curation of PDBBind refined set and general set. (b) An exemplar entry (PDB ID: 3UYT) retrieved after data curation that contains a highly bioactive and drug-like ligand

an 11-dimensional feature vector. Importantly, only β-atoms near the ligands-i.e., those automatically detected by AlphaSpace2-were retained to encourage the model to focus molecule generation on specific regions of the pocket rather than the entire cavity.

Following the G-SchNet approach [9], we sampled the growth trajectories of ligands surrounded by β-atoms using a breadth-first approach. Each trajectory involved multiple steps of placing atoms one-by-one onto the existing structures, starting from the ligand atom closest to the origin β-atom, analogous to the origin token in G-SchNet.

To address the scarcity of complex structures, we employed two types of augmentation techniques. First, different β-atoms were selected as origins, as ligand growth has no fixed ordering, which may help the generative model elongate compounds from any corner of a protein pocket. Second, although the traversal of the molecular graph was conducted in a breadth-first manner, the focal atom at each step was randomly selected from all available atoms. These on-the-fly augmentation strategies increased the number of trajectory samples by over 100-fold.

2.3 Training and Inference

The state representations are used for the subsequent prediction of the new atom type, e, and the bonds, $\boldsymbol{b}$, connecting the new atom to all existing atoms:

$$\hat{e}_t \sim \text{Softmax}(\text{Aggregate}(\text{MLP}^e(e; \tilde{L}_{t-1})))$$
$$\hat{\boldsymbol{b}}_t \sim \text{Softmax}(\text{MLP}^b(b; \tilde{L}_{t-1}, e_t))$$

$$(4)$$

where MLP^e and MLP^b denote multi-layer perceptrons (MLPs), while Aggregate refers to sum pooling over all existing ligand atoms. Since the state representation of the protein pocket remains static, it does not participate in the decision-making process.

Following the G-SchNet approach, we determine the position of the next atom by aggregating pairwise distance distributions relative to the preceding atoms, ensuring equivariance during the generation process.

$$r_t \sim \frac{1}{\alpha} \prod_{i=1}^{t-1} \text{MLP}^d(d_{i,t}; \tilde{L}_{t-1}, e_t, \boldsymbol{b}_t) \tag{5}$$

We fuzzified the distance value, d, by modeling it with a Gaussian distribution, $N(d, \sigma)$, and used this as the ground truth for the distance distribution to compute the loss. Cross-entropy loss functions were applied to predict the atomic type, bond types, and distances, denoted as $\mathcal{L}_e$, $\mathcal{L}_b$, and $\mathcal{L}_d$, respectively. The overall loss is the sum of these three components:

$$\mathcal{L} = \mathcal{L}_e + \mathcal{L}_b + \mathcal{L}_d \tag{6}$$

Although equivariance is maintained by computing pairwise distances, uncertainty arises at the early stages of the generation process, particularly when fewer than four atoms are present in the pocket. This is because multiple locations can simultaneously satisfy the inter-atomic distance constraints. While this early-stage uncertainty poses minimal challenges when generating molecular structures in the free space, it can cause problems inside pockets, such as deviations from the correct trajectory, steric clashes, or premature termination. To mitigate this, we initialized the generation with a seed structure consisting of more than four heavy atoms, along with the protein pocket, rather than starting with an empty pocket. For each protein pocket in the test set, we generated 20,000 samples and conducted further evaluations.

2.4   Evaluation Metrics

We selected widely adopted metrics to evaluate the properties of the generated molecules. Validity and Uniqueness measure the proportion of generated molecules with valid, non-redundant topological structures, as determined by RDKits molecular structure parser [1]. QED (Quantitative Estimate of Drug-likeness) evaluates the likelihood of a compound being a potential drug candidate [6]. The SA score (Synthetic Accessibility score) assesses the synthetic feasibility of a drug, ranging from 1 to 10, with lower values indicating easier synthesis [7]. Conformational stability is measured by the average root-mean-square deviation (RMSD) of molecular conformations before and after optimization using the MMFF94 force field [10].

To assess how well the generated molecules fit into the protein pocket, we compared the shape similarity (SS) between the atoms of the generated molecules and the β-atoms of the protein pocket. In order to examine the advantage of generated compound over reference ligands in the protein pockets, the improvement in shape similarity is calculated as follows:

$$I_{SS} = SS_{gen} - SS_{ref} \tag{7}$$

A positive I_{SS} represents a better geometric matching of generated compounds with the protein pocket than the reference ligands. And we used Smina [14], an user-friendly docking program based off AutoDock Vina [29], to estimate the affinity value (aff) of the generated molecules binding to the protein pocket. We computed the ligand efficiency (LE) of the generated molecules as the normalized binding affinity divided by the number of atoms. Ligand efficiency is widely used in structure-based drug design and optimization. The improvement of affinity and ligand efficiency for generated compounds over reference ligands are calculated as:

A positive I_{SS} indicates superior geometric alignment of generated compounds with the protein pocket compared to the reference ligands. We also employed Smina [14], a user-friendly docking tool based on AutoDock Vina [29], to estimate the binding affinity (aff) of the generated molecules to the protein pocket. Additionally, we calculated the ligand efficiency (LE), defined as the normalized binding affinity per atom. Ligand efficiency is a commonly used metric in structure-based drug design and optimization. The improvements in affinity and ligand efficiency of generated compounds over reference ligands are computed as:

$$\begin{aligned} I_{aff} &= aff_{ref} - aff_{gen} \\ I_{LE} &= LE_{ref} - LE_{gen} \end{aligned} \tag{8}$$

3 Results and Discussions

3.1 Modelling Protein-Binding Ligand Space

We analyzed the generated molecules within all protein pockets from the test set and compared their molecular properties to those of the reference ligands in the dataset (Fig. 3). The distributions of various molecular properties between the generated molecules and the reference ligands closely align, demonstrating that our model effectively captures the chemical and pharmaceutical characteristics of protein-binding compounds.

It is important for the generated molecules to have a stable conformation and fit well in the protein pocket. The averaged RMSD of the generated molecules before and after MMFF94 force filed optimization is 1.08Å(Fig. 4a). We computed the shape similarity between the β-atoms of the protein pocket and the generated molecules and compared it with that between the β-atoms and the known ligands (Fig. 4b). The majority of the generated molecules are less similar to the pocket in shape than the known ligands, but the difference is small. We also docked each generated molecule to its target pocket and found that generated molecules in near 25% of the test set protein pockets have a better averaged

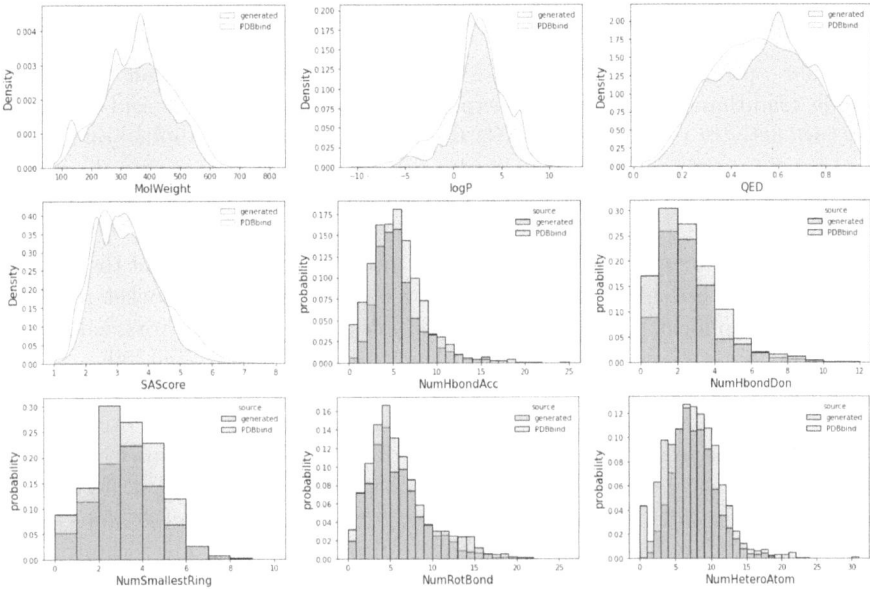

Fig. 3. Comparison of distributions of nine properties for molecules generated by our model and from the dataset: molecular weight, logP, QED, SA score, number of H-bond acceptors, number of H-bond donors, number of rings, number of rotable bonds and number of heteroatoms

docking scores than that of the redocked known ligands (Fig. 4c). Because the generated molecules are of a slightly smaller size than the known ligands, comparing the ligand efficiency is more proper. Nearly 45% of pockets have a higher average ligand efficiency for the generated molecules than that for the known ligands (Fig. 4d).

Ensuring that generated molecules adopt stable conformations and fit well within the protein pockets is essential. The average root-mean-square deviation (RMSD) of generated molecules before and after MMFF94 force field optimization was 1.08 (Fig. 4a). We also calculated the shape similarity between the β-atoms of the protein pockets and the generated molecules, comparing this to the shape similarity between the β-atoms and known ligands (Fig. 4b). While the generated molecules generally exhibit slightly lower shape similarity to the pockets compared to known ligands, the difference is minimal. Furthermore, docking simulations revealed that in approximately 25% of test set protein pockets, the generated molecules achieved better average docking scores than the redocked known ligands (Fig. 4c). Given that the generated molecules tend to be smaller than the known ligands, ligand efficiency provides a more appropriate comparison. Notably, nearly 45% of protein pockets showed higher average ligand efficiency for the generated molecules than for the known ligands (Fig. 4d).

3.2   Molecular Optimization Case Studies

Molecular optimization is a critical process in identifying potent lead compounds, traditionally reliant on the expertise of medicinal chemists and expensive structure-activity relationship (SAR) tests. In this study, we applied our model for automatic optimization of molecules in binding sites, validating the generated results against resolved complex structures and experimental data from the literature.

This process was guided by beta atoms in unoccupied regions of the pocket, which informed potential interactions between the ligand and pocket residues. The pharmacophoric features were encoded into beta feature vectors, calculated using AlphaSpace2 and the scoring function from AutoDock Vina [29].

We selected targets with reported potent binders and resolved crystal structures to evaluate whether our model could recapture key interactions within binding sites. We removed fragments involved in crucial interactions with pocket residues, using the remaining portions of known ligands as initial structures for our generative model to regrow. The therapeutic targets selected were Janus kinase 2 (JAK2), peptidylprolyl isomerase (hPin1), and Mycobacterium tuberculosis malate synthase (GlcB).

CASE 1. The first case examined JAK2 kinase and its inhibitor, phenyl-substituted indazole **2**, derived from a fragment-based approach (PDB ID: 3e63).

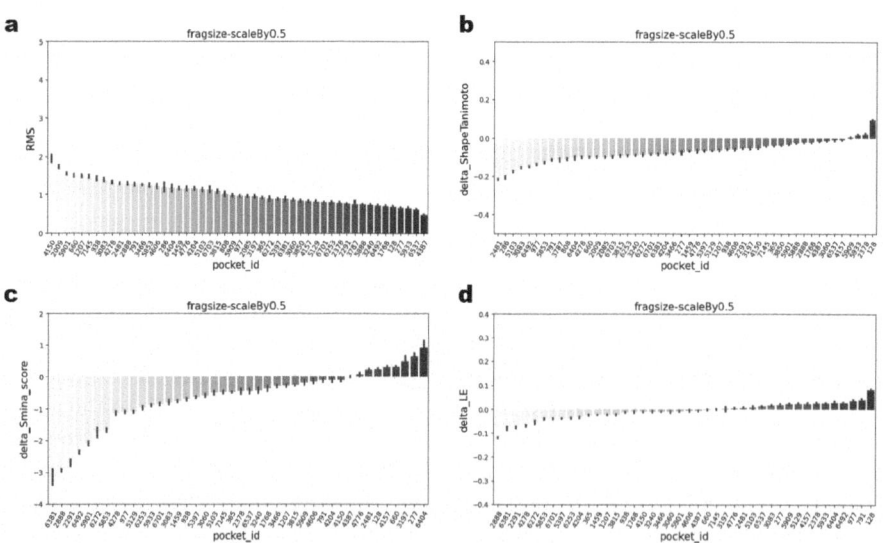

Fig. 4. Evaluation on the test set pockets. Distributions of (a) RMSD between conformations before and after MMFF94 force field optimization; (b) Improvement of shape Tanimoto index; (c) Improvement of docking scores and (d) Improvement of ligand efficiency

JAK2, a member of the Janus kinase family, plays a key role in signal transduction mediated by cytokines and cytokine-like hormones. Mutations in JAK2 lead to its constitutive activation, contributing to myeloproliferative neoplasms (MPNs), driving the development of selective JAK2 inhibitors. Compound **2** was an optimized version of bromoaminoindazole **1**, showing a 25-fold increase in potency with an IC_{50} of 1.6 μM. The crystal structure revealed that the 5-phenyl substituent interacts favorably with the p-loop and Val863 from the N-lobe of the catalytic domain [2].

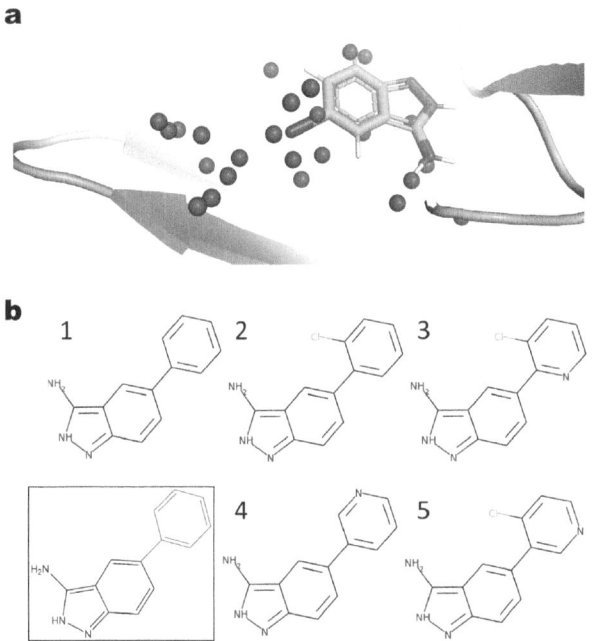

Fig. 5. Case study of optimization of JAK2 inhibitors. (a) The generation setting with beta atoms in magenta. (b) Top-5 recommended structures extended from the initial fragment by our model. The initial fragment is shown at the lower left corner, with the reference elaboration colored in red (Color figure online)

We tested whether our model could rediscover the phenyl ring critical for potency, using **2** with the phenyl ring removed as the initial structure (Fig. 5a). Our generator extended the structure into the beta atom region with suitable fragments, successfully recalling compound **2** as the top recommendation (Fig. 5b). Furthermore, the model suggested ortho-substitution with Cl in the six-membered rings, with the 2-chlorophenyl moiety being the second most frequent recommendation. This moiety has been experimentally tested, showing an IC_{50} of 0.37 μM, over a 100-fold potency increase compared to **1** [2].

CASE 2. The second case involved hPin1, a prolyl isomerase implicated in cell cycle regulation and linked to various pathologies, including cancer. Prolyl isomerases have also been shown to regulate immune cell functions. Previous studies identified potent inhibitors against hPin1 using traditional structure-based drug design [23], with a phenyl imidazole acid core forming hydrophobic interactions with multiple residues (L122, F134, M130, L61) and π-π interactions with H59. However, deep learning-based methods like DeepFrag failed to recall the phenyl imidazole moiety, instead proposing bulkier, less effective bicyclic rings (Fig. 6).

We used our model to optimize the ligand and rediscover the phenyl imidazole core, starting from the seed structure based on the complex (PDB ID: 2XP9). Our model successfully regenerated the original phenyl imidazole as the most frequent structure, while alternative moieties among the top-5 recommendations had similar volumes and properties: 4-phenol, pyridine, 4-chlorobenzene, and thiophene.

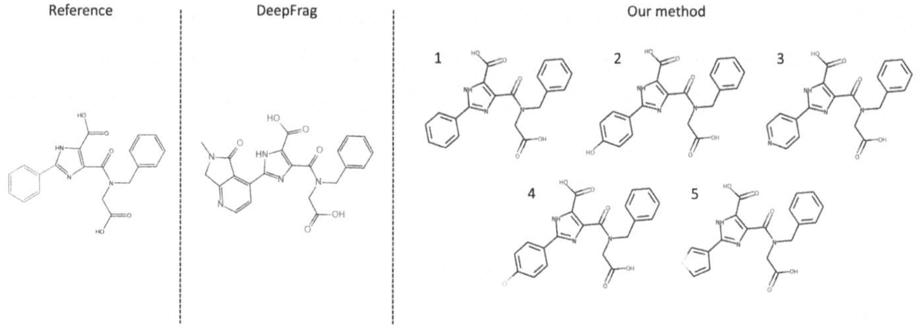

Fig. 6. Case study of optimization of hPin1 inhibitors. (left) The structure of the original inhibitor with the reference elaboration colored in red. (middle) The best results from DeepFrag. (right) Top-5 recommended structures extended from the initial fragment by our model (Color figure online)

CASE 3. The final validation case for our model involved the identification of inhibitors for malate synthase (GlcB) in Mycobacterium tuberculosis (Mtb). GlcB is a key enzyme in the glyoxylate shunt, a pathway critical for Mtb virulence, making it a promising pharmacological target. Krieger et al. identified a potent phenyl-diketo acid (PDKA) inhibitor, referred to as compound 4, and the crystal structure revealed a crucial face-on anion-π interaction between the Asp633 side chain and the phenyl ring of compound 4 [16]. The study suggested a strong requirement for an aromatic moiety, as evidenced by the lack of activity in aliphatic replacements for the phenyl ring. We employed our model to reproduce this key interaction with Asp633. To this end, we extracted the beta carbon atoms surrounding the ligand, using the PDKA scaffold-where the ortho-substituted phenyl ring was removed-as the starting structure for fragment extension (Fig. 7b). The model was then guided by the beta atoms in the ligand-free region to populate it with suitable fragments.

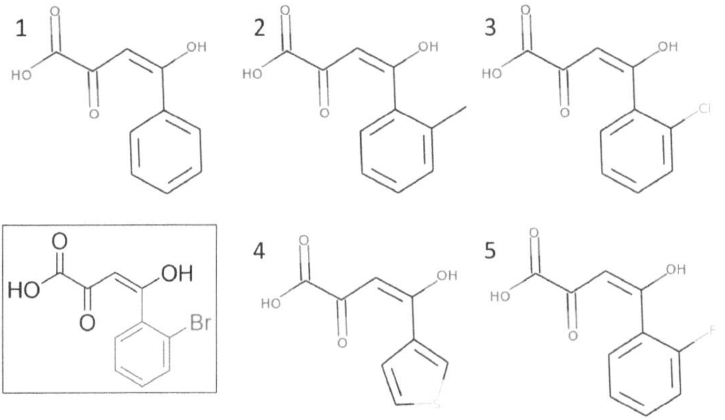

Fig. 7. Case study of optimization of GlcB inhibitors. Top-5 recommended structures extended from the initial fragment by our model. The initial fragment is shown at the lower left corner, with the reference elaboration colored in red (Color figure online)

We used our model to sample 20,000 times repetitively and filtered out invalid structures not recognized by RDKit. Our model successfully recalled the original benzene ring as the top recommendation and also proposed alternative ortho- and para-substitutions which were experimentally validated with bioactivity between 0.24–1.1 μM in the literature (Table 1). Although the Br at the ortho position did not appear, it was initially introduced to improve stability, with no significant effect on inhibitor binding [16]. The majority (93.2%) of the generated structures contained aromatic rings, with 70% being phenyl rings.

Table 1. Recommended structures with bio-activity supported by the literature. The experimental affinity (IC50 values) are from [16]

Compound	R	IC50 (μM)	Recommendation
PDKA	Ph	2.0	No. 1
1	2-MePh	1.1	No. 2
2	2-FPh	0.24	No. 5
3	2-ClPh	0.5	No. 3

3.3   Model Parameters Analysis

As described in Sect. 2.3, we used a fragment from a known binder in the test set protein pocket as the seed structure. Our generative model extended this structure by adding new atoms, guided by the surrounding beta atoms. We observed that using small fragments, containing 4, 5, or 6 heavy atoms, resulted in smaller structures compared to the known binders (Fig. 8a–c). The larger the known ligand, the greater the discrepancy. This suggests that starting with a small fragment makes it difficult for the model to extend the structure to fully occupy the binding site. This issue is partly due to high variability at the initial stages of generation, leading to final structures that differ from the reference binders. Additionally, fixed-sized fragments are unsuitable for pockets of varying volumes, as structures generated in large pockets deviate more from the reference compared to those in small pockets.

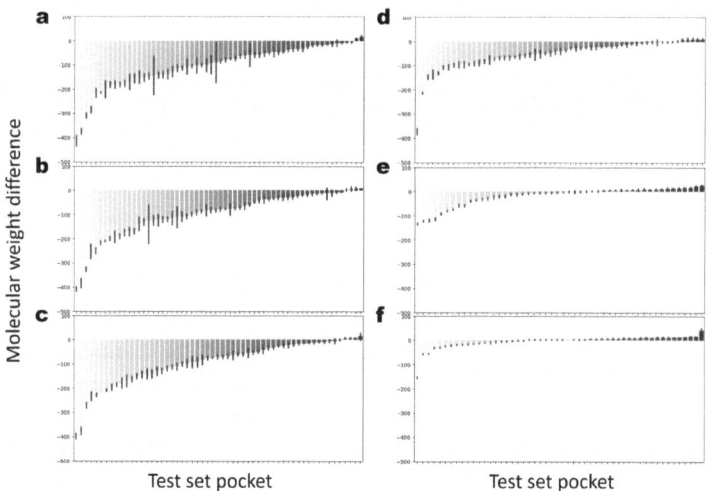

Fig. 8. Molecular weight differences between generated molecules and known ligands over all test set protein pockets. A negative molecular weight difference means that the generated molecule has a smaller size than the known ligand. The vertical black lines are standard deviations. (a-c) Molecular weight differences of the generated molecules starting from a seed fragment with 4, 5 and 6 heavy atoms, respectively. (d) Molecular weight differences of the generated molecules starting from a seed fragment with the size of 25%, 50% and 75% of the original size of the known binder, respectively

To ensure a fair comparison, we employed starting fragments proportional to the number of heavy atoms in the known binder for each pocket, testing three proportions: 25%, 50%, and 75%. The generated molecules were more comparable in size to the known binders (Fig. 8d–f), particularly at 50% and 75% proportions. We also found that larger starting fragments improved the validity of the final structures but reduced their uniqueness (Fig. 9), a reasonable trade-off. The overall distribution of QED and SA score deviations from the known ligands did not vary significantly across the different proportions. Consequently, we used a 50% fragment proportion for balanced comparisons with known ligands and optimized sampling efficiency.

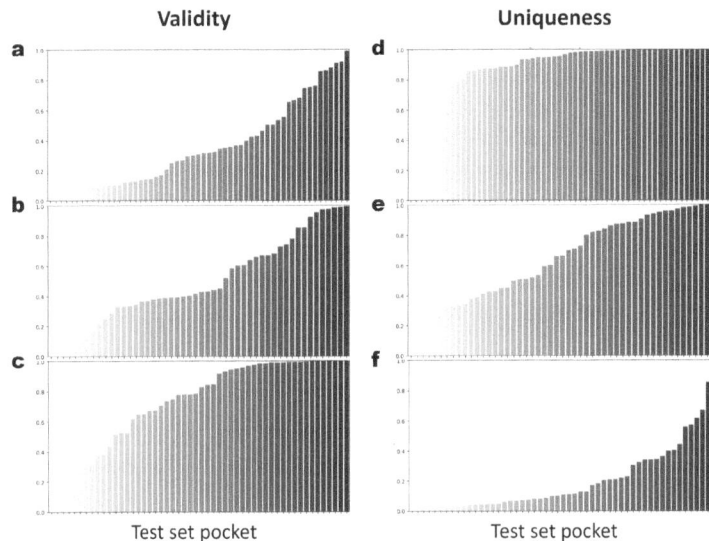

Fig. 9. Validity and uniqueness of generated molecules across all test set protein pockets. (a–c) Validity and uniqueness of the generated molecules starting from a seed fragment with 4, 5 and 6 heavy atoms, respectively. (d) Validity and uniqueness of the generated molecules starting from a seed fragment with the size of 25%, 50% and 75% of the original size of the known binder, respectively

As outlined in Sect. 2.3, our model employed temperature-based sampling, with low temperatures applied to atom types. We examined how temperature influenced sampling exhaustion by gradually increasing it and sampling 20,000 times at each temperature. As expected, higher temperatures led to an increase in accumulated structures and scaffolds. However, the exhaustion trend persisted, particularly in scaffold accumulation (Fig. 10). Higher temperatures flattened the accumulation curve more slowly, likely due to increased entropy and diminished model constraints, resulting in more random sampling and reduced adherence to the protein binding context.

Finally, we investigated how variations in seed structures affect the reproduction of molecular fragments that likely contribute to high binding affinity. Specifically, we provided the model with several shortened initial fragments and tested its ability to reconstruct the remaining portions extending from these truncated positions. This approach exposed the generative model to a broader region of the binding pocket, beyond the limited space defined by the beta atoms

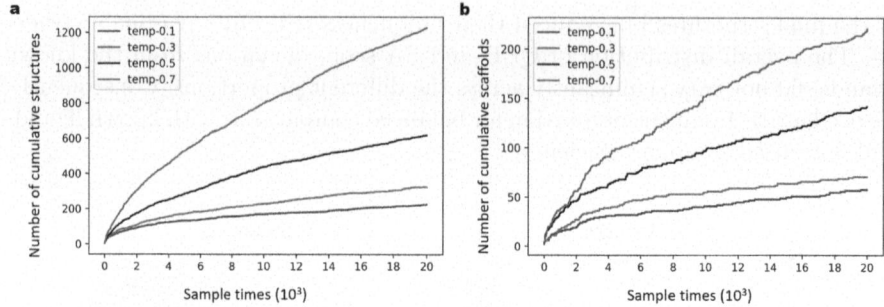

Fig. 10. Effects of varying sample temperatures. (a) The number of accumulated structures varies with sampling times under different temperatures. (b) The number of accumulated scaffolds varies with sampling times under different temperatures

surrounding the masked aromatic rings examined in Sect. 3.2. All other generation parameters were kept consistent with prior settings.

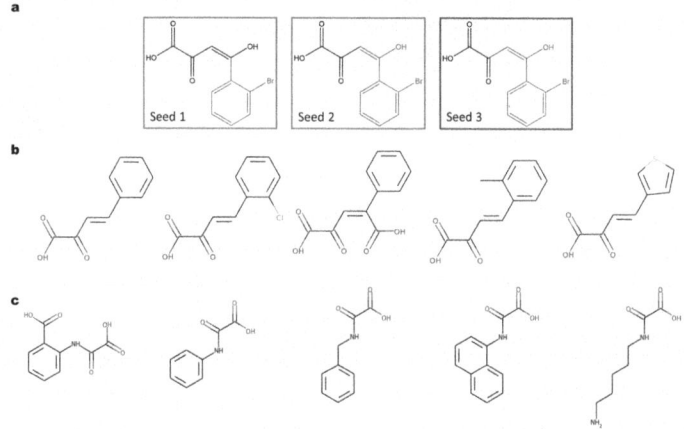

Fig. 11. Effects of lengths of seeding structures. (a) Three shortened initial fragments. (b) Structures elongated from the seed structure 2. (c) Structures elongated from the seed structure 3

Beginning with the GlcB protein and its PDKA inhibitor, we introduced three shortened initial fragments to the model and tasked it with extending from these points (Fig. 11a). As the region of exploration expanded, the uncertainty increased, prompting the generative model to explore different fragment combinations, which explains the steady rise in uniqueness. We deemed reproduction successful if the model could recall the phenyl ring, connected by an identical topological path length starting from the initial "open" atom, among the 5 most frequent scaffolds after sampling 10,000 molecules. Although the proportion of generated molecules containing a benzene ring declined significantly as the initial fragment was shortened (Table 2), the model successfully retrieved scaffolds similar to the original for the first two truncated fragments (see Fig. 11b for the second fragment).

Table 2. Performance of reproduction of molecular fragments that contribute to high binding affinity using different seed structures

Seed	Validity (%)	Uniqueness (%)	Ratio of single ring	Ratio of single aromatic ring	Ratio of phenyl ring
1	51.8	2.1	99.2	94.7	72.6
2	31.1	6.1	93.1	92.2	79.1
3	33.4	25.7	60.6	38.2	29.8

4   Conclusion

In this study, we introduced a novel SO(3)-equivariant generative model for structure-based drug design (SBDD), leveraging pseudo-ligand point-cloud representations of protein cavities to generate 3D molecules with stable conformations. By conditioning on receptor structures and utilizing autoregressive generation, our model captures the intricate chemical space of protein-binding ligands, offering a powerful approach for ligand optimization. Through evaluation on three therapeutically significant targets-Janus kinase 2 (JAK2), peptidylprolyl isomerase (hPin1), and Mycobacterium tuberculosis malate synthase-our model demonstrated its ability to rediscover key interaction moieties and identify alternative bioactive compounds supported by the literature.

The success of our model in proposing novel, bioactive ligands highlights its potential to streamline early-stage drug discovery. By enhancing the precision and efficiency of molecular design, this approach represents a significant step forward in data-driven drug discovery, particularly in addressing public health challenges. Our results demonstrate that generative models conditioned on receptor structures offer a promising new direction for advancing SBDD and facilitating the development of targeted therapeutics.

References

1. Rdkit: Open-source cheminformatics. https://www.rdkit.org
2. Antonysamy, S., Hirst, G., Park, F., Sprengeler, P., Stappenbeck, F., Steensma, R., Wilson, M., Wong, M.: Fragment-based discovery of JAK-2 inhibitors. Bioorg. Med. Chem. Lett. (2009). https://doi.org/10.1016/j.bmcl.2008.08.064
3. Arús-Pous, J., Patronov, A., Bjerrum, E.J., Tyrchan, C., Reymond, J.L., Chen, H., Engkvist, O.: Smiles-based deep generative scaffold decorator for de-novo drug design. J. Cheminform. **12** (5 2020). https://doi.org/10.1186/s13321-020-00441-8
4. Bagal, V., Aggarwal, R., Vinod, P.K., Priyakumar, U.D.: Molgpt: molecular generation using a transformer-decoder model. J. Chem. Inf. Model. (2021). https://doi.org/10.1021/acs.jcim.1c00600

5. Berman, H.M., et al.: The Protein Data Bank. Nucleic Acids Res. **28**(1), 235–242 (2000). https://doi.org/10.1093/nar/28.1.235

6. Bickerton, G.R., Paolini, G.V., Besnard, J., Muresan, S., Hopkins, A.L.: [qed] quantifying the chemical beauty of drugs. Nature Chemistry **4**, 90–98 (2012). https://doi.org/10.1038/nchem.1243

7. Ertl, P., Schuffenhauer, A.: Estimation of synthetic accessibility score of drug-like molecules based on molecular complexity and fragment contributions. J. Cheminformatics **1** (2009). https://doi.org/10.1186/1758-2946-1-8

8. Gebauer, N.W.A., Gastegger, M., Hessmann, S.S.P., Müller, K.R., Schütt, K.T.: Inverse design of 3d molecular structures with conditional generative neural networks. Nature Communications **13**(1) (Feb 2022). https://doi.org/10.1038/s41467-022-28526-y,

9. Gebauer, N.W., Gastegger, M., Schütt, K.T.: Symmetry-adapted generation of 3d point sets for the targeted discovery of molecules (2019)

10. Halgren, T.A.: Merck molecular force field. i. basis, form, scope, parameterization, and performance of mmff94. J. Comput. Chem. **17**(5-6), 490–519 (1996)

11. Imrie, F., Hadfield, T.E., Bradley, A.R., Deane, C.M.: [develop] deep generative design with 3d pharmacophoric constraints. Chem. Sci. **12**, 14577–14589 (2021). https://doi.org/10.1039/D1SC02436A

12. Jumper, J., Evans, R., Pritzel, A., Green, T., Figurnov, M., Ronneberger, O., Tunyasuvunakool, K., Bates, R., Žídek, A., Potapenko, A., et al.: Highly accurate protein structure prediction with alphafold. Nature **596**(7873), 583–589 (2021)

13. Katigbak, J., Li, H., Rooklin, D., Zhang, Y.: AlphaSpace 2.0: representing concave biomolecular surfaces using β-Clusters. J. Chem. Inf. Modeling **60**(3), 1494–1508 (2020)

14. Koes, D.R., Baumgartner, M.P., Camacho, C.J.: Lessons learned in empirical scoring with smina from the csar 2011 benchmarking exercise. J. Chem. Inf. Model. **53**(8), 1893–1904 (2013)

15. Kotsias, P.C., Arús-Pous, J., Chen, H., Engkvist, O., Tyrchan, C., Bjerrum, E.J.: Direct steering of de novo molecular generation with descriptor conditional recurrent neural networks. Nature Mach. Intell. **2**, 254–265 (2020). https://doi.org/10.1038/s42256-020-0174-5

16. Krieger, I.V., Freundlich, J.S., Gawandi, V.B., Roberts, J.P., Gawandi, V.B., Sun, Q., Owen, J.L., Fraile, M.T., Huss, S.I., Lavandera, J.L., Ioerger, T.R., Sacchettini, J.C.: Structure-Guided Discovery of Phenyl-diketo Acids as Potent Inhibitors of M. Tuberculosis Malate Synthase. Chemistry Biol. (2012). https://doi.org/10.1016/j.chembiol.2012.09.018

17. Li, Y., Hu, J., Wang, Y., Zhou, J., Zhang, L., Liu, Z.: Deepscaffold: A comprehensive tool for scaffold-based de novo drug discovery using deep learning. J. Chem. Inf. Modeling **60**, 77–91 (2020). https://doi.org/10.1021/acs.jcim.9b00727

18. Li, Y., Pei, J., Lai, L.: [deepligbuilder] structure-based de novo drug design using 3d deep generative models. Chem. Sci. (2021). https://doi.org/10.1039/d1sc04444c

19. Li, Y., Zhang, L., Liu, Z.: Multi-objective de novo drug design with conditional graph generative model. J. Cheminform. **10**, December 2018. https://doi.org/10.1186/s13321-018-0287-6

20. Lim, J., Hwang, S.Y., Moon, S., Kim, S., Kim, W.Y.: Scaffold-based molecular design with a graph generative model. Chem. Sci. **11**, 1153–1164 (2020). https://doi.org/10.1039/c9sc04503a

21. Liu, Z., Su, M., Han, L., Liu, J., Yang, Q., Li, Y., Wang, R.: Forging the Basis for Developing Protein-Ligand Interaction Scoring Functions. Acc. Chem. Res. (2017). https://doi.org/10.1021/acs.accounts.6b00491

22. Luttens, A., et al.: Ultralarge virtual screening identifies sars-cov-2 main pro-
    tease inhibitors with broad-spectrum activity against coronaviruses. J. Am. Chem.
    Soc. **144**, 2905–2920 (2022). https://doi.org/10.1021/jacs.1c08402. https://pubs.
    acs.org/doi/10.1021/jacs.1c08402
23. Potter, A., Oldfield, V., Nunns, C., Fromont, C., Ray, S., Northfield, C.J., Bryant,
    C.J., Scrace, S.F., Robinson, D., Matossova, N., Baker, L., Dokurno, P., Surgenor,
    A.E., Davis, B., Richardson, C.M., Murray, J.B., Moore, J.D.: Discovery of cell-
    active phenyl-imidazole pin1 inhibitors by structure-guided fragment evolution.
    Bioorganic Med. Chem. Lett. **20**(22), 6483–6488 (2010). https://doi.org/10.1016/
    j.bmcl.2010.09.063
24. Ragoza, M., Masuda, T., Koes, D.R.: [ligan] generating 3d molecules conditional
    on receptor binding sites with deep generative models, October 2021. https://doi.
    org/10.1039/d1sc05976a, arxiv:2110.15200
25. Ravindranath, P.A., Sanner, M.F.: Autosite: an automated approach for pseudo-
    ligands prediction-from ligand-binding sites identification to predicting key ligand
    atoms. Bioinformatics **32**(20), 3142–3149 (2016)
26. Rooklin, D., Wang, C., Katigbak, J., Arora, P.S., Zhang, Y.: AlphaSpace: fragment-
    centric topographical mapping to target protein-protein interaction interfaces. J.
    Chem. Inf. Model. (2015). https://doi.org/10.1021/acs.jcim.5b00103
27. Sadybekov, A.A., Sadybekov, A.V., Liu, Y., Iliopoulos-Tsoutsouvas, C., Huang,
    X.P., Pickett, J., Houser, B., Patel, N., Tran, N.K., Tong, F., Zvonok, N., Jain,
    M.K., Savych, O., Radchenko, D.S., Nikas, S.P., Petasis, N.A., Moroz, Y.S., Roth,
    B.L., Makriyannis, A., Katritch, V.: Synthon-based ligand discovery in virtual
    libraries of over 11 billion compounds. Nature (12 2021). https://doi.org/10.1038/
    s41586-021-04220-9, https://www.nature.com/articles/s41586-021-04220-9
28. Schütt, K., et al.: Schnet: a continuous-filter convolutional neural network for mod-
    eling quantum interactions. Advances in neural information processing systems **30**
    (2017)
29. Trott, O., Olson, A.J.: Autodock vina: improving the speed and accuracy of docking
    with a new scoring function, efficient optimization, and multithreading. J. Comput.
    Chem. (2009). https://doi.org/10.1002/jcc.21334
30. Xie, W., Wang, F., Li, Y., Lai, L., Pei, J.: Advances and challenges in de novo drug
    design using three-dimensional deep generative models. J. Chemical Inf. Modeling
31. Xu, M., Ran, T., Chen, H.: De Novo Molecule Design through the Molecular Gen-
    erative Model Conditioned by 3D Information of Protein Binding Sites (2021).
    https://doi.org/10.1021/acs.jcim.0c01494
32. Yang, Y., Zheng, S., Su, S., Zhao, C., Xu, J., Chen, H.: Syntalinker: automatic
    fragment linking with deep conditional transformer neural networks. Chem. Sci.
    11, 8312–8322 (8 2020). https://doi.org/10.1039/d0sc03126g
33. Zhang, J., Mercado, R., Engkvist, O., Chen, H.: Comparative study of deep gener-
    ative models on chemical space coverage, July 2021. https://doi.org/10.1021/acs.
    jcim.0c01328

Multi-channel Hypergraph Convolutional Network Predicts circRNA-Drug Sensitivity Associations

Chunjiang Yin, Tuo Jiang, Huan Liu, and Lingyun Luo[✉]

School of Computer Science, University of South China, Hengyang,
Hunan 421001, China
luoly@usc.edu.cn

Abstract. Recent studies indicate that variations in the expression of circular RNA (circRNA) can alter cellular drug sensitivity, which in turn significantly impacts drug efficacy and plays a crucial role in human health and disease treatment. Thus, predicting the associations between circRNA and drug sensitivity is essential. In this study, to enhance the prediction accuracy, we introduce a novel method named MHCDA that leverages graph convolutional networks and hypergraph convolutional networks to extract both local and global information of the circRNA-drug network. Specifically, MHCDA first constructs homogeneous graphs for circRNAs and drugs through similarity fusion networks, then obtain the representations of circRNAs and drugs using graph convolutional networks. On the other hand, we utilize hypergraph convolutional networks to extract more complex higher-order interactions between drugs and circRNAs, respectively. Utilizing Contrastive Learning to Analyze circRNA Feature Representations and Pharmacological Feature Representations Across Various Convolutional Architectures. Meanwhile, we utilize autoencoders to extract circRNA and drug features from the established associations between circRNAs and drugs. Finally, we integrate the various features obtained to predict the relationship between circRNA and drug sensitivity. Experiments reveal that the AUC and AUPR values of MHCDA are 0.918 and 0.929, respectively, surpassing those of other advanced models.

Keywords: circRNA-drug associations · Similarity network · HGNN

1 Introduction

Circular RNAs (circRNAs), a class of non-coding RNAs distinguished by their covalently closed circular shape, have been associated with the onset and progression of numerous diseases, such as neurological conditions, cancer, and cardiovascular disorders [1]. Evidence indicates that circRNA expression can significantly impact cellular sensitivity to drugs, thereby influencing drug efficacy. For instance, circ-AKT3 expression is elevated in cisplatin-resistant gastric cancer

© The Author(s), under exclusive license to Springer Nature Singapore Pte Ltd. 2025
Y. Zhang et al. (Eds.): CHIP 2024, CCIS 2433, pp. 130–146, 2025.
https://doi.org/10.1007/978-981-96-3752-2_9

cells [2], while circ-PVT1 enhances paclitaxel resistance in these cells. Therefore, elucidating the relationships between circRNAs and drug sensitivity is crucial for circRNA-focused drug discovery and therapeutic strategies.

Traditional biomedical experiments tend to be costly and time-consuming. Thus, it is essential to explore computational methods that can accurately predict the relationship between circular RNAs and drug sensitivity. Recently, graph neural networks (GNNs) have demonstrated strong performance in drug-gene interaction (DGI) prediction due to their ability to effectively represent relational data [4]. When using GNNs for prediction, the two primary approaches are based on local and global relationships to predict associations between drugs and RNA.

The local relationship-based approach involves using traditional graph convolutional network (GCN) methods for prediction. For example, Deng et al. [5] organized circRNA and drug sensitivity data and introduced the GATECDA prediction method, which is based on a graph attention autoencoder (GATE). Yang et al. [6] built upon Deng et al.'s groundwork with their study, MNGACDA, which integrates a node-level attention layer into a deep graph neural network architecture. Luo et al. [7] predicted circRNA-drug sensitivity by constructing a heterogeneous graph of drugs and circRNAs, employing dual-view learning, and utilizing a path-masking graph autoencoder [8]. Although they have achieved promising results, GCN has limitations. GCN is limited to aggregating information from neighboring nodes in a layer-wise manner, which hinders its ability to effectively capture higher-order correlations among nodes.

To overcome the limitations of Graph Convolutional Networks (GCNs), researchers have begun utilizing Hypergraph Neural Networks (HGNNs) [9] to explore higher-order relationships between drugs and RNA from a global relational perspective [10]. Liu et al. [11] proposed an HGNN-based method called HGNNLDA, which predicts sensitivity associations between lncRNAs and drugs. HGNNLDA models associations as a bipartite graph of lncRNAs and drugs, constructing a hypergraph for each. Hu et al. [12] utilized hypergraphs to capture higher-order relationships between mRNA and drugs, employing hypergraph convolutional network methods and contrastive learning to predict mRNA-drug sensitivity. Although they have achieved promising results, some limitations still persist. They only utilize associations between drugs and RNA, neglecting the rich information inherent in interactions among drugs and RNAs [13].

In this study, we present a novel computational model called MHCDA, which integrates Graph Convolutional Networks (GCNs) and hypergraph convolutional networks to identify associations between circular RNAs (circRNAs) and drug sensitivity. First, MHCDA utilizes various data sources related to circRNAs and drugs to construct integrated similarity networks for circRNA-circRNA and drug-drug pairs, as well as networks that illustrate circRNA-drug sensitivity associations. Next, we use Graph Convolutional Networks (GCNs) to derive latent representations for circRNAs and drugs based on their similarity graphs. To explore higher-order relationships between these entities, we employ a hypergraph convolutional network for modeling. We then implement contrastive learning to enhance information interaction between the hypergraphs and GCNs, ensuring consistency in learned features across various convolutions. Recognizing the importance of established associations between circRNAs and drugs, MHCDA employs a variational autoencoder to extract nonlinear features from these associations, effectively integrating prior knowledge into the prediction process. Finally, we evaluate the composite embedding features and utilize the model's training outcomes for predictions. Experimental results indicate that MHCDA outperforms the other four models across all performance metrics. Therefore, it can serve as an effective computational tool for identifying novel circRNA-drug associations.

2   Materials and Methods

We obtained the datasets from Ref. [5]. In Ref. [5], Deng et al. gathered circRNA–drug sensitivity associations from the circRic database, with drug sensitivity data sourced from the GDSC database [14]. The dataset comprises 404 circRNAs, 250 drugs, and 80,076 associations. We extracted associations with a false discovery rate (FDR) of less than 0.05, resulting in 4,134 associations involving 271 circRNAs and 218 drugs. Based on these associations, we constructed an association matrix $A_{cd} \in R^{271 \times 218}$. For any element A_{ij} in A_{cd}, if $A_{ij} = 1$, it indicates that circRNA i is associated with the sensitivity of drug j; otherwise, $A_{ij} = 0$. To obtain more circRNA and drug data, we screened the host gene sequences of circRNAs from the National Center for Biotechnology Information (NCBI) gene database and specifically retrieved the structural information of drugs from the PubChem database [15].

2.1   Similarity Calculation

CircRNA Similarity. Similar to previous studies [5], we utilize the sequence similarity between host genes to quantify circRNA similarity, calculated using the Levenshtein distance. The results are represented as a matrix CSS $\in R^{M \times M}$, where M represents the total number of circRNAs.

Drug Similarity. Since the structural information of drugs significantly impacts their function, it is feasible to use this information when constructing drug similarity. First, we extract the structural information of drugs from the PubChem database and calculate each drug's topological fingerprint using RDKit [16]. Next, we use the Tanimoto method to calculate the structural similarity between the drugs. Finally, we output the drug similarity matrix DSS $\in R^{N \times N}$, where N indicates the total number of drugs.

GIP Kernel Similarity of CircRNAs and Drugs. Although we obtained the sequence similarity of circRNAs, not all pairs exhibit this similarity, resulting in sparsity and insufficient informational content in the constructed circRNA sequence similarity matrix. To address this issue, we employ Gaussian interaction profile (GIP) kernel similarity as complementary information [17]. The similarity of circRNAs based on the GIP kernel is determined from the circRNA–drug sensitivity association matrix, using the formula below:

$$\text{CGS}(c_i, c_j) = \exp(-\gamma_c \|\text{IP}(c_i) - \text{IP}(c_j)\|^2)$$

$$\gamma_c = \alpha_c / \left(\frac{1}{N_c} \sum_{i=1}^{N_c} \|\text{IP}(c_i)\|^2 \right) \tag{1}$$

The Gaussian kernel function measures the correlation between nodes by calculating their Euclidean distances, using these values to represent the network's topological structure. Here, $\text{CGS} \in R^{M \times M}$, and $\text{IP}(c_i)$ represents the respective column of circRNA c_i in the circRNA–drug association matrix. The parameter γ_c controls the kernel bandwidth. The parameter α_c is set to 1, consistent with previous research. In the circRNA-drug sensitivity association network A,N_c represents the total number of circRNAs. Likewise, we calculate the GIP kernel similarity matrix for the drugs.

Similarity Fusion As described above, we assess the similarities between circRNAs and drugs from multiple perspectives. To create a comprehensive similarity matrix, it is essential to integrate the similarity matrices from different perspectives. The updated circRNA similarity matrix is constructed as follows:

$$CS_{ij} = \begin{cases} \frac{(CSS_{ij} + CGS_{ij})}{2} & , if \quad CSS_{ij} \neq 0 \\ CGS_{ij} & , otherwise \end{cases} \tag{2}$$

In a similar manner, the comprehensive similarity matrix for drugs is calculated as follows:

$$DS_{ij} = \begin{cases} \frac{(DSS_{ij} + DGS_{ij})}{2}, & \text{if } DSS_{ij} \neq 0 \\ DGS_{ij}, & \text{otherwise} \end{cases} \tag{3}$$

3   Methods

In this study, we introduce a novel computational model called MHCDA, which integrates graph convolutional networks and hypergraph convolutional networks to predict circRNA-drug associations. The overall design of our model is depicted in Fig. 1. The MHCDA model is implemented through the following steps:

Step 1: As previously mentioned, we constructed the adjacency matrix A_{cd} for circRNAs and drugs, along with the drug similarity matrix DS and the circRNA similarity matrix CS. For CS and DS we obtain only the top 25 neighbors ranked by similarity values, removing the others. The drug hypergraph matrix H_{d-d} and the circRNA hypergraph matrix H_{c-c} are constructed based on CS and DS, respectively.

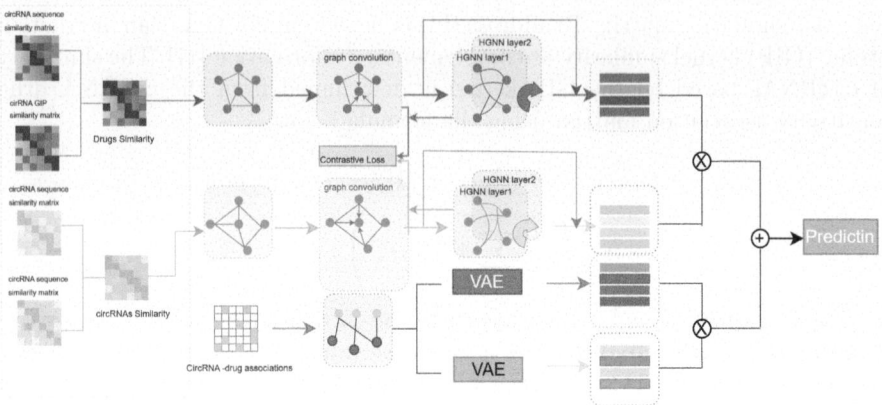

Fig. 1. The flow chart of MHCDA for predicting circRNA-drug sensitivity associations.

Step 2: Learn the embedded representations of circRNAs and drugs using GraphConv [18] and HGNN [9] based on CS and DS, respectively. On the other hand, we also use VAE [19] to learn additional representations of circRNAs and drugs by leveraging the association matrix A.

Step 3:Obtain the final representations of circRNAs and drugs and use the inner product operation to calculate the final circRNA-drug sensitivity score matrix. The predicted circRNA–drug sensitivity associations are ranked based on the final scores.

3.1 Graph Convolutional Network for circRNA/Drug Similarities

We use a circRNA graph and a drug graph to represent the similarities of circR-NAs and drugs, respectively. The two graphs were constructed using KNN. In the Drug graph, nodes represent drugs, and edges are defined as follows:

$$A_d(i,j) = \begin{cases} \text{if the circRNA } i \text{ and } j \text{ are the} \\ k\text{-nearest neighbors of each other,} \\ 0 \text{ otherwise,} \end{cases} \tag{4}$$

The matrix A_d represents the adjacency matrix of the drug graph DS. The parameter k is a hyperparameter that determines the number of connections in the graph. The circRNA graph CS can be constructed similarly, with its adjacency matrix denoted as A_c.

To extract output from the similarity matrix, we employ the graph convolution operator from prior research [18] to learn vector representations of circRNAs and drugs from the similarity graphs. For a drug, the learnable embedding vector is denoted as $x_i \in \mathbb{R}^{d \times d}$. To obtain information from the drug similarity graph, we define it as follows:

$$x_i^{(l)} = \sigma\left(W_1 x_i^{(l-1)} + W_2 \sum_{j \in N(i)} x_j^{(l-1)}\right) \tag{5}$$

Here, σ represents the non-linear activation function, and $x^{(l-1)}$ denotes the embedding vector of node i at the $(l-1)$-th layer, and $x_i^0 = x_1$. W_1 and W_2 are two learnable parameter matrices. Similarly, the circRNA representations can be derived from the circRNA-similarity graph

3.2 Hypergraph Convolution Network for CircRNA/Drug Similarities

In this section, we utilize hypergraph convolutional techniques to capture the complex patterns of high-order neighborhood structures within the circRNA-drug hypergraph. Subsequently, the embedding results of circRNAs and drugs are used in subsequent calculations.

Construction of the Hypergraph. A hypergraph is a specific kind of graph where, unlike a standard graph that connects only two vertices with an edge, an edge can link multiple vertices. In a hypergraph, an edge can connect more than one node and is therefore called a hyperedge. Similar to standard graph representations, a hypergraph is typically defined as $G = (V, E)$, where V represents the set of vertices, and E represents the set of hyperedges. Let the hypergraph $G = (V, E)$, where $V = \{v_1, v_2, v_3, \ldots, v_n\}$ is the set of nodes, and $E = \{e_1, e_2, e_3, \ldots, e_m\}$ is the set of hyperedges. The adjacency matrix of the hypergraph G, denoted as $H \in \mathbb{R}^{|V| \times |E|}$, is defined as follows:

$$H(v, e) = \begin{cases} 1, v \in e \\ 0, v \notin e \end{cases}. \tag{6}$$

If the hyperedge e_j includes the vertex v_i, then $H(v_i, e_j) = 1$; otherwise, it is 0. There are $n(d)$ drugs, and we construct $n(d)$ hyperedges for the hypergraph by gathering each drug along with its K most similar drugs. Hence, the drug hypergraph contains $n(d)$ hyperedges. We constructed two hypergraphs: Hypergraph H_{d-d} is based on drug similarity, and Hypergraph H_{c-c} is based on RNA similarity.

Construction of Hypergraph Convolution Neural Network. In Sect. 2, we obtained the feature representations of circRNA and drug using graph convolution [18]. To further explore their deeper and more complex relationships, we use hypergraph convolution to update the feature representations of circRNA and drug. The hypergraph convolution is defined as follows:

$$\text{Hconv}(\mathbf{H}, \mathbf{X}|\mathbf{W}) = \sigma\left((\mathbf{D^v})^{-\frac{1}{2}} \mathbf{H} (\mathbf{D^e})^{-1} \mathbf{H^T} (\mathbf{D^v})^{-\frac{1}{2}} \mathbf{X} \mathbf{W}\right) \tag{7}$$

where D_v and D_e represent the diagonal degree matrices for vertices and hyperedges, respectively. Vertex features are denoted by X, while W represents the learnable weight matrix. Additionally, T denotes the transposition operator.

The HGNN used in this work has two hypergraph convolution layers. Taking drug as an example, the hypergraph convolution for each layer can be expressed as follows:

$$X_d^{(l)} = \mathrm{Hconv}\left(\mathbf{H}_{d-d}, \mathbf{X_d}^{(l-1)} \middle| \mathbf{W}^{(l-1)}\right) \tag{8}$$

where $X^{(t-1)}$ is the drug representation vector at the $(l-1)$-th layer. W is the learnable weight matrix.

To effectively learn features of circRNAs and drugs from the hypergraph to identify their associations, we implement loss constraints based on the circRNA-drug scoring matrices derived from it. The following provides a comprehensive description of these loss constraints.

$$l_h = -M_{\mathrm{ij}}\left[A_{cd}\log\sigma\left(X_d\right) + (1 - A_{cd})\log\left(1 - \sigma\left(X_d\right)\right)\right] \tag{9}$$

In this context, A_{cd} represents the known correlation matrix. The matrix M_{ij} is an indicator matrix where $M_{ij} = 1$ if the association between the ith circRNA and the jth drug is present in the training set, and $M_{ij} = 0$ otherwise.

To efficiently obtain the desired node features, we apply contrastive learning to different views of drugs and circRNAs. Different views of the same circRNA or drug are considered positive sample pairs, while views of different circRNAs or drugs are treated as negative sample pairs [20]. During the gradient update process, the model enhances similarity among positive samples while simultaneously increasing dissimilarity among negative samples after learning the discriminative representations of circRNAs and drugs. The contrastive loss for hypergraphs representing pharmacological features is defined as follows:

$$l_i^{(d)} = \sum_{i=1}^{N}\sum_{l=1}^{M} - \log \frac{\exp\left(sim(\mathbf{X}_{n,m}^{(d)}, \mathbf{x}_{n,m}^{(d)})/\tau\right)}{\sum_{i'=1}^{N}\exp\left(sim(\mathbf{X}_{n,m}^{(d)}, \mathbf{x}_{n',m}^{(d)})/\tau\right)} \tag{10}$$

where $sim(\cdot)$ represents the cosine similarity function, and τ is the tunable temperature hyperparameter used to adjust the scale of the softmax function.

3.3   Residual Connection

After convolution by the hypergraph, we obtained feature representations for drugs and circRNAs, respectively. To alleviate over-smoothing during layer aggregation and emphasize the importance of central nodes, we introduce residual connections in the neighbor aggregation process [24]. The information propagation method for the residual connection from layer $(l-1)$ to layer l is defined as follows:

$$\begin{cases} e_{j,l}^{(c)} = x_{j,l}^{(c)} + X_{j,l}^{(c)} + e_{j,l-1}^{(c)} \\ e_{i,l}^{(d)} = x_{i,l}^{(d)} + X_{i,l}^{(d)} + e_{i,l-1}^{(d)} \end{cases} \tag{11}$$

The inner product was utilized to predict the associated preference scores for circRNA c_i and drug d_j as as follows:

$$\Psi^{(c)} = \sum_{l=0}^{L} E_{j,l}^{(c)}, \Psi^{(d)} = \sum_{l=0}^{L} E_{i,l}^{(d)}, CD_h = \Psi_j^{(c)T} \Psi_i^{(d)} \tag{12}$$

3.4 Variational Auto-Encoder–Based Learning of CircRNA and Drug Features

According to previous studies, known information is often crucial in forecasting. Therefore, MHCDA adopts a variational auto-encoder (VAE) to learn the nonlinear key features of circRNA and drugs. Using the established circRNA–drug association matrix A_{cd}, we take circRNA as an example. The initial features of circRNA, derived from the known circRNA–drug associations, are input into a variational autoencoder to obtain the drug's nonlinear key features, as follows:

$$x_d' = f(A_{cd}W_{cd} + b_{cd}) \tag{13}$$

where, W_{cd} denotes the weight and b_{cd} represents the bias, while f denotes a nonlinear activation function that allows our model to effectively approximate complex nonlinear functions [21].

Next, based on the obtained feature x_d', two independent fully connected layers are employed to compute the mean μ_{m_cd} and variance σ_{cd} of the feature, as follows:

$$\mu_d = \tanh(x_d'W_{\mu d} + b_{\mu d}) \tag{14}$$

$$\sigma_d = \tanh(x_d'W_{\sigma d} + b_{\sigma d}). \tag{15}$$

where $W_{\mu d}$, $W_{\sigma d}$, $b_{\mu d}$, and $b_{\sigma d}$ are the learnable weights and biases. Finally, the key features of the drug are calculated using the following equation:

$$d_v = u_d + \sigma_d \odot \varepsilon \tag{16}$$

where, σ represents a random vector σ ($\sigma \sim N(0, 1)$) sampled from the standard normal distribution, and "$\odot$" denotes element-wise multiplication. After obtaining the key feature of the circRNA and drug, the prediction score of circRNA–drug associations based on the VAE is calculated as follows:

$$CD_v = sigmoid\left(x_d'd_v^T\right). \tag{17}$$

The loss constraints for the VAE component are specified as follows:

$$l_v = -M_{ij}\left[A_{cd}log\sigma(CD_v) + (1 - A_{cd})\log(1 - \sigma(CD_v))\right]$$
$$- \left(\text{KL}\left(q\left(d_v|CD_v\right)\|p\left(d_v\right)\right) + \text{KL}\left(q\left(d_v|CD_V\right)\|p\left(d_v\right)\right)\right). \tag{18}$$

The final prediction score CD is obtained by summing CDh and CDv

$$CD = CD_v + CD_h \tag{19}$$

The loss constraints for the final prediction are specified as follows:

$$l_r = -M_{ij} \left[A_{cd} log\sigma\left((CD)\right) + (1 - A_{cd})\log\left(1 - \sigma(CD)\right)\right]. \tag{20}$$

Then, the total losses of the model is as follows:

$$l = l_r + l_h + \beta l_i + \alpha l_v \tag{21}$$

4   Experiments and Results

4.1   Baselines

As mentioned in Ref. [5], the currently available computational methods for predicting circRNA-drug sensitivity associations are limited. To validate the effectiveness of MHCDA, we list and compare several classic methods. A brief description of these models is provided below:

GATECDA [5]: The computational model GATECDA, based on GATE, employs a graph attention autoencoder to extract low-dimensional representations of circRNAs and drugs, aiming to predict circRNA-drug sensitivity associations. GATECDA is believed to be the first research achievement to successfully predict circRNA-drug sensitivity.

MNGACDA [6]: This study presents a computational approach to forecast the associations between circRNA and drug sensitivity. The proposed approach employs a graph autoencoder with node-level attention to derive embedding representations for both circRNAs and drugs from diverse multimodal networks. Subsequently, it employs an inner-product decoder to estimate the association scores linking circRNAs to drug sensitivities.

LAGCN [32]: This methodology integrates known drug-disease associations, disease-disease similarities, and drug-drug similarities into a heterogeneous network, utilizing graph convolution to predict drug-disease associations.

GraphCDA [23]: Concatenated coherent paragraph: The proposed model utilizes Graph Attention Networks (GAT) [30] and Graph Convolutional Networks (GCN) to generate node embedding representations. Following this, a random forest approach is used to link circRNA with diseases.

Table 1. Performance comparison based on 5-CV

Method	AUC	AUPR	F1-score	Accuracy	Recall	Precision
MHCDA	**0.918**	**0.929**	**0.852**	**0.850**	**0.863**	**0.846**
MNGACDA	0.907	0.916	0.841	0845	0.823	0.823
GATECDA	0.890	0.898	0.820	0.815	0.845	0.845
LAGCN	0.887	0.889	0.835	0.833	0.848	0.848
HRAPHCDA	0.827	0.851	0.779	0.785	0.821	0.826

Figure 2(a) shows a comparison of the AUC values averaged over five validations for several models. Among these, MHCDA achieved the highest AUC value
of 0.9188. Figure 2(b) presents a comparison of the AUPR values, with MHCDA
again achieving the highest value. Additionally, other performance metrics, such
as accuracy, precision, recall, and F1 score, are presented in Table 1.

4.2   Parameter Sensitivity Analysis

The following parameters are included in MHCDA:(1) the number of layers n
in the HGNN,(2) the embedding dimension F of the hidden layer, and (3) the
influence of k-nearest neighbors.

The number of HGNN layers greatly impacts the model's predictive performance and generalization ability. Increasing the number of HGNN layers can
aggregate more node information; however, stacking too many layers may cause
overfitting or oversmoothing. On the other hand, too few HGNN layers can result
in underfitting. Therefore, determining the optimal number of HGNN layers is
essential. As illustrated in Fig. 3, he optimal values for AUC and AUPR are
obtained when n is set to 2.

Different embedding dimensions, represented as F, can significantly influence the model's predictive performance, training efficiency, and generalization
ability. To clarify the effect of hidden layer embedding dimension F on model
performance, we tested various dimensions to identify the optimal F. As shown
in Fig. 4, both AUC and AUPR reach their optimal values when F = 128.

In constructing the circRNA and drug homogeneous graphs, we employed
the KNN algorithm; therefore, it is essential to explore the impact of k-nearest

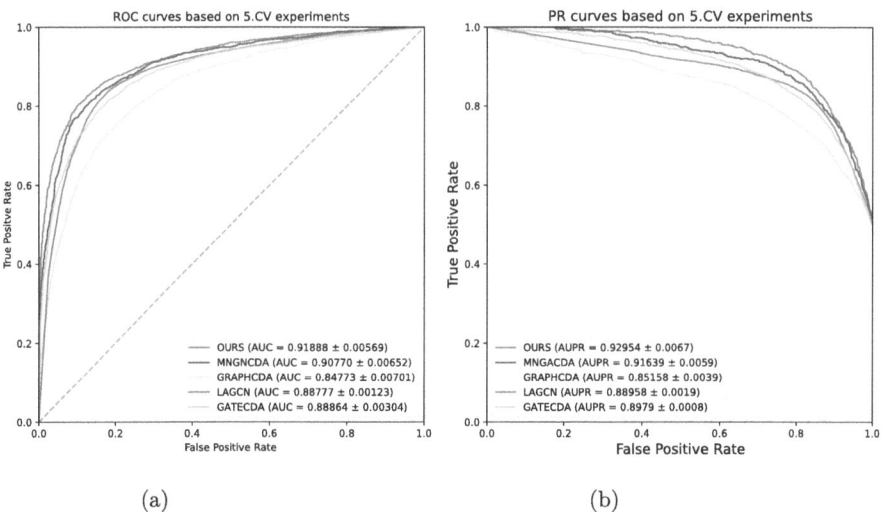

(a)   (b)

Fig. 2. ROC and PR curves based on 5-CV experiment.

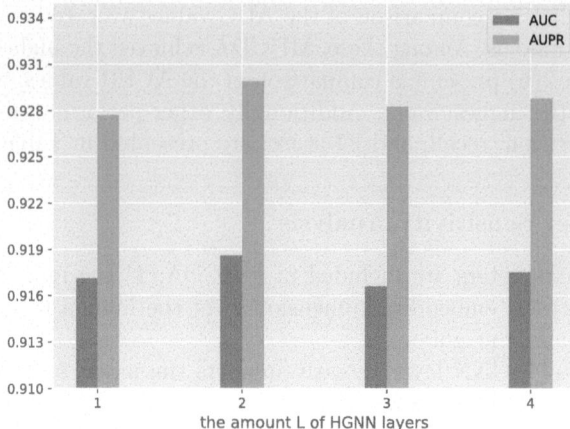

Fig. 3. Parameter sensitivity analysis for the number of layers n.

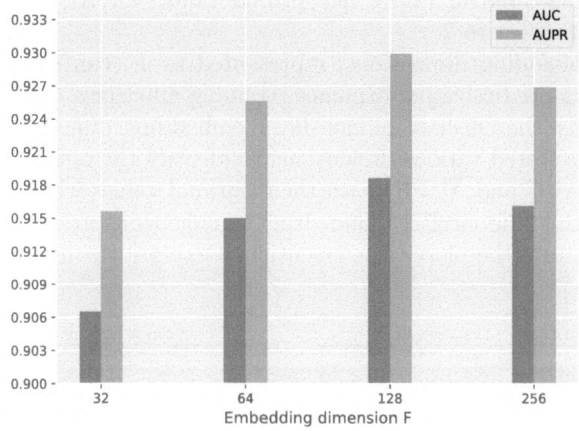

Fig. 4. Parameter sensitivity analysis for the embedding dimension F.

neighbors. As shown in Fig. 5, we selected the optimal k from the set 10, 15, 20, 25, 30. The influence of k-nearest neighbors on the model is not significant.

4.3   Ablation Tests

Our model MHCDA derives features of drugs and circRNAs by processing information from both the similarity network and the association network, leading to the implementation of two distinct embedding computation modules. MHCDA-ass extracts features exclusively from the association network, while MHCDA-sim obtains features solely from the similarity network of circRNA and drug fusion. To evaluate the importance of each module, we established multiple model variants and performed random ablation experiments.

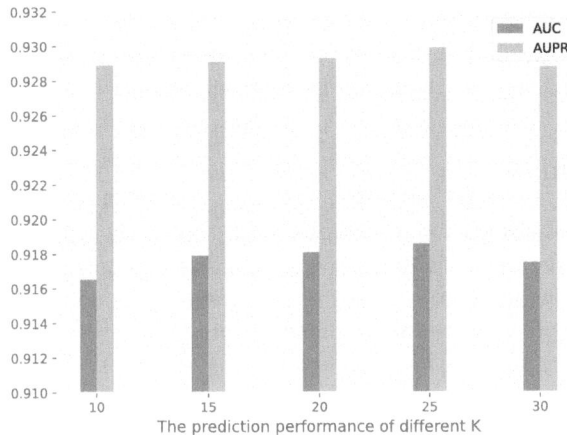

Fig. 5. Parameter sensitivity analysis for the number of heads T.

MHCDA−GraphConv model: The GraphConv [18] operation was removed from the model, while other modules were retained.

MHCDA−Hgnn model: Retain the original model backbone and exclude the HGNN layer from the original framework.

MHCDA−Res model: Retain the core structure of the model while eliminating residual connections from the original framework.

To ensure fairness in the comparison, we performed a consistent experimental setup for all methods. As shown in Table 2, we summarize the following conclusions: the AUC and AUPR values of MHCDA are consistently higher than those of MHCDA-asso and MHCDA-sim, illustrating the effectiveness of integrating diverse modal networks to enhance model performance. As shown in Table 2, compared to MHCDA, the MHCDA-GraphConv model slightly outperforms in accuracy, but its other metrics are significantly worse. This suggests that the GraphConv module is effective in enhancing model performance. The performance of the MHCDA-HGNN model is also worse than that of MHCDA, implying that the HGNN combiner module can effectively capture deeper relationships

Table 2. Ablation tests

Method	AUC	AUPR	F1-score	Accuracy	Recall
MHCDA	**0.918**	**0.929**	**0.852**	0.850	**0.863**
MHCDA-Asso	0.912	0.925	0.846	0.843	0.837
MHCDA-Sim	0.915	0.926	0.847	0.844	0.856
MHCDA-GraphConv	0.917	0.927	0.850	**0.852**	0.840
MHCDA-Hgnn	0.912	0.922	0.846	0.843	0.835
MHCDA-Residual	0.914	0.924	0.846	0.839	0.857

within node features. The performance metrics of the MHCDA-Residual model fall short in all aspects, indicating that the introduction of the residual module improves the efficiency of training a deep neural network.

5 Case Studies

To enhance the credibility of our experimental results, we utilized all established associations in the GDSC [14] dataset for training purposes. Subsequently, we generated a prediction matrix based on our model's outcomes. This approach ensures that our predictions are grounded in comprehensive training data, there by bolstering the reliability and validity of our findings. We then identified predicted new associations by searching another independent database, CTRP [26].

Specifically, we conducted a case study on the drugs PAC-1 [25] and Piperlong–umine [22]. After selecting the top 20 circRNAs with the highest scores among the predicted associations for each drug, we validated them in the CTRP dataset.

PAC-1 is a compound with potential anticancer activity, being investigated as a therapeutic agent for cancer treatment, particularly in promoting tumor cell apoptosis (programmed cell death) [27]. We list the top 20 predicted PAC-1-associated circRNAs in Table 3 and have confirmed the presence of 15 of them in the CTRP dataset.

Table 3. The Top 20 circRNAs associated with the drug PAC-1

Ranking	circRNA	Evidence	Ranking	circRNA	Evidence
1	VIM	CTRP	11	ANP32B	CTRP
2	MEF2D	CTRP	12	SPARC	CTRP
3	POLR2A	CTRP	13	AHNAK	CTRP
4	SPINT2	Nonsignificant	14	TCOF1	CTRP
5	LTBP1	Nonsignificant	15	FKBP10	CTRP
6	COL1A1	CTRP	16	DBN1	Nonsignificant
7	CTTN	CTRP	17	ADPGK	Nonsignificant
8	COL1A2	CTRP	18	ENO2	Nonsignificant
9	ASPH	CTRP	19	CRIM1	CTRP
10	ILF3	CTRP	20	COL6A2	CTRP

Concurrently, Piperlongumine selectively targets various tumor cells, including those from colon, ovarian, and liver cancers, without adversely affecting normal cells or causing significant toxic side effects [28]. In Table 4, we present the top 20 predicted Piperlongumine-related circRNAs, with 17 of these circRNAs identified in the CTRP.

Table 4. Prediction of top 20 circRNAs related to Piperlongumine

Ranking	circRNA	Evidence	Ranking	circRNA	Evidence
1	POLR2A	CTRP	11	CUX1	CTRP
2	ANP32B	CTRP	12	HSP90BA	CTRP
3	COL1A1	CTRP	13	DCBLD2	CTRP
4	VIM	CTRP	14	THBS1	CTRP
5	COL5A1	CTRP	15	MEF2D	CTRP
6	ACTB	Nonsignificant	16	SFPQ	CTRP
7	ENO2	Nonsignificant	17	EHBP1L1	CTRP
8	EFEMP1	CTRP	18	MYH9	CTRP
9	PTMS	CTRP	19	PLOD1	CTRP
10	CPIM1	CTRP	20	COL6A2	CTRP

Table 5. Prediction of the top 10 circRNAs related to the new drugs Crizotinib and MG-132

	Erlotinib			Crizotinib	
Rank	circRNAs	Evidence	Rank	Energy	circRNAs
1	POLR2A	Nonsignificant	1	VIM	CTRP
2	ENO2	CTRP	2	ADPGK	CTRP
3	FBLN1	Nonsignificant	3	SPINT2	CTRP
4	VIM	CTRP	4	COL6A2	CTRP
5	KRT19	CTRP	5	ENO2	Nonsignificant
6	PTMS	Nonsignificant	6	ANP32B	CTRP
7	ADPGK	Nonsignificant	7	FBLN1	CTRP
8	DHRS2	Nonsignificant	8	POLR2A	CTRP
9	ASPH	Nonsignificant	9	MEF2D	CTRP
10	ANKRD36	Nonsignificant	10	BPTF	CTRP

From the dataset, we selected two drugs, Erlotinib and Crizotinib, each associated with only one circRNA, for conducting de novo testing. This step aims to further evaluate the predictive capability of our model regarding circRNAs and their sensitivity to new drugs. We removed the only known associations of these two drugs with circRNAs and treated them as unknown drugs. This approach allowed us to demonstrate the model's potential in identifying new therapeutic candidates in cancer treatment. Erlotinib is a targeted therapeutic agent that works by inhibiting the epidermal growth factor receptor (EGFR) on tumor cells, thereby blocking the proliferation and division of malignant cells [31]. Crizotinib is another targeted therapeutic agent that has been shown to significantly prolong progression-free survival in some patients with advanced NSCLC. This drug belongs to the class of multi-kinase inhibitors, which inhibit specific kinase activities to halt the growth and spread of cancer cells [29]. As shown in Table 5, four of the top ten predicted circRNAs associated with erlotinib have been validated in circRic, while nine of the top ten circRNAs related to crizotinib have been confirmed in circRic as well.

6   Discussions and Conclusions

Recent studies indicate that circular RNAs (circRNAs) have a substantial impact on drug sensitivity. Predicting associations between circRNAs and drug sensitivity can aid in drug discovery, ultimately enhancing disease treatment. In this study, we introduce a novel computational model called MHCDA to predict associations between circRNAs and drugs. Initially, we convert the circRNA similarity matrix and drug similarity matrix into homogeneous graphs. Subsequently, we employ graph convolutional networks to extract meaningful feature embeddings from the circRNA and drug similarity graphs. These embeddings serve as inputs for the subsequent layer, where we utilize hypergraph convolutional networks to extract additional feature embeddings from the constructed hypergraphs of drugs and circRNAs. Next, MHCDA employs a variational autoencoder (VAE) to learn the nonlinear key features of circRNAs and drugs. Finally, we integrate the learned features of circRNAs and drugs to uncover their associations. We tested our model on the human circRNA–disease association dataset, demonstrating that it outperforms state-of-the-art methods in identifying previously undiscovered circRNA–drug associations.

   Although the proposed method demonstrates competitive performance in predicting circRNA–drug associations, it has some limitations. It must be recognized that the number of circRNAs associated with drug sensitivity that we have identified to date is limited, potentially introducing bias into the prediction outcomes. Integrating more experimentally validated circRNA–drug sensitivity associations would enhance the reliability of the predictions. In future research, we intend to incorporate additional sources of biomedical data to develop more comprehensive similarity measures. Additionally, the proposed method relies on pre-existing relationships for drug prediction. For new drugs absent from the dataset, they must be treated as isolated nodes, which leads to unsatisfactory results. Future research should therefore focus on deeply integrating relationship-based and feature-based prediction methods. For example, drug structures can be used to derive features for predicting new drugs, rather than only extracting structural similarities from existing datasets. However, current results remain suboptimal, requiring further refinement. Additionally, we have designed a graph convolutional layer within the model to extract information based on circRNA and drug similarities. The effectiveness of the graph convolutional layer depends on the graph defined by the KNN algorithm. However, as the hyperparameter K increases, it may introduce some noise, potentially interfering with our prediction results. Despite exploring various approaches to address this issue, the results were not statistically significant. We will further investigate this issue in future research. Conversely, when constructing hypergraphs, is it feasible to create heterogeneous hypergraphs with nodes beyond circRNAs or drugs? All these aspects require continuous improvement in future research. Finally, current predictive methods for examining the relationship between circular RNAs and drug sensitivity are limited. Additional efforts are essential to advance research in this area.

References

1. Salzman, J., Gawad, C., Wang, P.L., Lacayo, N., Brown, P.O.: Circular rnas are the predominant transcript isoform from hundreds of human genes in diverse cell types. PLoS ONE **7**(2), e30733 (2012)
2. Wang, C.C., Han, C.D., Zhao, Q., Chen, X.: Circular rnas and complex diseases: from experimental results to computational models. Briefings Bioinform. **22**(6), bbab286 (2021)
3. Tao, W., Liu, Y., Lin, X., Song, B., Zeng, X.: Prediction of multi-relational drug–gene interaction via dynamic hypergraph contrastive learning. Briefings Bioinform. **24**(6), bbad371 (2023)
4. Zhou, J., Cui, G., Hu, S., Zhang, Z., Yang, C., Liu, Z., Wang, L., Li, C., Sun, M.: Graph neural networks: a review of methods and applications. AI open **1**, 57–81 (2020)
5. Deng, L., Liu, Z., Qian, Y., Zhang, J.: Predicting circrna-drug sensitivity associations via graph attention auto-encoder. BMC Bioinform. **23**(1), 160 (2022)
6. Yang, B., Chen, H.: Predicting circrna-drug sensitivity associations by learning multimodal networks using graph auto-encoders and attention mechanism. Briefings Bioinform. **24**(1), bbac596 (2023)
7. Luo, Y., Deng, L.: Dpmgcda: Deciphering circrna–drug sensitivity associations with dual perspective learning and path-masked graph autoencoder. J. Chem. Inform. Modeling (2024)
8. Zhong, Y., Shen, C., Xi, X., Luo, Y., Ding, P., Luo, L.: Multitask joint learning with graph autoencoders for predicting potential mirna-drug associations. Artif. Intell. Med. **145**, 102665 (2023)
9. Feng, Y., You, H., Zhang, Z., Ji, R., Gao, Y.: Hypergraph neural networks. In: Proceedings of the AAAI Conference on Artificial Intelligence, vol. 33, pp. 3558–3565 (2019)
10. Ruan, D., et al.: Exploring complex and heterogeneous correlations on hypergraph for the prediction of drug-target interactions. Patterns **2**(12) (2021)
11. Liu, D., Li, X., Zhang, L., Hu, X., Zhang, J., Liu, Z., Deng, L.: Hgnnlda: predicting lncrna-drug sensitivity associations via a dual channel hypergraph neural network. IEEE/ACM Trans. Comput. Biology Bioinform. (2023)
12. Hu, X., Dong, Y., Zhang, J., Deng, L.: Hgclmda: predicting mrna-drug sensitivity associations via hypergraph contrastive learning. J. Chem. Inf. Model. **63**(18), 5936–5946 (2023)
13. Liang, X., Guo, M., Jiang, L., Fu, Y., Zhang, P., Chen, Y.: Predicting mirna-disease associations by combining graph and hypergraph convolutional network. Interdisciplinary Sciences: Computational Life Sciences, pp. 1–15 (2024)
14. Yang, W., et al.: Genomics of drug sensitivity in cancer (gdsc): a resource for therapeutic biomarker discovery in cancer cells. Nucleic Acids Res. **41**(D1), D955–D961 (2012)

15. Rangwala, S.H., et al.: Accessing ncbi data using the ncbi sequence viewer and genome data viewer (gdv). Genome Res. **31**(1), 159–169 (2021)

16. Landrum, G., et al.: Rdkit: a software suite for cheminformatics, computational chemistry, and predictive modeling. Greg Landrum **8**(31.10), 5281 (2013)

17. Van Laarhoven, T., Nabuurs, S.B., Marchiori, E.: Gaussian interaction profile kernels for predicting drug-target interaction. Bioinformatics **27**(21), 3036–3043 (2011)

18. Morris, C., et al.: Weisfeiler and leman go neural: Higher-order graph neural networks. In: Proceedings of the AAAI conference on artificial intelligence, vol. 33, pp. 4602–4609 (2019)

19. Kingma, D.P.: Auto-encoding variational bayes. arXiv preprint arXiv:1312.6114 (2013)

20. Oord, A.v.d., Li, Y., Vinyals, O.: Representation learning with contrastive predictive coding. arXiv preprint arXiv:1807.03748 (2018)

21. Gardner, M.W., Dorling, S.: Artificial neural networks (the multilayer perceptron)-a review of applications in the atmospheric sciences. Atmos. Environ. **32**(14–15), 2627–2636 (1998)

22. Li, D., Yang, Y., Lai, R., Wu, L.: Status of chemical constituents and pharmacological activities of piper longum l. Chin. J. Clin. Pharmacol. **33**(6), 565–569 (2017)

23. Dai, Q., Liu, Z., Wang, Z., Duan, X., Guo, M.: Graphcda: a hybrid graph representation learning framework based on gcn and gat for predicting disease-associated circrnas. Briefings Bioinform. **23**(5), bbac379 (2022)

24. He, K., Zhang, X., Ren, S., Sun, J.: Deep residual learning for image recognition. In: Proceedings of the IEEE Conference on Computer Vision and Pattern Recognition, pp. 770–778 (2016)

25. Peterson, Q.P., Goode, D.R., West, D.C., Ramsey, K.N., Lee, J.J., Hergenrother, P.J.: Pac-1 activates procaspase-3 in vitro through relief of zinc-mediated inhibition. J. Mol. Biol. **388**(1), 144–158 (2009)

26. Rees, M.G., Seashore-Ludlow, B., Cheah, J.H., Adams, D.J., Price, E.V., Gill, S., Javaid, S., Coletti, M.E., Jones, V.L., Bodycombe, N.E., et al.: Correlating chemical sensitivity and basal gene expression reveals mechanism of action. Nat. Chem. Biol. **12**(2), 109–116 (2016)

27. S Roth, H., J Hergenrother, P.: Derivatives of procaspase-activating compound 1 (pac-1) and their anticancer activities. Current Med. Chemistry **23**(3), 201–241 (2016)

28. Shankar, D.B., et al.: Abt-869, a multitargeted receptor tyrosine kinase inhibitor: inhibition of flt3 phosphorylation and signaling in acute myeloid leukemia. Blood **109**(8), 3400–3408 (2007)

29. Shaw, A.T., Yasothan, U., Kirkpatrick, P.: Crizotinib. Nature reviews Drug discovery **10**(12) (2011)

30. Veličković, P., Cucurull, G., Casanova, A., Romero, A., Lio, P., Bengio, Y.: Graph attention networks. arXiv preprint arXiv:1710.10903 (2017)

31. Yang, Z., Hackshaw, A., Feng, Q., Fu, X., Zhang, Y., Mao, C., Tang, J.: Comparison of gefitinib, erlotinib and afatinib in non-small cell lung cancer: a meta-analysis. Int. J. Cancer **140**(12), 2805–2819 (2017)

32. Yu, Z., Huang, F., Zhao, X., Xiao, W., Zhang, W.: Predicting drug–disease associations through layer attention graph convolutional network. Briefings Bioinform. **22**(4), bbaa243 (2021)

Knowledge Enhancement with LLMs for Few-Shot Medical Relation Extraction

Kunli Zhang, Yunlong Li, Pengcheng Wu, Yuting Li, Chenghao Zhang, and Hongying Zan[✉]

School of Computer Science and Artificial Intelligence, Zhengzhou University, 450001 Henan, China
iehyzan@zzu.edu.cn

Abstract. The purpose of relational extraction is to extract the relational triples in a given text. Recent work shows that Large Language Models(LLMs) achieve excellent performance in information extraction, especially in the few-shot learning. An important challenge in the medical field is the long-tail problem, which has not received much attention in the context of LLMs. Therefore, we propose a novel approach, the **K**nowledge **E**nhancement-**Prompt**ed **R**elationship **E**xtraction (KE-PromptRE), to improve the performance of LLM for long-tail problems of relationship extraction in the medical domain. KE-PromptRE transforms labeled data in the medical domain into generative data accepted by LLM and infuses it into LLM to enhance LLM's performance in the medical domain. In addition, we use Curriculum Learning (CL) to infuse knowledge data into LLM in batches according to difficulty to improve the performance of LLM on the relation extraction. The results showed that our approach performed 9.5% and 2.3% above baseline on the Critical Illness entities and relationships Corpus (CIC) and Chinese Medical Information Extraction (CMeIE) datasets.

Keywords: Medical field · Relational extraction · LLM · Knowledge Enhancement · Curriculum Learning

1 Introduction

Relation Extraction (RE) [1,2], as an important task in the field of Natural Language Processing (NLP), is aimed at extracting entities and relationships between entities from semi-structured and unstructured documents. With the development of data, the medical field information data is developing very rapidly [3]. However, the large amount of semi-structured and unstructured data is not easily analyzed and processed directly [4,5].

Traditional deep learning methods perform poorly in medical long-tail relationship extraction, in recent years, Large Language Models (LLMs) such as GPT3.5 [6], GPT4 [7] have shown extremely excellent capabilities in natural language processing problems such as context recognition and question and answer. However, due to differences between sequence labeling and generative

© The Author(s), under exclusive license to Springer Nature Singapore Pte Ltd. 2025
Y. Zhang et al. (Eds.): CHIP 2024, CCIS 2433, pp. 147–160, 2025.
https://doi.org/10.1007/978-981-96-3752-2_10

tasks, LLMs face specific challenges in handling relation extraction tasks. Data annotation in the medical field requires certain expertise and involves patient privacy and ethical issues, which makes the data in the medical field characterized by long-tailed distribution, high cost, and not easy to share. Based on the data characteristics of the medical field, it is more suitable for Few-Shot Relation Extraction (FSRE). FSRE [8] can train a model with excellent generalization ability with limited training data.

Existing LLMs [9] are used for general purpose scenarios and do not perform well in the medical field. As shown in Fig. 1, the LLM cannot recognize the relationship between breast cancer and ER due to the lack of relevant medical knowledge. To address this issue, we propose a novel knowledge enhancement approach, Knowledge Enhancement - Prompt Relation Extraction (KE-PromptRE). This method converts relevant medical domain knowledge into generative data compatible with LLMs and uses the converted data to fine-tune the LLM, enabling it to better master medical knowledge.

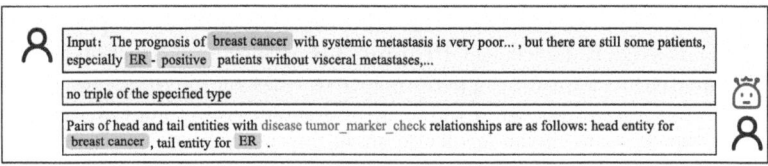

Fig. 1. Sample on the failure of LLMs to recognize relations

In this paper, we investigate the performance of LLMs in the medical domain and fully incorporate the generalization capabilities of the LLM and the knowledge base. Relation extraction is defined as a structured text generation task, and the model's performance about triple extraction in new types of samples is improved by a few-shot samples. To enhance the LLM's performance in medical domain, we employ Curriculum Learning (CL) [10], which enables more effective learning by ordering training data by difficulty. We categorize natural language processing tasks into simple and complex groups based on the output text complexity, then introduce these tasks to the LLM in stages to further improve its performance.

The main contributions of this work are summarized as follows:

- We propose KE-PromptRE, which converts existing annotated medical data into generative data compatible with large language models (LLMs). This method infuses medical knowledge into the LLM, enhancing its performance in medical domain.
- We categorize medical data by output complexity using a Curriculum Learning (CL) approach. We infuse data to the LLM in stages, improving its performance on relational extraction.
- Compared to GPT-3.5 and GPT-4, the method proposed in this paper is more cost-effective and performs better in medical domain. We validate our

approach on datasets Critical Illness entities and relationships Corpus (CIC) [11] and Chinese Medical Information Extraction(CMeIE) [12], achieving performance that surpasses GPT-3.5 and GPT-4. Ablation experiments further demonstrate a 10.

2   Related Work

Deep learning-based relational extraction has achieved notable success [13]. However, significant challenges remain in complex real-world applications. Traditional deep learning methods struggle with few-shot learning, limiting their effectiveness in addressing issues like data scarcity and long-tail distributions [14]. Recently, large language models (LLMs) have demonstrated strong performance in relation extraction tasks [15,16], and have also shown considerable capability in few-shot and zero-shot scenarios [17,18].

Relationship extraction methods are typically divided into two categories based on their approach [19]: pipeline-based methods [20,21] and joint extraction methods [22]. Pipeline-based methods perform relationship extraction in stages, first identifying entities (e_1, e_2, ..., e_n) and then classifying relationships for each entity pair (e_i, e_j) with potential connections. These models generally consist of feature extractors and relationship classifiers. While pipeline-based approaches are straightforward to implement [23], they suffer from issues such as error accumulation, entity redundancy, and a lack of integration between the two tasks, leading to increased errors.

Medical domain labeled data suffers from uneven distribution and high costs, which has led Labrak et al. [24] to explore the use of large language models (LLMs) for automatic annotation. However, since LLMs perform poorly in specific domains and suffer from hallucination issues [25], some scholars [26,27] have employed knowledge enhancement methods to generate more effective prototype representations by integrating external knowledge with text features. External knowledge can be classified into unstructured text and structured knowledge graphs based on its format [28]. Integrating such knowledge into LLMs has been shown to enhance their effectiveness [29,30]. Therefore, we propose KE-PromptRE, which enhances the performance of LLMs in the medical domain by injecting external knowledge into the model.

3   Methodology

The general architecture of our approach is shown in Fig. 2. First, the collected annotated medical domain data is transformed into generative data that can be accepted by the LLM through **knowledge acquisition**. Next, the medical domain knowledge is injected into the LLM via LoRA fine-tuning through **knowledge injection**. Finally, the relationships within the text to be annotated are extracted through **knowledge inference**. In the following sections, we will introduce each of these three modules in detail.

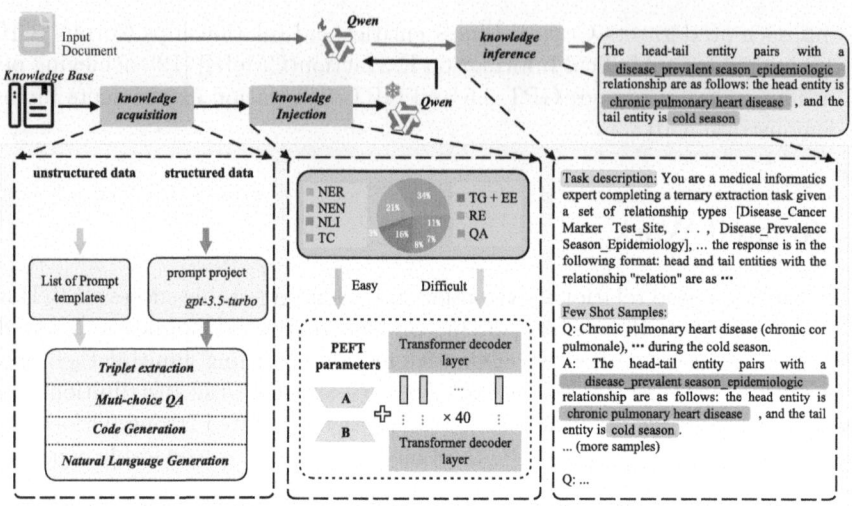

Fig. 2. The structural diagram of the model illustrates three phases. The first phase involves transforming unstructured and structured medical domain data into a format accepted by the LLM. The second phase injects the acquired knowledge into the model through CL. The final phase extracts the relationships within the sentences through reasoning

3.1   Knowledge Acquisition

The main sources of medical knowledge include structured datasets and unstructured datasets. These sources are transformed into generative data consisting of prompted learning templates and answers. This format is easily accepted by LLMs. Therefore, we constructed specific template sets for datasets with different tasks, with larger datasets corresponding to a larger number of templates. Since task diversity, instruction diversity, and data quality are factors that affect the model generalization ability and knowledge learning effect, we construct datasets that follow the principle of multiple instructions and multiple templates. For unstructured and structured data, we construct instruction sets in two ways: labeled data translation and knowledge distillation.

(1) Unstructured Data

Labeled datasets consist of annotated textual information. To enhance the diversity and richness of the training data for the LLM, different cue templates are used to transform them into various natural language processing tasks. These tasks include multiple-choice, ternary extraction, and natural language generation, among others.

The process of data translation is presented as an example of a relational triple extraction task. The original input x is modified into a textual prompt $x^{'}$ with slots by the prompt function $f_{prompt}(.)$, which is then fed into the language model, which probabilistically fills the information to be filled in the templates to generate the result $\hat{y}$ containing the expected triples as follows.

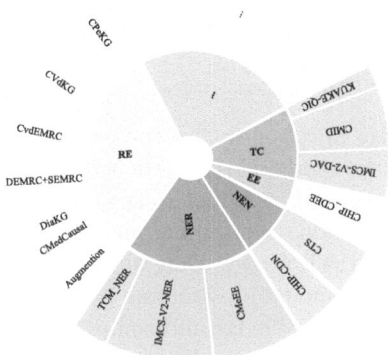

Fig. 3. Model injection statistics, the width of the semicircle indicates the amount of data

A template t is randomly selected from the set T of templates for this task, and t contains three slots, where $[X_1]$ and $[X_2]$ are from the original input x and $[Z]$ is from the original output y, as shown in Eq. 1.

$$text = t + [X_2] + triple : [X_1] + Answer : [Z] \tag{1}$$

For the sample Eq. 1, the result after input and template splicing x': "In the following passage, identify the [complication, synonym, pathologic typing, differential diagnosis, related (symptom)] triplet: respiratory diseases can have extra-pulmonary manifestations, and bronchopulmonary carcinoma can cause pestle and mortar fingers. Answer:"

(2) Structured Data

For the knowledge base, the pediatric triplet from CMeKG [31] was selected as a seed and GPT-3.5 was used to generate the corresponding triplet interpretation. To generate high-quality data, restrictions must be included in the prompt template, as well as the use of the more common relation types. For example, given a triplet <bronchopulmonary cancer, complications, pestle finger>, a sentence is generated based on this triplet to describe the synonym relationship between bronchopulmonary cancer and Pestle finger. Where bronchopulmonary cancer and the Pestle finger are the head entity and tail entity respectively, the sentence must contain the head and tail entities, and the relationship "complications" can be included only in the semantics, not necessarily in the sentence.

Due to the existence of many forms of medically labeled data, we collected several common NLP task datasets to aid in model training from Prompt-CBLUE [31] and Huatuo-26M [32] and expanded on the PromptCBLUE instruction template collection. Among them, the PromptCBLUE dataset contains tasks such as classification, structured information extraction, and natural language reasoning. The collected data is presented in Fig. 3, and these collected structured and unstructured data are transformed into generative tasks according to a variety of prompt templates.

3.2   Knowledge Injection

The process of knowledge injection is also the process of supervised fine-tuning to make the output of the model close to the expected knowledge by calculating the evaluation metrics of the model rouge-1, rouge-2, rouge-l, and bleu-4. Specifically, a parameter module containing medical knowledge is trained based on the WINGPT2-14B-CHAT model using the LoRA parameter efficient fine-tuning technique. Since the model pre-training parameters are associated with a large amount of generalized knowledge and comprehension. Therefore, we retain the pre-training parameters of the model and improve the performance of the model in extracting relational triplets by LoRA fine-tuning. As shown in Eq. 2. LoRA fine-tuning freezes most of the parameters and trains only a fraction of them.

$$h = W_0 x + \Delta W x = W_0 x + B A x \tag{2}$$

The W_0 is frozen, does not receive gradient updates, and only fine-tunes the A and B matrices, which ultimately reduces the number of parameters in the model fine-tuning and achieves the same effect as the full-parameter fine-tuning.

The loss imbalance caused by presenting all data to the model at once can hinder the convergence of more complex NLP tasks. To address this, we adopt a staged supervised instruction fine-tuning strategy based on CL, allowing the LLM to learn medical knowledge from simple to complex tasks, thereby achieving better performance in the medical domain. As shown in Table 1, we categorize tasks into easy and difficult categories based on the complexity of their outputs. Table 1 lists the difficulty classification for each task.

Table 1. Curriculum Learning Difficulty Classification

Task	Numbers of Task	difficulty
Named Entity Recognition (NER)	80,911	easy
Natural Language Inference (NLI)	54,188	easy
Named Entity Normalization (NEN)	15,000	easy
Text Categorization (TC)	12,254	easy
Relationship Extraction (RE)	153,045	difficult
Event Extraction (EE)	1,971	difficult
Text Generation (TG)	3,705	difficult
Question and Answer (QA)	79,800	difficult

3.3   Knowledge Inference

This phase defines relational extraction as a conditional text generation task. Given a sequence of contexts $X = [c_1, c_2, ...c_n]$ containing n characters, and a structured sequence $Y = [y_1, y_2, ..., y_m]$ containing a collection of triplets T, join the prompts P. The goal is to maximize the conditional probability of the following autoregressive formula as shown in Eq. 3.

$$\theta(Y|X, P) = \prod_{i=1}^{m} p_\theta(y_i|X, P, y < i) \tag{3}$$

where θ is a parameter that contains the language knowledge and the original LLM, which is frozen in the prompt learning phase. To maximize the probability $p_\theta(Y|X, P)$, the prompt template is divided into two parts: the task description and the few-shot prompt. As shown in Fig. 4, the task description restricts the output and helps guide the model to output formatted target text, and multiple labeled samples are added to the current input text to acquire knowledge from the language model without adjusting the model parameters.

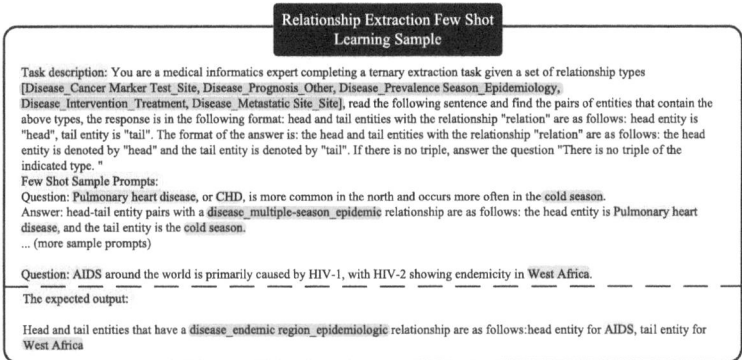

Fig. 4. Sample model inference, which includes a task description, a description of the few-shot sample prompts, and the expected outputs

4   Experiments

In this section, we discuss the experimental data for the validation part, experimental settings, comparison experiment, and ablation experiments.

4.1   Dataset

In this paper, two datasets are used to evaluate few-shot relationship extraction. (1) CIC [11], a dataset focused on relationship extraction of entities related to critical illnesses, including lung, liver, and breast cancers, with data sourced from medical books, specialized medical websites, and disease knowledge bases. (2) CMeIE [12], released as part of the CHIP 2020 evaluation task, contains a corpus derived from clinical pediatrics and obstetrics. To address the long-tail problem, we select five relationship types from both datasets for comparison in the relationship extraction results.

4.2 Experimental Settings

In the experiment, our parameters are set as follows: lora_alpha is set to 16, Learning_rate is set to $5e-5$, batch_size is set to 2, and f16 is used for acceleration. Since the WINGPT-14B-CHAT model is trained on Chinese medical data, the original parameter number is 14B, and the corresponding instruction set is about 400,000, the lora_rank is selected as 8. The fine-tuning phase adopts the stage 3 optimization strategy of a mixture of precision training, gradient checkpoints, and deepspeed to reduce graphic memory consumption.

4.3 Comparison Experiment

In the experimental phase, we conducted comparative experiments on selecting hyperparameters to select the most suitable hyperparameters for the relation extraction task. Comparisons with other LLMs on zero-shot and few-shot tasks demonstrate the effectiveness of our approach.

In the few-shot testing stage, the hyperparameters affecting the inference performance are Temperature, Top_p, Top_k, and Repetition_penalty, which are used to control the degree of randomness of the generated characters. In this paper, we analyze the test effects under different settings for a zero-shot scenario with CIC data, as shown in Table 2. When the degree of randomness is increased (one or more of Temperature, Top_p, and Top_k are increased), the performance of the model decreases to varying degrees, with the greatest impact being on top_p. The F1 value of the model also decreases when the repetition penalty factor, repetition_penalty, is increased. This suggests that the relational extraction task is more suited to the rigorous specification of parameter settings and allows for the generation of duplicate text.

The data for the experiments are CMF-RED relational triple extractions, which are used for testing separately according to the relation types. To avoid knowledge leaking, there is no intersection between the relation types used for testing and the training data relation types. Since the output of the LLM is natural language text, the output is further mapped to the triples and evaluated in terms of F1 values. Table 3 shows the experimental results of the KE-PromptRE method and other models on the CMF-RED dataset, testing CIC and CMeIE data with zero and few-shot. The results show that KE-PromptRE outperforms existing LLMs on the medical few-shot relationship extraction task with the highest F1 value. The method improves on WINGPT-14B-CHAT, suggesting that domain knowledge and LLM can be combined in the fine-tuning phase to improve its performance for a specific task (relation extraction). In addition,

Table 2. Impact of hyperparameters on relational extraction tasks

Temperature	Top_p	Top_k	Repetition_penalty	F1
0.5	0.5	5	1.0	**0.528**
0.5	0.8	5	1.0	0.468(0.06↓)
0.5	0.5	5	1.1	0.493(0.035↓)
0.5	0.5	50	1.0	0.510(0.018↓)
0.95	0.8	5	1.0	0.440(0.088↓)
0.95	0.8	50	1.0	0.399(0.129↓)
0.95	0.8	50	1.1	0.377(0.151↓)
0.95	0.5	5	1.0	0.510(0.018↓)

5w1s has higher accuracy and lower recall than 5w0s, probably because the model has a maximum output length of 4096 and can only output a limited number of results.

Table 3. Experimental results of the KE-PromptRE method on the CMF-RED dataset

Dataset	Model	Precision(0 s/1 s)	Recall(0 s/1 s)	F1(0 s/1 s)
CIC	Baichuan2-13B-CHAT [33]	-/0.135	-/0.115	-/0.124
	WINGPT-7B-CHAT	0.123/0.118	0.071/0.082	0.09/0.097
	WINGPT-14B-CHAT	0.345/0.335	0.193/0.318	0.247/0.326
	GPT-3.5 [6]	0.159/0.290	0.113/0.253	0.132/0.270
	GPT-4 [7]	0.338/0.426	0.253/0.406	0.289/0.415
	KE-PromptRE	**0.505/0.545**	**0.553/0.479**	**0.528/0.510**
CMeIE	Baichuan2-13B-CHAT [33]	-/0.152	-/0.204	-/0.174
	WINGPT-7B-CHAT	0.055/0.034	0.076/0.137	0.064/0.055
	WINGPT-14B-CHAT	0.269/0.349	0.168/0.288	0.207/0.315
	GPT-3.5 [6]	0.164/0.286	0.124/0.235	0.141/0.258
	GPT-4 [7]	0.313/0.372	0.262/0.393	0.285/0.382
	KE-PromptRE	**0.396/0.411**	**0.458/0.399**	**0.424/0.405**

In addition to the selected 5 types of long-tail relationships, we also experimentally validate the other relationships. The results are shown in Fig 5, if the actual number of that relation in the text is less, its F1 value is lower. This is due to the phenomenon that LLM produces a misjudgement every time the relationship is interrogated.

Validation of our dataset using others' methods. Among them, RelationPrompt [34] introduces the Zero-Shot Relation Triplet Extraction (ZeroRTE) task setup and designs a structured prompt template for generating synthetic relation

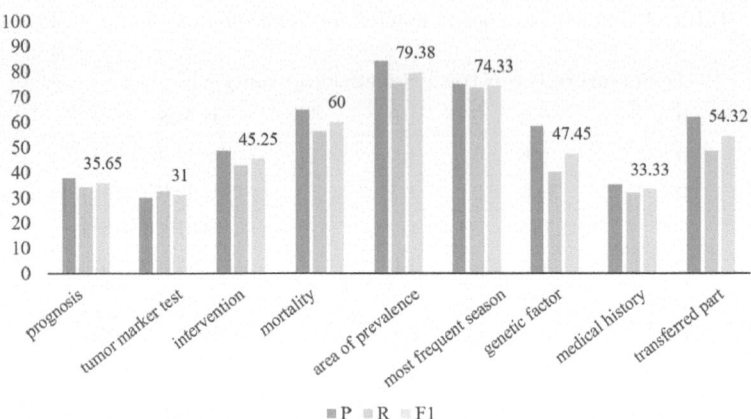

Fig. 5. KE-PromptRE method for extracting each type of F1 value on a task in a relational triple extraction

samples. ZETT [35] uses the T5 model to first match relationship types to sentences with each other, and then extract the entities in the sentences (Table 4).

4.4   Ablation Experiments

To determine the effect of knowledge injection and CL on the final experimental results, we conduct ablation experiments on the CIC dataset for both domain knowledge injection as well as CL components used in this paper. CL impact: in Table 5, -CL indicates that the recognition effect is reduced by 2.1% by direct knowledge injection without dividing it according to difficulty. Domain knowledge injection impact: In Table 5, -Knowledge Injection indicates that the model is not enhanced with knowledge and lacks domain knowledge, and its recognition results are reduced by 7.6%. The ablation experiments show that both CL, as well as domain knowledge injection, affect the final results of the model. These findings demonstrate that the domain knowledge injection method as well as the CL method in this paper can significantly enhance the accuracy of model recognition.

Table 4. Comparison experiment of the KE-PromptRE method on the CMF-RED dataset

	CIC			CMeIE		
Model	Precision	Recall	F1	Precision	Recall	F1
RelationPrompt [34]	0.386	0.327	0.354	0.357	0.298	0.325
ZETT [35]	0.411	0.384	0.397	0.365	0.342	0.353
KE-PromptRE	**0.505**	**0.553**	**0.528**	**0.396**	**0.458**	**0.424**

Table 5. Ablation Experiments of the KE-PromptRE method on the CIC

Method	Precision	Recall	F1
KE-PromptRE	0.545	0.479	0.510
-CL	0.516	0.465	0.489
-Knowledge Injection	0.430	0.382	0.405

5   Conclusion

In this work, we perform relational extraction on medical domain texts and propose the KE-Prompt approach to address the hallucination problem caused by the lack of medical domain knowledge in LLMs. The results on a few-shot test dataset with new relation types demonstrate that our method effectively combines the generalization ability of LLMs with medical knowledge, leading to improved performance in few-shot relation triple extraction. Experimental results on the Few-RED dataset show a performance improvement of 0.28 in the F1 score for the relational triple extraction task with the base model. Additionally, ablation experiments identify optimal hyperparameter settings for this task, suggesting that combining a knowledge base with an LLM is a feasible approach for few-shot relational triple extraction.

Although the domain knowledge enhancement method improves model performance, it has certain limitations. Future work will focus on exploring how the model learns new knowledge, such as the efficient fine-tuning of DoRA parameters, to prevent the model from forgetting previously learned knowledge during the learning process. We hope this work will advance relational extraction in the medical field and contribute to the development of related areas.

Acknowledgements. We appreciate the constructive feedback from the anonymous reviewers and the support provided for this research by the following projects: Science and Technology Tackling Project of Henan Provincial Science and Technology Department (202102AA100021), and the Science and Technology Innovation 2030-"New Generation of Artificial Intelligence" Major Project under Grant No. 2021ZD0111000.

References

1. Zelenko, D., Aone, C., Richardella, A.: Kernel methods for relation extraction. J. Mach. Learn. Res. **3**, 1083–1106 (2003)
2. Bunescu, R., Mooney, R.: A shortest path dependency kernel for relation extraction. In: Proceedings of Human Language Technology Conference and Conference on Empirical Methods in Natural Language Processing, pp. 724–731 (2005)
3. Hong, L., Lin, J., Li, S., Wan, F., Yang, H., Jiang, T., Zhao, D., Zeng, J.: A novel machine learning framework for automated biomedical relation extraction from large-scale literature repositories. Nature Mach. Intell. **2**(6), 347–355 (2020)

4. Luo, L., Yang, Z., Cao, M., Wang, L., Zhang, Y., Lin, H.: A neural network-based joint learning approach for biomedical entity and relation extraction from biomedical literature. J. Biomed. Inform. **103**, 103384–103384 (2020)
5. Lu, Y., Liu, Q., Dai, D., Xiao, X., Lin, H., Han, X., Sun, L., Wu, H.: Unified structure generation for universal information extraction, arXiv e-prints (2022) arXiv–2203
6. Achiam, J., et al.: Gpt-4 technical report, arXiv preprint arXiv:2303.08774 (2023)
7. Ouyang, L., Wu, J., Jiang, X., Almeida, D., Wainwright, C., Mishkin, P., Zhang, C., Agarwal, S., Slama, K., Ray, A., et al.: Training language models to follow instructions with human feedback. Adv. Neural. Inf. Process. Syst. **35**, 27730–27744 (2022)
8. Han, X., et al.: Fewrel: a large-scale supervised few-shot relation classification dataset with state-of-the-art evaluation. In: Proceedings of the 2018 Conference on Empirical Methods in Natural Language Processing, pp. 4803–4809 (2018)
9. Thirunavukarasu, A.J., Ting, D.S.J., Elangovan, K., Gutierrez, L., Tan, T.F., Ting, D.S.W.: Large language models in medicine. Nat. Med. **29**(8), 1930–1940 (2023)
10. Yuan, S., Yang, D., Liang, J., Li, Z., Liu, J., Huang, J., Xiao, Y.: Generative entity typing with curriculum learning. In: Proceedings of the 2022 Conference on Empirical Methods in Natural Language Processing, pp. 3061–3073 (2022)
11. Zhang, K., Zhang, C., Zhang, W., Zan, H.: Corpus construction of critical illness entities and relationships. In: Workshop on Chinese Lexical Semantics, pp. 61–75. Springer (2023)
12. Guan, T., Zan, H., Zhou, X., Xu, H., Zhang, K.: Cmeie: construction and evaluation of chinese medical information extraction dataset, in: Natural Language Processing and Chinese Computing: 9th CCF International Conference, NLPCC 2020, Zhengzhou, China, October 14–18, 2020, Proceedings, Part I 9, pp. 270–282. Springer (2020)
13. Tang, W., Xu, B., Zhao, Y., Mao, Z., Liu, Y., Liao, Y., Xie, H.: Unirel: unified representation and interaction for joint relational triple extraction. In: Proceedings of the 2022 Conference on Empirical Methods in Natural Language Processing, pp. 7087–7099 (2022)
14. Wang, Q., Zhou, K., Qiao, Q., Li, Y., Li, Q.: Improving unsupervised relation extraction by augmenting diverse sentence pairs. In: Proceedings of the 2023 Conference on Empirical Methods in Natural Language Processing, pp. 12136–12147 (2023)
15. Duan, J., Liao, X., An, Y., Wang, J.: Keyee: enhancing low-resource generative event extraction with auxiliary keyword sub-prompt. Big Data Mining Anal. **7**(2), 547–560 (2024)
16. Li, G., Xu, Z., Shang, Z., Liu, J., Ji, K., Guo, Y.: Empirical analysis of dialogue relation extraction with large language models, arXiv preprint arXiv:2404.17802 (2024)
17. Li, G., Wang, P., Liu, J., Guo, Y., Ji, K., Shang, Z., Xu, Z.: Meta in-context learning makes large language models better zero and few-shot relation extractors, arXiv preprint arXiv:2404.17807 (2024)
18. Liu, Y., Peng, X., Du, T., Yin, J., Liu, W., Zhang, X.: Era-cot: improving chain-of-thought through entity relationship analysis, arXiv preprint arXiv:2403.06932 (2024)
19. Nguyen, T.H., Grishman, R.: Relation extraction: Perspective from convolutional neural networks. In: Proceedings of the 1st Workshop on Vector Space Modeling for Natural Language Processing, pp. 39–48 (2015)

20. Zeng, D., Liu, K., Lai, S., Zhou, G., Zhao, J.: Relation classification via convolutional deep neural network. In: Proceedings of COLING 2014, the 25th International Conference on Computational Linguistics: Technical Papers, pp. 2335–2344 (2014)

21. Socher, R., Huval, B., Manning, C.D., Ng, A.Y.: Semantic compositionality through recursive matrix-vector spaces. In: Proceedings of the 2012 Joint Conference on Empirical Methods in Natural Language Processing and Computational Natural Language Learning, pp. 1201–1211 (2012)

22. Miwa, M., Sasaki, Y.: Modeling joint entity and relation extraction with table representation. In: Proceedings of the 2014 Conference on Empirical Methods in Natural Language Processing (EMNLP), pp. 1858–1869 (2014)

23. Z. Zhong, D. Chen, A frustratingly easy approach for entity and relation extraction, in: Proceedings of the 2021 Conference of the North American Chapter of the Association for Computational Linguistics: Human Language Technologies, 2021, pp. 50–61

24. Labrak, Y., Rouvier, M., Dufour, R.: A zero-shot and few-shot study of instruction-finetuned large language models applied to clinical and biomedical tasks. In: Proceedings of the 2024 Joint International Conference on Computational Linguistics, Language Resources and Evaluation (LREC-COLING 2024), pp. 2049–2066 (2024)

25. Li, G., Ke, W., Wang, P., Xu, Z., Ji, K., Liu, J., Shang, Z., Luo, Q.: Unlocking instructive in-context learning with tabular prompting for relational triple extraction, in: Proceedings of the 2024 Joint International Conference on Computational Linguistics, Language Resources and Evaluation (LREC-COLING 2024), pp. 17131–17143 (2024)

26. Zhang, K., Gutiérrez, B.J., Su, Y.: Aligning instruction tasks unlocks large language models as zero-shot relation extractors. In: Findings of the Association for Computational Linguistics: ACL 2023, pp. 794–812 (2023)

27. Mo, Y., et al.: C-icl: contrastive in-context learning for information extraction, arXiv preprint arXiv:2402.11254 (2024)

28. Wadhwa, S., Amir, S., Wallace, B.C.: Revisiting relation extraction in the era of large language models. In: Proceedings of the Conference. Association for Computational Linguistics. Meeting, Vol. 2023, pp. 15566–15589 (2023)

29. Roy, A., Pan, S.: Incorporating medical knowledge in bert for clinical relation extraction. In: Proceedings of the 2021 Conference on Empirical Methods in Natural Language Processing, pp. 5357–5366 (2021)

30. Tang, X., Su, Q., Wang, J., Deng, Z.: Chisiec: an information extraction corpus for ancient Chinese history. In: Proceedings of the 2024 Joint International Conference on Computational Linguistics, Language Resources and Evaluation (LREC-COLING 2024), pp. 3192–3202 (2024)

31. Zhu, W., Wang, X., Zheng, H., Chen, M., Tang, B.: Promptcblue: a Chinese prompt tuning benchmark for the medical domain, arXiv preprint arXiv:2310.14151 (2023)

32. Li, J., et al.: Huatuo-26m, a large-scale chinese medical qa dataset, arXiv preprint arXiv:2305.01526 (2023)

33. Yang, A., et al.: Baichuan 2: Open large-scale language models, arXiv preprint arXiv:2309.10305 (2023)

34. Chia, Y.K., Bing, L., Poria, S., Si, L.: Relationprompt: leveraging prompts to generate synthetic data for zero-shot relation triplet extraction. In: Findings of the Association for Computational Linguistics: ACL 2022, pp. 45–57 (2022)

35. Kim, B., Iso, H., Bhutani, N., Hruschka, E., Nakashole, N., Mitchell, T.: Zero-shot triplet extraction by template infilling, in: Proceedings of the 13th International Joint Conference on Natural Language Processing and the 3rd Conference of the Asia-Pacific Chapter of the Association for Computational Linguistics (Volume 1: Long Papers), pp. 272–284 (2023)

A Review of Drug-Target Interaction Prediction Methods

Jieyi Yu[1], Yin Wang[1,2], and Jungang Lou[1(✉)]

[1] College of Information Engineering, Huzhou University, Huzhou 313000, Zhejiang, China
ljg@zjhu.edu.cn
[2] Zhejiang SightedIn MediTec. Ltd., Huzhou 313000, Zhejiang, China

Abstract. Drug-target interaction prediction can help researchers understand the mechanism of action of drugs and discover new drug targets, and even assist researchers in designing more effective drug therapeutic regimens, which will be of great significance to drug development. In recent years, computer-aided technology has been better applied in various fields, and the paper will discuss drug-target interaction prediction methods: molecular docking, ligand-based, text mining, and feature-based methods in the context of computer-aided technology. The paper mainly discusses and elaborates on the feature-based techniques and analyzes each type of method's principles, advantages, and disadvantages. At the same time, the paper also discusses the problems and challenges faced by drug-target interaction prediction, including its dataset, cold-start, and model design problems. Finally, deep learning technology will still play a great potential for application in this field and briefly point out the direction and trend of future research.

Keyword: Drug-target interaction prediction · Features extraction · Deep learning · Artificial intelligence

1 Introduction

Drug development and discovery have always been a core task in pharmaceuticals, while the interaction between drugs and biomolecules is one of the most important factors determining the efficacy and safety of drugs. The drug discovery process is generally divided into two phases: early discovery and development [1]. In the early discovery stage, scientists need to identify the target of drug action, search for potentially active compounds, and screen drug candidates [2]. In the early discovery phase, scientists need to identify the target, search for potentially active compounds, and screen drug candidates. Once the drug candidates are identified, the R&D process will enter the development phase, including preclinical studies and clinical trials, in which the drug-target interaction studies play an irreplaceable and critical role in this process. The main objective of predicting drug-target interaction (DTI) is to discover potential drugs that can interact with specific proteins, which will be crucial for drug repositioning, side effect prediction, multi-pharmacology, and drug resistance studies (Fig. 1).

© The Author(s), under exclusive license to Springer Nature Singapore Pte Ltd. 2025
Y. Zhang et al. (Eds.): CHIP 2024, CCIS 2433, pp. 161–195, 2025.
https://doi.org/10.1007/978-981-96-3752-2_11

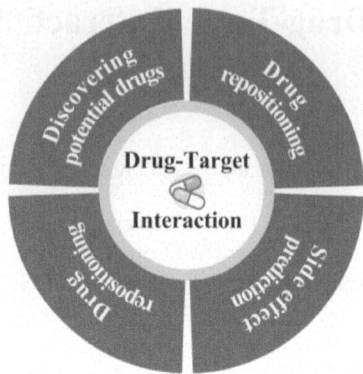

Fig. 1. Predicting the role of drug-target interactions

For a drug to be effective, it needs to bind to a biomolecule with a specific function in the organism, and this biomolecule is the target of the drug. The majority of targets that interact with drugs are proteins, with a small number of nucleic acids and sugars. At the same time, the strength and stability of the interaction depend on the structural and functional relationship between the drug molecule and the target. After the drug interacts with the target, it will lead to structural or functional changes in the target, which will have a therapeutic effect on the treatment or alleviation of the disease [3] to achieve the treatment or alleviation of the disease [6]. The drug will have a therapeutic effect on the target by interacting with it.

The most direct way for researchers to understand the pairwise interaction between the drug to be tested and the target pair is to validate it through biological experiments, which, as one of the most traditional methods, involves not only in vitro but also in vivo experiments, such as cell cultures, animal experiments, and clinical trials [7]. During traditional biological experiments, researchers can directly measure the biological activity or potency of the drug-target pair to be tested, and use the results as an indicator of whether the drug-target pair has an interaction. However, because of the shortcomings of this traditional validation method, such as low precision, high cost, and a lot of time [8]. However, because of the shortcomings of this traditional validation method, such as low accuracy, high cost, and long lead time, this traditional bioassay method has encountered great challenges in the process of new drug discovery and development.

2   Drug-Target Interaction Prediction in Computers

In recent years, the processing power and algorithms of computers have been continuously upgraded, and computer-aided technology has been better applied in various fields. As early as in the 1980s, a new technology closely related to basic pharmacy theories has been developed, i.e., computer-aided drug design (CADD). CADD is a cross-discipline combining computer technology and drug research. Through molecular simulation, chemical computation, machine learning, and other technical means, it can rapidly predict and analyze the information on molecular structure, properties, and behaviors and further calculate the strength of the interaction between the drug-target pairs to be predicted or the existence of interactions, to assist researchers in searching for the potential targets of the drugs, so that drug research can be more efficient and accurate. Research more efficiently and accurately. For this reason, computer-aided technology has become an important supplement to drug-target interaction prediction, providing a fast, low-cost, and efficient prediction strategy for drug-target interaction prediction [9]. The computer-assisted technology has become an important complement to drug-target interaction prediction, providing a fast, cost-effective and efficient prediction strategy for drug-target interaction prediction (Fig. 2).

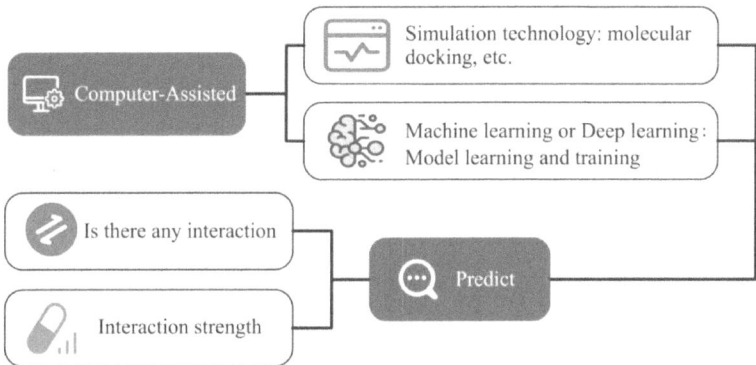

Fig. 2. Computer-assisted prediction of drug-target interactions

3   Drug-Target Interaction Prediction Methods

In this paper, under the premise of computer-assisted prediction techniques, we will broadly categorize the methods into four types of methods based on the type of data and application scenarios of drugs and targets [12]: molecular docking-based methods, ligand-based methods, text mining-based methods & feature-based methods.

3.1   Methods Based on Molecular Docking

The molecular docking method is through the simulation modeling of the three-dimensional structure of the drug molecule and the target, and then uses the algorithm to simulate the binding process between them, in the binding process, it will analyze the drug molecule and the target one by one in the binding process of the interaction ability and the binding site and other information, and finally through the model of the scoring function to predict the degree of interaction and the effect of the interaction between the drug and the target. In practical application, molecular docking methods can be divided into many kinds, and for example, there are Rarey [13]. DOCK method proposed by Rarey et al., Gohlkes [14] et al. and the DrugScore method and the SCORE method proposed by Wang et al. [15] proposed SCORE method. Among these methods, the molecular docking methods can be further categorized into flexible docking, semi-flexible docking, and rigid docking based on their docking modes, as the DOCK method mentioned earlier is flexible docking. The conceptual diagram of molecular docking-based methods is shown in Fig. 3.

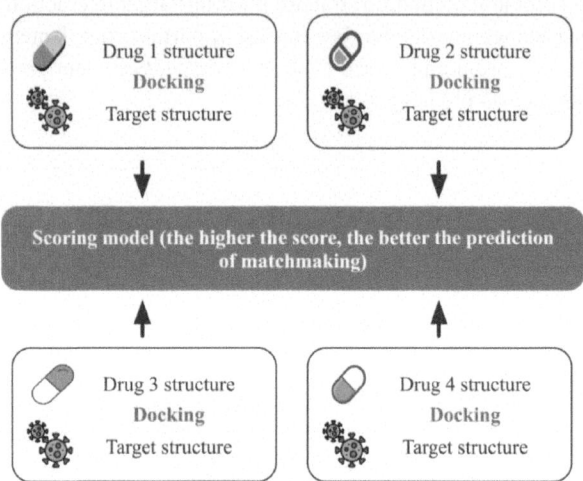

Fig. 3. DTI prediction method based on molecular docking

The molecular docking method predicts the interaction between drug-target pairs through docking technology, screening, and designing more active and selective drugs for researchers, which will effectively improve the therapeutic efficacy of drugs and reduce unnecessary drug side effects for patients. Besides, the research process of molecular docking between drugs and targets can help scientists understand the structure and function of target proteins and reveal the mechanism of drug action to a certain extent. Even though the molecular docking method has made some progress in both theory and practical application, it still faces some challenges, such as the affinity prediction between drug and target, which is precisely because the affinity prediction ability is seriously dependent on the structure and model scoring function of the drug and target, resulting in the affinity prediction results being deeply affected by its structure and model, and is prone to large deviations during the prediction process, therefore, researchers Therefore, researchers need to establish a more accurate and comprehensive computational model in subsequent studies to improve the accuracy and effectiveness of model prediction.

3.2 Ligand-Based Approaches

In pharmacology, a receptor is a biomolecule composed of glycoproteins or lipoproteins, which are found in the cell membrane, cytoplasm, or nucleus. Different receptors have different structures and conformations and are targeted in drug-target interaction predictions. A ligand, on the other hand, is a substance that recognizes and binds to the receptor, which is the drug in drug-target interaction prediction [16]. Ligand-based approaches are, therefore, the most effective way to predict drug-target interactions.

Thus, the ligand-based approach utilizes information about known ligands to predict the interaction between a candidate ligand and a specific target. The approach focuses on studying the nature and structure of the drug molecules themselves, as well as their interactions with the target, such as their chemical structure, charge distribution, and binding modalities [17]. The process does not require much information about the specific target. In short, the principle of the method is to compare the candidate ligands with the known ligands of the target and evaluate the interaction between the candidate ligands and the target by comparing the similarity between the candidate ligands and the known ligands [19]. A conceptual visualization of the ligand-based approach is shown in Fig. 4.

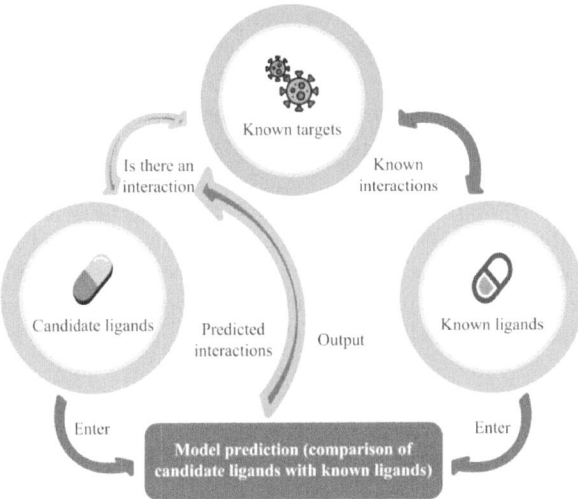

Fig. 4. Ligand-based DTI prediction methods

Ligand-based methods can be categorized into three main types: structural similarity, pharmacophore modeling, and quantitative structure-activity relationships (QSAR), among which quantitative structure-activity relationships (QSAR) methods dominated early drug design. QSAR can effectively screen drug molecules when the target structure is unknown and has the advantages of low computational effort and good predictive ability. QSAR can effectively screen drug molecules when the target structure is unknown, and it has the advantages of small computational volume and good prediction ability. However, one of the major doubts about this method is that it cannot give the physical meaning of the regression equation, which cannot help people understand the mechanism of action of drugs and targets. In addition, although more and more potential drug targets and ligands have been discovered, screening suitable active ligands from millions of small molecule compounds for different targets is still a considerable workload and challenge, especially when the number of known ligands for the target is insufficient, which will greatly reduce the accuracy of its prediction results.

3.3 Text Mining Based Approach

Text mining is a technique that can extract important information from a large amount of scattered, unstructured data, and it can extract drug-target interaction information from a large number of documents and databases by constructing a knowledge base and analyzing keywords and semantic information in text data infer and discover potential drug-target interactions [20]. It can infer and discover potential drug-target interactions by building a knowledge base, extracting drug-target interactions from a large number of documents and databases, and analyzing keywords and semantic information in textual data, and the process usually involves document summarization, information retrieval, entity recognition, and relationship extraction [21]. The process usually includes document summarization, information retrieval, entity recognition, and relationship extraction. In 2010, Von Eichborn J. [23] et al. constructed a PROMISCUOUS database for network-based drug repositioning by using data mining methods such as text mining to obtain drug-target and protein-protein interaction information to build and analyze networks responsible for polypharmacology, providing a new starting point for drug repositioning.

However, due to the ever-changing paradigm, text mining models will require higher maintenance to effectively extract information about drug-target pair interactions, and as drug-disease interactions become more complex, network-based models will also require more effective link prediction algorithms to improve model accuracy, or else the effectiveness of these models will begin to decline.

3.4 Feature-Based Approach

Drug-target interaction prediction is currently a field that makes extensive use of machine learning and deep learning. Numerous studies have demonstrated that feature-engineered models are an effective strategy for drug-target interaction prediction, and the method is gradually gaining advantages in this area [24, 25]. In this area, the technique is progressively demonstrating its benefits. A variety of data types, including drug molecule structure, target sequence, and drug-target binding modalities, may be described using the feature-based method and then fed into a model network for learning, analysis, and prediction. Figure 5 displays the feature-based approach's flowchart.

The feature-based approach is described in simple language by inputting the drug and target information into the designed model through certain descriptions, and the model will be processed by feature engineering and then input into the predictor for the prediction of drug-target pair interaction. Such an approach can realize the effective integration of drug and target information, allowing researchers to more comprehensively understand the interaction mechanism between drugs and target proteins the models of the feature-based approach are usually designed using techniques such as machine learning and deep learning, which makes it easy for us to find that artificial intelligence plays an indispensable role in the prediction of drug-target interactions [26].

Definition of Tasks. In the prediction of drug-target interactions based on the feature approach, it is first necessary to define this prediction task and confirm the nature of its task. In recent years, related research work has shown that this task can be categorized

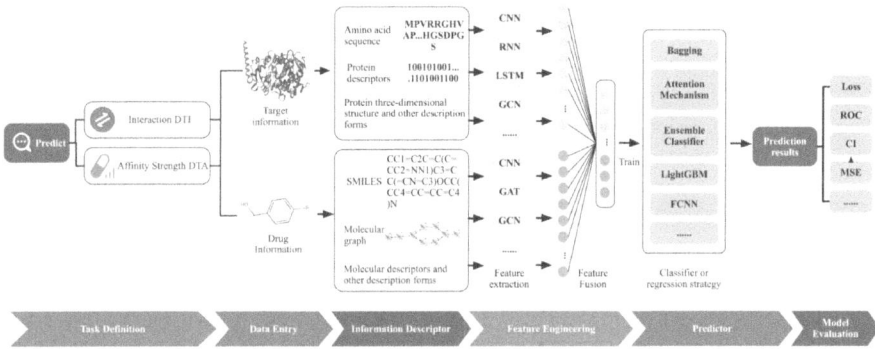

Fig. 5. Feature-based prediction method

into categorical prediction and regression prediction based on the type of model output variables. The categorical prediction of drug-target interaction (DTI) aims to predict whether or not there is an interaction between a drug and a target, and the goal of this task is to categorize samples into interactions and non-interactions using a classification algorithm. In contrast, regression prediction of drug-target interactions aims to predict the strength of the interaction between the drug and the target, i.e., drug-target binding affinity (DTA), which is usually achieved by regression modeling such that the resultant output is a continuous binding affinity value. Table 1. organizes the types of prediction tasks corresponding to different drug-target interaction prediction models.

Data Entry. The drug-target interaction prediction model requires a large amount of drug and target information as data input for the model, and its main role is to provide data support for the model. For this reason, researchers need to find suitable drug-target databases as data inputs before constructing the model to provide clues and guidance for drug screening and drug design. General drug-target databases contain a large amount of experimental data, such as structural information on drug compounds, biological activity data, structural information on target proteins, etc. Table 2. below will briefly organize the contents of some public databases.

Among them, the BindingDB database is the more widely used DTI database in predicting drug-target interactions. In addition to this, many researchers use some relatively small datasets to reach model convergence quickly, such as the Davis dataset and the KIBA dataset.

Information Descriptors Since drug and target information exist in various forms, it is necessary to integrate drug and target information and describe them to form relevant descriptors before using them as inputs to the model. Currently, drug descriptors include Simplified Molecular Input Specification for Linearity (SMILES), molecular descriptors, molecular diagrams, etc., while target descriptors include amino acid sequences, protein descriptors, three-dimensional structures of proteins, etc.

Molecular descriptors of drugs are commonly used to represent mathematical descriptions of chemical molecular structures and are widely used in drug design and

Table 1. Types of drug-target interaction prediction tasks

Forecasting task type	Author	Model
Categorical and regression forecasting	Öztürk H [28] etc.	DeepDTA
	Öztürk H [29] etc.	WideDTA
Classification projections	Lee I [30] et al.	DeepConv-DTI
	Wang SD [31] etc.	LDCNN-DTI
	Wei LS [32] etc.	MDL-CPI
	Zheng S [33] etc.	DrugVQA
	Hyeoncheol Cho [34] etc.	InteractionNet
	Zhang S [35] etc	SAG-DTA
	Zhao Q [36] etc.	HyperAttentionDTI
	Huang K [37] etc.	MolTrans
	L Chen[38] etc.	TransformerCPI
	E Zixuan [39] etc.	GSL-DTI
regression prediction	Jiang MJ [40] etc	DGraphDTA
	Guo BJ [41] etc.	FeatNN
	Li Y [42] etc.	DeepAtom
	Yuni Zeng [43] etc.	MATT_DTI
	L Zheng [44] etc.	OnionNet
	Nguyen [45] etc.	GraphDTA
	Ziduo Yang [46] etc.	MoleculeNet
	Zhang [47] etc.	GPCNDTA

development to describe and compare both the structural features and the physical or chemical properties of molecules. The main principle of molecular description is to convert the structural information of a molecule into a series of binary or digitized fingerprint descriptors, which can be analyzed and compared to enable drug classification or similarity comparison. For this reason, molecular descriptors are also known as molecular fingerprints, and common molecular fingerprints include MACCS fingerprints, ECFPs fingerprints, PubChem fingerprints, and so on. Molecular descriptors have the characteristics of simplicity and efficiency, which make them easy for computer processing and analysis, and are suitable for large-scale comparison and classification of drug molecules and even for structural similarity analysis of drug candidates to excavate compounds with similar structural features, but in some cases, other important biological information may also be neglected, resulting in the accuracy of the model being affected.

At the same time, drugs need to bind to specific targets in the organism to produce biological effects. Most of the targets are proteins with a few nucleic acids and sugars, and there is an urgent need to predict the protein's primary structure (amino acid sequence) due to the limitations of experimentally analyzing the protein structure. Amino acid

Table 2. Drug-target database

Database name	Web address	Thrust
DrugBank [48]	https://go.drugbank.com/	The library combines bioinformatics and chemoinformatics databases of drug data and target information and contains 11,912 pharmaceutical small molecules, of which 4,224 are FDA-approved
SIDER [49]	http://sideeffects.embl.de/	This repository contains information on adverse reactions for marketed drugs, 139756 drugs side effect relationships
PubChem [50]	https://publichem.ncbi.nlm.nih.gov	The library is an open access chemical database from the US Institutes of Health that stores the results of bioactivity testing of small molecules and other compounds
ChEMBL [51]	https://www.ebi.ac.uk/chembl/	The library is a free online database developed by the European Bioinformatics Institute (EBI) that provides literature-based data on the biological activity of targets and compounds
KEGG [52]	https://www.genome.jp/kegg/	The library integrates databases of genomic, chemical, and systemic functional information, storing drugs, compounds, pathway information, and more
SuperTarget [53]	https://ng ghttps://ndc.cncb.ac.cn/databasecommons/database/id	The library contains drug-related data such as side effects, medical indications, drug metabolism, etc., with a total of 330,000 interactions
HPRD [54]	http://www.hprd.org/	The library stores a database of human target interaction information and contains 41,327 interactions between 30,047 target entities
UniProtKB [55]	https://www.uniprot.org/	The library is an informative target database containing amino acid sequence information for 564,277 targets

(*continued*)

Table 2. (*continued*)

Database name	Web address	Thrust
PDB [56]	http://www.wwpdb.org/	The library collects databases on the structure of biological macromolecules, representing three-dimensional data in two-dimensional form
TTD [57]	http://bidd.nus.edu.sg/group/ttd/ttd.asp	The library is a database of amino acid target sequences, diseases, pathway information, etc., and contains close to 40,000 drug molecules
Pfam [58]	http://pfam.xfam.org/	The library is a database developed for protein families and contains information on protein annotation, sequence comparison, and more
BindingDB [59]	https://www.bindingdb.org/bind/index.jsp	The library provides a large amount of activity data of small molecules acting on various proteins, as well as information on the affinities of their interactions

sequences are composed of 20 different amino acids arranged in a specific order and are usually represented by sequence coding or numerical coding, i.e., the amino acid sequence is directly represented by a string of letters or converted into numerical form. Amino acid sequences directly determine the three-dimensional structure of proteins, and the structure of proteins is closely related to their function so that the amino acid sequences can be used to identify active and binding sites on the surface of proteins and thus predict the drug molecules with which they may interact.

Feature Engineering. The input biological information of drugs and targets is described and represented as feature vectors and needs to be feature extracted and input into the training model for training before it can be used to predict the interactions between drugs and targets. In DTI, feature extraction is between data input and model training, connecting the original data and model input, and is the premise and foundation of model training, so whether effective information can be extracted from the original data will directly affect the performance and prediction effect of the model.

In the early stage of research, researchers usually choose common machine learning algorithms as the design of the model, and well-known machine learning algorithms include Support Vector Machines (SVM), Random Forest, Neural Networks, and so on. For example, Li [60] et al. extracted the PSSM features of proteins from amino acid sequences, transformed the drug chemical structures into substructural fingerprints, and developed a classifier with discriminative vector machines to predict DTI.

    As deep learning technology has already made significant progress in the biomedical field, a series of deep learning-based application strategies for disease diagnosis, protein design, and medical image recognition have been developed by researchers. Here, to improve the accuracy of the prediction model, researchers have been using more and more efficient and complex feature extractors in addition to the classical ones, such as convolutional neural networks (CNN), recurrent neural networks (RNN), long and short-term memory networks (LSTM), and deep learning techniques (DLM). RNN), long short-term memory (LSTM), graph convolutional networks (GCN), graph attention networks (GAT), and so on. There are many advantages of deep learning-based feature extractors, which can handle high dimensional and complex input data while enhancing the performance and interpretability of the model, for example, the network structure of CNN is always good at extracting information about local patterns and location invariant patterns, while the RNN structure is better at capturing long term dependencies, and at the same time, the graph network structure is much better at learning the input data from graph structures. Information. For this reason, more and more researchers choose to use deep learning algorithms for prediction, such as Rifaioglu [61]. The MDeePred model proposed by et al. uses circular molecular fingerprints to represent compounds and constructs multiple types of protein features, including amino acid sequences, structures, and physicochemical properties, and then utilizes CNNs and feed-forward neural networks, respectively, to make predictions after extracting the feature vectors of the drug and the target. The positive cause model enriches the integrated information from different perspectives by constructing multi-channel input feature vectors so that it will be expected to provide the MDeePred model with the ability to implicitly learn the intrinsic features of drugs.

    Meanwhile, with the application of graph structure models in various fields, researchers have also paid attention to the application of graph structure to drug-target interaction prediction models, and some deep learning networks based on graph structure and new algorithms have emerged. Jiang [40] et al. proposed the DGraphDTA model to extract feature representations of drugs and targets from molecular and protein graphs, respectively, using GNN to predict binding affinity. The model constructs graphs based on SMILES descriptors of drug molecules and also constructs protein contact graphs for protein sequences. After obtaining the two graphs, the model will be fed into two GNN networks to extract the representations, and finally, the representations will be connected for affinity prediction. The innovation of this method is the introduction of a new graph to represent proteins, allowing a better description of their structure and characterization.

    To describe the interaction between drugs and targets more comprehensively, feature extraction is followed by combining features from different data sources and feature extraction methods, i.e., feature fusion, and its method enables the model to predict drug-target interactions more accurately. Meanwhile, in previous DTI predictions, the structure of a drug or protein is embedded using only its information without considering the global features of other molecules. Song [62] et al. proposed a deep learning-based multi-scale interaction feature fusion method for predicting DTI, which uses two feature extraction channels to obtain global feature-based interactions and local substructure feature-based interactions and fuses these two features to generate the final encoded interaction features for more accurate prediction, thus obtaining the probability scores for predicting DTI.

Meanwhile, other researchers have chosen to introduce algorithms such as attention mechanisms to enhance the interpretability of the model, for example, Zhao [63] et al. proposed a deep learning-based end-to-end model, AttentionDTA, which uses a one-dimensional convolutional neural network (1D-CNN) to extract abstract information about drugs and proteins and associates an attention mechanism to predict the binding affinity of the DTI, by using the attention mechanism to consider which subsequences in the protein are more important for the drug, and which subsequences in the drug are more important. In order to enhance drug target affinity prediction performance, Zhang [47] et al. also developed intramolecular and intermolecular cross-attention mechanisms. The intramolecular cross-attention mechanism effectively fuses various modal data pertaining to the same biomolecule, while the intermolecular cross-attention mechanism enables information interaction between various biomolecules in the attention space. This allows the model to obtain enhanced features with multimodal information and effectively improves the model prediction accuracy, stability, and reliability.

Predictors serve as the core components in drug-target interaction prediction models, while classifiers and regression strategies are, in turn, commonly used predictors in the classification task and regression task of the models, and they are often used to classify and quantitatively predict the relationships between drug-target pairs. The ability of the classifier to classify drug-target interactions after learning and analyzing the extracted features and fused information makes the classifier play a crucial role in the classification task, while the regression strategy also has a significant impact on the accuracy of the regression task.

In the classification task of drug-target interaction prediction models, researchers usually use predictors based on machine learning algorithms, such as the Su [64] et al. further optimized this approach by proposing the LG-DTI model, which obtains global representations of the drug and target through a semi-supervised network and combines these features into a final representation of the drug and target through a tandem aggregation function, and finally, inputs these combined features into a Random Forest classifier to perform DTI prediction, whose results show that on multiple datasets and evaluation metrics, the LG-DTI outperforms other baseline methods. As the accuracy of models has increased, researchers have combined multiple types of protein features with drug features to make model predictions more accurate, such as the PreDTI proposed by S. M. Hasan Mahmud et al. [65] For example, the PreDTIs prediction method proposed by S. M. Hasan Mahmud et al. uses MACCS fingerprinting, PsePSSM, PseAAC, and DC to extract chemical structure features of drugs and sequence features of proteins and combines these features to form a drug-target dataset, which is then inputted into a LightGBM classifier to predict the interactions. This approach effectively combines multiple feature extraction techniques and improves the predictive performance of the classifier.

In order to improve the generalization performance of the model, Zhang [66] et al. employed the SMOTE algorithm to randomly undersample and oversample the unbalanced samples. This was done because, despite the use of more sophisticated and comprehensive algorithms in the prediction model, the researchers still ran into issues with unbalanced sample data categories, which caused some degradation of the model performance. In order to find the best features that reflect the drug-target pairings, they also employed LightGBM to eliminate noise from the data. Lastly, the model will use a deep stacking integrated classifier that consists of GRU, DNN, SVM, XGBoost, and LR to predict the DTIs. By combining multilevel and multi-modeling, this method increases the model's resilience and prediction accuracy.

In recent years, many researchers have successfully categorized pictures by fully connected networks, which have achieved some applications in the field of image recognition, and this has allowed scholars designing predictive models for drug-target interactions to find new ideas for model design. For example, Cheng [67]. The IIFDTI model proposed by Cheng et al. employs GAT and CNN for modeling and feature extraction of drug and target, respectively, and then inputs the obtained interaction feature information into the fully connected network for DTI prediction after splicing with the independent feature information, and their experimental results on multiple datasets show that IIFDTI has a significant improvement in the metrics such as AUC, AUPR, precision, and recall compared to the state-of-the-art methods. There is a significant improvement.

The fully connected layer mentioned in the IIFDTI model is a fundamental component in neural networks, where each neuron of the structure is connected to almost all the neurons of the previous layer, which can process the input features and make classification predictions. It is also worth mentioning that the fully connected layer can map the input features to the target category space through linear transformations and nonlinear activation functions, which will make the fully connected layer not only suitable for classification tasks but also for regression tasks. Then, in the regression task of drug-target interaction prediction modeling, only the activation function of the output layer needs to be removed, and linear activation function or other suitable activation function for regression (e.g., ReLU) is used, and the fully connected layer can directly output continuous values to satisfy the needs of the regression task.

In practical regression tasks, researchers usually still use regression strategies for task prediction. For example, Pu [68] et al. proposed the DeepFusionDTA model, which utilizes sequence and structural information to generate a fusion feature map of candidate proteins and drug pairs and performs regression prediction based on an integrated learning strategy of bagging. The approach combines the advantages of various algorithms, inefficient feature abstraction, and regression computation and achieves excellent results. While Mei S [69] et al. simplified the computational model for drug-target interaction prediction based on the potential drug perturbations of relevant genes and signaling pathways by representing the drug-target profile as a binary vector to describe the presence or absence of genes and simply combining the target profiles of the two drugs into a single feature vector to describe the drug pairs, and lastly, to minimize the potential effect of noise, they chose the model with L2 regularized logistic regression as the base learner.

In reviewing the scientific achievements of researchers, it is not difficult to find that drug-target interaction prediction models are gradually evolving from simple network structures to complex integrated learning or deep learning models, and this series of improvements not only improves the prediction performance of the models but also improves the reliability of the results, which provides a more effective and reliable tool for drug discovery and the design of disease treatment programs. The following is a brief overview of the popular models in feature-based methods, and Table 3. will list some of the feature prediction methods based on deep learning.

Table 3. Deep learning-based feature prediction methods

Author	Model	Feature extraction	Summarize
Zheng [33] etc.	DrugVQA	CNN, RNN	Proteins are represented using two-dimensional distance maps of monomer structures and drugs are represented with molecular linear symbols that follow a visual question-and-answer paradigm to predict their interactions. To efficiently train the system, a dynamic attention convolutional neural network is also introduced to learn fixed-size representations from variable-length distance maps, and a self-attentive sequence model is introduced to automatically extract semantic features from linear symbols
Cho [34] et al.	InteractionNet	GNN	The method predicts drug-target binding constants using a special GNN model, a framework that learns intramolecular covalent bonds and intermolecular noncovalent interactions for proteins and ligands, respectively. Learning is performed by independent covalent and noncovalent convolutional layers, which facilitates the evaluation of the contribution of each convolutional step to the prediction of dissociation constants and the graph construction strategy for analyzing noncovalent interactions

(continued)

Table 3. (*continued*)

Author	Model	Feature extraction	Summarize
Huang K [37] etc.	MolTrans	Transformer, self-attention	The model is based on the Transformer structure of molecular interactions, and its interaction module consists of two main layers: an interaction tensor for modeling the interactions of pairs of substructures and a CNN layer for extracting the interaction maps of neighborhood interactions
L Chen [38] etc.	TransformerCPI	CNN, GCN, self-attention	Inspired by Transformer's powerful ability to capture features between two sequences, the authors predicted CPI by modifying the Transformer architecture to treat compounds and proteins as two sequences, and retaining Transformer's decoder and modifying its encoder and final linear layer
Li [42] etc.	DeepAtom	CNN	The DeepAtom model is constructed to predict drug-target affinity by drawing on lightweight 3D CNN models such as ShuffleNet and Xception
Zeng [43] etc.	MATT_DTI	CNN	The model proposes a multi-attention module MATT_DTI on the basis of CNN, which extracts the interaction information and gives the prediction results through the multi-head attention module and the fully connected layer

(*continued*)

Table 3. (*continued*)

Author	Model	Feature extraction	Summarize
Nguyen [45] etc.	GraphDTA	CNN, GCN, GAT, GIN, GAT-GCN	The proposed GraphDTA model represents pairs of drugs as graphs and uses graph neural networks to predict drug-target affinity
Lin [66] et al.	DeepGs	CNN, GAT, Bi-GRU	The authors present DeepGs, a new end-to-end learning framework that uses deep neural networks to extract information from amino acids and SMILES sequences, and distributed representations of amino acids and SMILES sequences using Smi2Vec and Prot2Ve coding techniques
E Zixuan [39] etc.	GSL-DTI	GCN	The model employs an automated graph structure learning approach that utilizes filter gates on the DPP affinity score and relies on the classification loss of the downstream task to guide the learning of the structure of the underlying DPP network, which translates the prediction of drug-target interactions into a node classification problem based on the learned DPP network

(*continued*)

Table 3. (*continued*)

Author	Model	Feature extraction	Summarize
Qian Y [71] etc.	CAT-CPI	CNN, Transformer	The authors learn local features of molecular images by using CNNs and then capture the semantic relationships of these features using the Transformer encoder. The model utilizes a k-gram based approach to extract features of protein sequences and obtains the semantic relationships of subsequences using the Transformer encoder. In addition, a feature re-learning (FR) module is constructed to learn the interaction features of compounds and proteins
Z Yang [72] etc.	MGraphDTA	GNN, CNN	The authors propose a deep multiscale graph neural network for DTA prediction based on chemical intuition, by introducing dense connectivity in the GNN and constructing an ultra-deep GNN with 27 graph convolutional layers and capturing both the local and overall structure of compounds

(*continued*)

Table 3. (*continued*)

Author	Model	Feature extraction	Summarize
J Zhang [73] etc.	IMAEN	GNN, CNN	IMAEN is an interpretable molecular enhancement model for drug-target interaction prediction. The model employs a molecular enhancement mechanism to fully aggregate molecular node neighborhood information, especially for nodes with fewer neighbors. In addition, an interpretable stacked convolutional coding module is designed to process protein sequences from a multi-scale and multi-level interpretable perspective
Ingoo Lee [30] etc.	DeepConv-DTI	CNN	The model captures the local residue patterns of proteins involved in DTI and convolves amino acid subsequences of varying lengths to capture the local residue patterns of generalized protein classes when CNN is used on the original protein sequence

Indicators and Related Tools for Model Assessment. Model evaluation indexes are quantitative measures used to assess the performance and validity of models, which can provide objective and quantitative criteria to evaluate the accuracy, stability, and applicability of models. For this reason, researchers need to measure the results of drug-target interaction prediction models with assessment metrics, which can provide a more comprehensive understanding of the performance characteristics of the model and also enable effective improvement and optimization of the model to provide a scientific basis for drug discovery and development. Table 4. below will organize some of the model evaluation indexes.

In the above table, CI and MSE are usually used as evaluation metrics for regression tasks, and the rest of the evaluation metrics are for classification tasks. Meanwhile, there are also a large number of coding tools that can generate information descriptors for drugs and targets to assist researchers in converting drug- and target-related information into feature representations, and these tools have been widely used in bioinformatics;

Table 4. Model evaluation indicators

Norm	Descriptive	Formulas	Range of values
F1 Score	Combining the precision and recall of the model is the harmonic mean of precision and recall	$F1 = \frac{2 \times Precision \times Recall}{Precision + Recall}$	[0, 1]
Loss rate (Loss)	Refers to the error of the model during training, usually measured by a loss function, indicating the difference between the model's predictions and the true labels	/	[0, ∞]
Threshold	In binary classification models, a critical value used to determine the predicted probability or score	/	[0, 1]
Sensitivity	Also known as the true case rate, it represents the proportion of positive cases that the model successfully predicts. Where. *TP* is the number of actual positive cases and predicted positive cases; *FN* is the number of actual positive cases and predicted negative cases	$Sensitivity = \frac{TP}{TP+FN}$	[0, 1]
Specificity	Also known as the true negative case rate, it represents the percentage of negative cases that the model successfully predicts. Where. *TN* is the number of actual negative cases that are predicted to be negative; *FP* is the number of actual negative cases that are predicted to be positive cases	$Sensitivity = \frac{TN}{TN+FP}$	[0, 1]

(continued)

Table 4. (*continued*)

Norm	Descriptive	Formulas	Range of values
Precision	denotes the proportion of all samples that were predicted by the model to be positive cases that were actually positive cases	$Precision = \frac{TP}{TP+FP}$	[0, 1]
Recall	denotes the proportion of all samples that are actually positive cases that the model successfully predicts as positive	$Recall = \frac{TP}{TP+FN}$	[0, 1]
ROC Curve (Receiver Operating Characteristic Curve)	Curves plotted with true case rate on the vertical axis and false positive case rate on the horizontal axis are used to evaluate the performance of the binary classification model	/	[0, 1]
AUC value (Area Under the ROC Curve)	The area under the ROC curve, used to compare the performance of different models, the larger the AUC value, the better the model performance	/	[0, 1]
Consistency (CI)	A metric for evaluating the performance of a ranking model that measures the agreement between the relative order predicted by the model and the actual observations	/	[0, 1]
Mean Square Error (MSE)	A measure of the performance of a regression model that represents the average squared error between the predicted and true values of the model, where y_i is the true value, and $\hat{y}_i$ is the predicted value	$MSE = \frac{1}{n}\sum_{i=1}^{n}(y_i - \hat{y}_i)^2$	[0, 1]

therefore, Table 5. will record the contents of some tools used to generate information descriptors for drugs or targets. In addition, Table 6. also lists the contents of some commonly used tools for protein structure analysis and prediction.

Table 5. Information descriptor generation tools for drugs and targets

Artifact	Link (on a website)	Summary
RDKit [74]	http://www.rdkit.org	It is a toolkit for generating various descriptors for compounds, running on various operating systems
CDK [75]	http://cdk.github.io	The software needs to be installed under Linux, and can calculate 16 kinds of molecular fingerprints
PaDEL-Descriptor [76]	http://www.yapcwsoft.com/dd/ padeldescriptor	A software that calculates molecular descriptors and fingerprints for 12 types of fingerprints
ChemDes [77]	http://www.scbdd.com/chemdes/ list-fingerprints	It is a Web platform that provides format conversion, descriptor calculation, fingerprint generation, similarity calculation, and other functions
PyDPI [78]	http://sourceforge.net/projects/ pydpicao/	The software serves DTI and allows the calculation of molecular descriptors of drugs and structural and physicochemical properties of proteins
Rcpi [79]	http://www.yapcwsoft.com/dd/ padeldescriptor	This is a software that calculates molecular descriptors and fingerprints for 1875 descriptors and 12 types of fingerprints

Feature-based methods can utilize many different forms of data for prediction and have the advantages of good prediction and better interpretability, but because feature engineering is often more complex in the construction process, there are shortcomings such as higher computational costs, in addition to this, the model still exists an imbalance between positive and negative samples, which will lead to the emergence of assessment bias or overfitting phenomenon, which will make the accuracy of the model Decrease.

Table 6. Protein structure analysis and prediction tools

artifact	link (on a website)	summary
SWISS-MODEL [80]	https://swissmodel.expasy.org	is a fully automated protein structure homology modeling server that uses sequence homology to infer the 3D structure of proteins
phyre2 [81]	http://www.sbg.bio.ic.ac.uk/phyre2/html/page.cgi?id=index	is an online tool that enables prediction and analysis of protein structure, function and variation
AlphaFold [82]	https://alphafold.com	AlphaFold is an AI system developed by Google DeepMind that predicts the 3D structure of proteins based on their amino acid sequences, and the AlphaFold DB is open to over 200 million protein structure predictions
PyMOL [83]	https://www.pymol.org	This is a program that can be used in Structural Biology It is an open source visualization tool for visualizing the structure of protein molecules
SignalP 6.0 [84]	https://services.healthtech.dtu.dk/services/SignalP-6.0	It is the most widely used online prediction tool for signal peptides in amino acid sequences, predicting signal peptide cleavage sites in bacterial and eukaryotic amino acid sequences
YLoc [85]	https://abi-services.cs.uni-tuebingen.de/yloc/webloc.cgi	It is an online tool mainly used for protein subcellular localization prediction
Cell-PLoc [86]	http://www.csbio.sjtu.edu.cn/bioinf/Cell-PLoc-2	The tool is mainly used to predict the subcellular localization of proteins in different organisms
ESPript [87]	https://espript.ibcp.fr/ESPript/cgi-bin/ESPript.cgi	An online tool for aligned sequence display that adds the secondary structure of a protein, in addition to displaying conserved regions of the sequence

(*continued*)

Table 6. (*continued*)

artifact	link (on a website)	summary
IBS [88]	http://ibs.biocuckoo.org/usergu ide.php	This is an online tool for mapping the structure of gene-protein sequences
Jalview [89]	https://www.jalview.org	This is a one-to-many sequence alignment visualization and editing analysis software, which can be used to view and edit aligned sequences, as well as to perform related phylogenetic and principal component analyses, and even to check molecular structures and annotations

4   Summary and Outlook

It is not difficult to find that there are many kinds of drug-target interaction prediction methods, and each method has its advantages and disadvantages and corresponding application scenarios, for this reason, in the actual study, researchers need to choose the appropriate method or combination of methods according to the specific problem to achieve the best prediction effect of the model.

4.1   Comparison of DTI Forecasting Methods

It can be seen that when it is necessary to accurately predict the binding mode of a drug and its target, the molecular docking-based method is one of the best choices to maintain a high accuracy rate. However, often, the three-dimensional structure of the target protein is not available during the research process, and at this time, if you want to understand the drug-target interactions, the ligand-based approach will highlight its advantages over the molecular docking approach because the approach can effectively reduce the structural requirements. In the early stages of drug discovery, text mining can quickly discover some new drug-target pairs, and with the emergence of large and complex data sets, the prediction effect of the former will be reduced, but the feature-based machine learning methods are usually able to deal with structural and biometric data at the same time, and are also applicable to a variety of different types of data sources so that the prediction results will also be more accurate.

Simply put, when faced with complex drug-target relationships, traditional methods may not be sufficient to capture all potential interactions, while feature-based methods can effectively improve prediction accuracy through the comprehensive modeling of multiple features, this is because when the data volume is huge, and the feature dimensions are complex, deep learning can automatically extract the features and model them efficiently, which enables the prediction model to achieve higher prediction accuracy. Meanwhile, if the dataset is smaller or the feature design is simpler, the traditional machine learning method may have an advantage over the deep learning method because of its extensive and more complex training and learning.

Based on the classification of drug-target interaction prediction methods in this paper, molecular docking-based methods, ligand-based methods, text mining-based methods, and feature-based methods are briefly sorted out according to the principles, advantages, and disadvantages of each method, as shown in Table 7. below.

The more advanced models in the current feature-based approach were compared for their performance, and these models were also mostly used as baseline models by the researchers, and their experimental results are shown in Table 8. below.

From the experimental results, it can be seen that on the Davis dataset, MolTrans performs best in the classification task, and MGraphDTA slightly outperforms the other models in the regression task in terms of CI and MSE metrics, especially GraphDTA.The best model on the Human dataset is CAT-DTI, which achieves an AUC of 0.984, indicating that the prediction accuracy on the classification task is relatively high, outperforming the earlier GraphDTA and MGraphDTA.On the BindingDB dataset, the classification performance of DrugBAN and CAT-DTI is closer, with AUCs of 0.961 and 0.960, respectively, which are both better than the other models. Overall, the performance of different models is affected by the dataset and task type, but the new deep learning models outperform the earlier models on complex data. The comparative ROC curves of the models in the three datasets in Table 8. are shown in Fig. 6.

4.2   Issues and Challenges of DTI Forecasting Methods

In recent years, artificial intelligence technology has been developing at such an amazing rate that even though deep learning models have, to some extent, led to an improvement in the accuracy and validity of drug-target interaction prediction models, there are still certain problems and challenges in the field of drug-target interaction prediction.

Data Set Issues. In drug-target interaction prediction methods, the prediction problem is usually abstracted as a simple binary classification task, but in known drug-target interaction data, there are usually far more negative samples than positive samples, which can easily lead to an imbalance problem in the data [91], i.e., there is a situation in which the positive samples are incorrectly predicted to be negative samples, and such a bias will make the model easy to overfit the negative class of samples and neglect the positive class of characteristics of the samples, thus affecting model performance degradation and risk of misclassification. Specifically, the model may learn that in most cases, there is no interaction between the drug and the target, and does not know the specific representation of the interaction, which will make it possible to always judge the prediction of drug-target interaction as 'no interaction' resulting in inaccurate predictions, especially for the small number of positive samples. This leads to inaccurate model predictions, especially for a small number of positive samples. In addition, drug-target interaction data are usually sparse [92], i.e., there is only a small amount of known interaction information, which makes it difficult for the model to learn effective features from a limited number of positive samples and is accompanied by the phenomenon of overfitting the known data [93], which leads to a decrease in the ability to generalize to the unknown data, and thus affects the accuracy and reliability of the model. Therefore, how to solve the

Table 7. Comparison of DTI prediction methods

Methodologies	Principle	Vantage	Drawbacks	Application
A molecular docking-based approach	Predicting interactions by analysing and comparing three-dimensional structural information of drug molecules and targets	Higher accuracy for virtual screening	The requirements for structural data for drugs and targets are high, and the results suffer when there is a lack of high-quality structural data	It is suitable for cases where the structural information of the target is more complete and the drug molecule is simpler
Ligand-based approach	Information about known ligands is used to predict interactions between new ligands and specific targets	Easy to use and highly interpretable	The structural information of the target may be neglected, and the accuracy is relatively low and the efficiency is low	Only the structure of the ligand is known, but not the structure of the target
Text mining based approach	Identification and extraction of drug-target interaction information by natural language processing techniques	Being able to access a large amount of information quickly helps to discover new associations	Limited by the quality and coverage of literature and databases	Scenarios where you want to quickly discover information about potential interactions based on an existing drug-target knowledge graph or database
Feature-based approach	Information about drugs and target proteins are combined and predicted by artificial intelligence techniques such as machine learning	Can be able to utilize multiple types of data with high prediction accuracy	Higher requirements for data quality and model design, more computational resources, time-consuming, and lower interpretability	Sufficient characterisation data for drugs and targets, or large-scale datasets, are required

problem of data imbalance and sparsity in the subsequent model design is an important direction.

However, it is easy to predict that when data sets are integrated, certain new issues may surface. The primary issue is that data integration will make data more complex. However, most of the time, researchers are unable to determine which information is

Table 8. Comparison of model performance

Data set	Model	Particular year	AUC	CI	MSE	Type of forecast
Davis	GraphDTA [45]	2020	/	0.893	0.229	regression (statistics)
	MolTrans [37]	2021	0.905	/	/	categorization
	MGraphDTA [72]	2022	/	0.900	0.207	regression (statistics)
	DrugBAN [90]	2023	0.875	/	/	categorization
	IMAEN [73]	2024	/	0.905	0.211	regression (statistics)
Human	GraphDTA [45]	2020	0.959	/	/	categorization
	MGraphDTA [72]	2022	0.982	/	/	categorization
	CAT-DTI [71]	2024	0.984	/	/	categorization
BingdingDB	GraphDTA [45]	2020	0.950	/	/	categorization
	MolTrans [37]	2021	0.915	/	/	categorization
	DrugBAN [90]	2023	0.961	/	/	categorization
	CAT-DTI[71]	2024	0.960	/	/	categorization

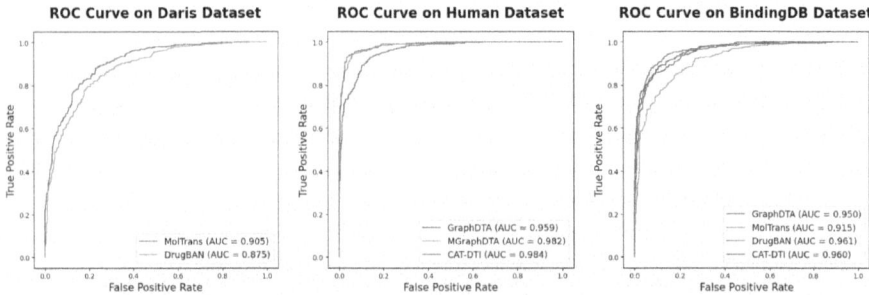

Fig. 6. Comparison of ROC curves of different models for each dataset

most crucial and essential for predicting drug-drug interactions, which information may contribute less to the prediction task, and—most importantly—how data integration tightens data constraints [94]. For this reason, researchers can improve the quality and consistency of the data by doing certain preprocessing operations on the data set, such as undersampling techniques that can effectively improve the quality and consistency of the data and, thus, the accuracy of the prediction model. Among them, Rayhan [95] and others proposed that the data imbalance problem can be dealt with by the clustering undersampling technique (CUS). A FastUS algorithm was proposed by S M Hasan Mahmud [65] to address the imbalance issue in the dataset. This algorithm is based on the undersampling technique in drug-target interaction prediction, which typically eliminates majority data samples that are similar to minority samples while maintaining the distance between the majority data samples and minority samples. The created balanced dataset gets more divisible while the choice restrictions are made clearer by using majority data samples that are similar to the minority class samples and keeping the majority class samples that are farther away from the minority class samples. Of course, in addition to pre-processing the data, the data imbalance problem can also be solved by unsupervised learning and other techniques, and solving the dataset problem with a more advanced network structure is also the direction of future research.

Cold-Start Problems. In machine learning or deep learning models, the cold-start problem is usually faced, and the cold-start scenario in drug-target interaction prediction refers to the problem that when the model is faced with a new drug or target, the prediction model lacks sufficient information or training data, which results in the model showing poor performance or failing to make effective predictions when predicting interactions between new drugs or new targets. This is because the performance of predictive models is highly dependent on a priori knowledge, such as information about the interactions between drugs and targets as well as their feature representations, etc. Once a new drug or target is encountered, due to the lack of relevant historical data, the traditional model may not be able to make accurate predictions or even to effectively evaluate the potential interactions between new drugs and targets. In brief, if the model is based on a recommendation algorithm for drug-target interaction prediction based on the similarity of drug molecules, the model cannot learn effectively from similar historical data when there is no known drug similar to the new drug molecule in the database of known drug-target interactions or when the new drug molecule may be significantly different from the known drug molecule. In addition to this, new drugs or new targets may often have unique molecular structures or unseen protein families, but since there are no drugs or targets with similar structures in the dataset, the model may lack the ability to represent the features of the new drug or target, which may make the model unable to adequately capture the important information of these new drugs or targets, resulting in the model's training effect due to incomplete or inaccurate feature representations This results in poor training effect of the model due to incomplete or inaccurate feature representation, and even accompanied by the phenomenon of overfitting.

In drug-target interaction prediction research, many researchers have adopted different strategies to alleviate the effects of the cold-start problem and improve the predictive ability of drug-target interaction prediction models when facing new drugs or new targets. Among them, unsupervised learning can be used to automatically extract useful features from a large amount of unlabelled data to help models learn more efficiently in the absence of explicit labels, such as the DeepCPI [96] model, which uses unsupervised representation learning to learn implicit but expressive low-dimensional features of compounds and proteins from large amounts of unlabelled data. Although a drug or target representation can be learned in an unsupervised manner, it still lacks interaction information, which is crucial for drug-target interactions. The C2P2 approach proposed by

Nguyen [97] and others migrate knowledge of intermolecular interactions learned from compound-compound interactions and protein-protein interactions to CPI prediction by transferring the intramolecular interaction information into unsupervised pre-training to enhance the feature representation in the task. In addition to this, the DrugBAN model proposed by Bai [90] et al. embeds a domain adaptation technique called CDAN, which can minimize the difference in the distribution of the model between different datasets by adjusting the internal representation of the model to better cope with the challenge of the different distributions of the training and test data in cross-domain prediction. Here, we can believe that in the future, more optimized methods can be used to learn the representation of compounds and proteins, such as migration learning and generative adversarial networks, making the cold-start problem better solved and that this will become a future trend in prediction.

Model Design Issues. Deep learning has been applied extensively in many different domains in recent years. Many researchers have created feature vectors representing the biological information of target proteins or medicinal compounds using deep learning models, and they have subsequently used these feature vectors to train deep neural networks. For instance, Chen [95] and others suggested the SupDTI self-supervised learning-enhanced end-to-end learning framework, which improves prediction performance, after being motivated by the success of the self-supervised learning (SSL) algorithm and arguing that the algorithm could use the input data itself as supervision. Deep learning can process complex data and enable automatic feature extraction and multimodal data fusion it also has advantages such as end-to-end learning, which will make deep learning a major trend for future prediction tasks.

It is also worth mentioning that the molecular mechanisms of drug-drug interactions are often overlooked or drowned in a flood of information precisely because the model is trained to be a black box, while its internal workings are difficult to explain and understand, and the prediction results are difficult to interpret biologically, leaving the model lacking in transparency, interpretability, and trustworthiness, and unable to pinpoint which factors contribute to the interactions well enough, and also unable to indicate which specific subsequences in a protein are the best binding sites. However, understanding the mechanism of action of a drug is one of the core goals of drug discovery and development, and interpretability plays an important role in clinical decision support. The lack of interpretability of such a deep learning or machine learning model in making predictions can leave drug developers unaware of which atoms, molecular fragments, or amino acids play a decisive role in the binding of a drug to its target, and it is difficult to guide the optimization of a drug's structure to the point that they may feel distrustful of the decision-making process of the model and thus be reluctant to perform experimental validation based on the predicted results. Therefore, if the model can provide interpretability, researchers can understand how the model arrives at its conclusions and thus increase their trust in the predicted results. This has also led researchers to introduce attention mechanisms to models in an attempt to address the problem of interpretability to increase the interpretability of models. To help researchers better understand the DTIs, the MINN-DTI [99] model, for instance, uses multiple heads of attention for drugs and targets, calculates the weights of each atom and amino acid residue in the target and drug molecules to determine their importance in the prediction, and visualizes their attention weights to highlight important target atoms and amino acid residues. This will ease the investigation of drug structure-effect relationships and mechanisms of action, as well as aid researchers in developing a more thorough understanding of DTI. In addition, DrugBAN effectively improves the interpretability of the model by using pairwise interaction modules composed of bilinear attention networks to learn the local interaction representations of drug-target pairs and by using pairwise bilinear attention graphs to visualize the contribution of each substructure to the final prediction results.

It can be seen that although the main goal of drug-target interaction prediction is to accurately predict the existence or strength of drug-target interactions, increasing the interpretability of the model can improve the usefulness and application prospects of the model. At the same time, to maintain the accuracy of the model, the introduction of the attention mechanism and the mapping of the attention weights to protein sequences and drug atoms can enable the model to provide biological insights to explain the nature of the interaction, which is also a better way to explain the current and future research. However, it is not difficult to find out that there is still a lack of a unified standard to evaluate the interpretability of the model, and improving the interpretability of the model will undoubtedly become a major challenge, and with the continuous optimization of the drug-target interaction prediction model, the design of the model will be accompanied by a certain degree of complexity, and how to design the model to achieve the greatest optimization should be a matter of careful consideration for the researcher in the process of research. The design of the model to achieve maximum optimization should also be a careful consideration for the researchers during the research process.

The emerging artificial intelligence technologies, especially generative adversarial networks (GANs), provide new ideas to solve the limitations of traditional model design, such as the GGANDTI model and BGANDTI model proposed by Ma [100], which solve the problems of limited data size and feature consistency and feature homogeneity and information balance problem in the network, providing a new solution for the models to obtain better performance. This is precisely because GANs can extend existing datasets by generating virtual drug-target interaction data, which provides new solutions to the cold-start problem and the problem of data scarcity. Currently, unsupervised learning frameworks for accurate prediction of molecular properties and drug targets have been constructed by researchers [101], which will make us realize that unsupervised learning techniques also show great potential in drug-target interaction prediction because they do not rely on labeled data and can learn potential patterns from unlabelled data, and their algorithms can also mine the implicit relationships between drugs and targets, improving the scalability of the model. In addition to this, language models excel in the field of natural language processing, where they can learn deep representations from such sequences, which makes them also passable for sequence modeling of drug SMILES representations and target protein sequences and are effective in capturing potential relationships between drugs and targets. The ConPLex [102] model, for instance, is a pre-trained protein language model that finds proteins and possible drug molecules in a common feature space and learns to differentiate genuine drugs from similar non-binding "decoy" molecules. This leads to both specificity to decoy compounds and a high degree of accuracy. This enables very sensitive computational drug screening, which in turn promotes effective drug development. It excels in accuracy, broad flexibility to unknown data, and specificity to the decoy compounds.

Finally, we believe that the drug discovery process will become more and more intelligent with the continuous development of deep learning technologies. Emerging technologies such as GANs, unsupervised learning techniques, and large language models will become the core tools in the prediction of drug-target interactions, and they can be combined as new modules to achieve more accurate and efficient drug screening and design, accelerating the intelligent development of drug discovery.

5 Conclusion

Predicting drug-target interactions is a crucial step in the drug discovery and development process, which is important for both drug design and drug therapy initiatives. The principles of several drug-target interaction prediction techniques are compiled and examined in this study under the framework of computer-aided technology. A brief assessment of the benefits and drawbacks of each technique is also included. Even though drug-target interaction prediction has advanced, there are still a lot of issues and difficulties, like unbalanced datasets, cold-start scenarios, and low model interpretability, among others. Nevertheless, we continue to think that as artificial intelligence continues to advance, deep learning technology will have a significant role in drug-target interaction prediction.In the future, we will need to continue to explore new prediction methods and techniques, work on solving existing problems, and continue to improve the drug development process to make greater contributions to human health.

References

1. Shardlow, C.E., Generaux, G.T., MacLauchlin, C.C., et al.: Utilizing drug-drug interaction prediction tools during drug development: enhanced decision making based on clinical risk. Drug Metab. Dispos. **39**(11), 2076–2084 (2011)
2. Li, F., Hu, Q., Xiong, R., et al.: Deep learning-based drug design method. Nature Mag. **43**(5), 383–390 (2021)
3. Masoudi-Nejad, A., Mousavian, Z., Bozorgmehr, J.H.: Drug-target and disease networks: polypharmacology in the post-genomic era. In silico pharmacology **1**, 1–4 (2013)
4. Yıldırım, M.A., Goh, K.I., Cusick, M.E., et al.: Drug-target network. Nat. Biotechnol. **25**(10), 1119–1126 (2007)
5. Torchilin, V.P.: Drug targeting. Eur. J. Pharm. Sci. **11**, S81–S91 (2000)
6. Dejori, M., Schuermann, B., Stetter, M.: Hunting drug targets by systems-level modeling of gene expression profiles. IEEE Trans. Nanobiosci. **3**(3), 180–191 (2004)
7. Kai, T.A.N., Yongjie, L.I., Haiming, P.A.N., et al.: Research on drug target prediction method based on multi-information integration. J. Guangxi Normal Univ. (Nat. Sci. Edition) **40**(2), 91–102 (2022)
8. Li, Y.C., You, Z.H., Yu, C.Q., et al.: PPAEDTI: personalized propagation auto-encoder model for predicting drug-target interactions. IEEE J. Biomed. Health Inform. **27**(1), 573–582 (2022)
9. Veselovsky, A.V., Ivanov, A.S.: Strategy of computer-aided drug design. Current Drug Targets-Infectious Disorders **3**(1), 33–40 (2003)

10. Macalino, S.J.Y., Gosu, V., Hong, S., et al.: Role of computer-aided drug design in modern drug discovery. Arch. Pharmacal Res. **38**, 1686–1701 (2015)
11. Kore, P.P., Mutha, M.M., Antre, R.V., et al. Computer-aided drug design: an innovative tool for modeling (2012)
12. Sharma, A., Rani, R.: BE-DTI': Ensemble framework for drug target interaction prediction using dimensionality reduction and active learning. Comput. Methods Programs Biomed. **165**, 151–162 (2018)
13. Rarey, M., Kramer, B., Lengauer, T., et al.: A fast flexible docking method using an incremental construction algorithm. J. Mol. Biol. **261**(3), 470–489 (1996)
14. Gohlke, H., Hendlich, M., Klebe, G.: Knowledge-based scoring function to predict protein-ligand interactions. J. Mol. Biol. **295**(2), 337–356 (2000)
15. Wang, R., Lai, L., Wang, S.: Further development and validation of empirical scoring functions for structure-based binding affinity prediction. J. Comput. Aided Mol. Des. **16**, 11–26 (2002)
16. Shi, H., Liu, S., Chen, J., et al.: Predicting drug-target interactions using Lasso with random forest based on evolutionary information and chemical structure. Genomics **111**(6), 1839–1852 (2019)
17. Cleves, A.E., Jain, A.N.: Robust ligand-based modeling of the biological targets of known drugs. J. Med. Chem. **49**(10), 2921–2938 (2006)
18. Shaikh, F., Tai, H.K., Desai, N., et al.: LigTMap: ligand and structure-based target identification and activity prediction for small molecular compounds. J. Cheminform. **13**(1), 44 (2021)
19. Dudek, A.Z., Arodz, T., Gálvez, J.: Computational methods in developing quantitative structure-activity relationships (QSAR): a review. Comb. Chem. High Throughput Screening **9**(3), 213–228 (2006)
20. Joshy, A., Kasyap, G.C., Reddy, P.D., et al.: Drug target interaction prediction using graph convolution-based neural fingerprinting. In: 2022 IEEE 19th India Council International Conference (INDICON), pp. 1-6. IEEE (2022)
21. Masoudi-Sobhanzadeh, Y., Omidi, Y., Amanlou, M., et al.: Drug databases and their contributions to drug repurposing. Genomics **112**(2), 1087–1095 (2020)
22. Fleuren, W.W.M., Alkema, W.: Application of text mining in the biomedical domain. Methods **74**, 97–106 (2015)
23. Von Eichborn, J., Murgueitio, M.S., Dunkel, M., et al.: PROMISCUOUS: a database for network-based drug-repositioning. Nucleic Acids Res. **39**(suppl_1), D1060-D1066 (2010)
24. Yang, C., Chen, E.A., Zhang, Y.: Protein-ligand docking in the machine-learning era. Molecules **27**(14), 4568 (2022)
25. Yamanishi, Y.; Chemogenomic approaches to infer drug-target interaction networks. Data Mining Syst. Biol. Methods Protocols, 97–113 (2013)
26. Ezzat, A., Wu, M., Li, X.L., et al.: Computational prediction of drug-target interactions using chemogenomic approaches: an empirical survey. Brief. Bioinform. **20**(4), 1337–1357 (2019)
27. Zhang, W., Chen, Y., Liu, F., et al.: Predicting potential drug-drug interactions by integrating chemical, biological, phenotypic, and network data. BMC Bioinformatics **18**, 1–12 (2017)
28. Öztürk, H., Özgür, A., Ozkirimli, E.: DeepDTA: deep drug-target binding affinity prediction. Bioinformatics **34**(17), i821–i829 (2018)
29. Öztürk, H., Ozkirimli, E., Özgür, A.: WideDTA: prediction of drug-target binding affinity. arXiv preprint arXiv:1902.04166 (2019)
30. Lee, I., Keum, J., Nam, H.: DeepConv-DTI: prediction of drug-target interactions via deep learning with convolution on protein sequences. PLoS Comput. Biol. **15**(6), e1007129 (2019)

31. Wang, S., Du, Z., Ding, M., et al.: LDCNN-DTI: a novel light deep convolutional neural network for drug-target interaction predictions. In: 2020 IEEE International Conference on Bioinformatics and biomedicine (BIBM), pp. 1132–1136. IEEE (2020)

32. Wei, L., Long, W., Wei, L.: Mdl-cpi: Multi-view deep learning model for compound-protein interaction prediction. Methods **204**, 418–427 (2022)

33. Zheng, S., Li, Y., Chen, S., et al.: Predicting drug-protein interaction using quasi-visual question answering system. Nat. Mach. Intell. **2**(2), 134–140 (2020)

34. Cho, H., Lee, E.K., Choi, I.S.: Layer-wise relevance propagation of InteractionNet explains protein-ligand interactions at the atom level. Sci. Rep. **10**(1), 21155 (2020)

35. Zhang, S., Jiang, M., Wang, S., Wang, X., Wei, Z., Li, Z.: SAG-DTA: prediction of drug-target affinity using self-attention graph network. Int. J. Mol. Sci. **22**(16), 8993 (2021)

36. Zhao, Q., Zhao, H., Zheng, K., Wang, J.: HyperAttentionDTI: improving drug-protein interaction prediction by sequence-based deep learning with an attention mechanism. Bioinformatics **38**(3), 655–662 (2022)

37. Huang, K., Xiao, C., Glass, L.M., et al.: MolTrans: molecular interaction transformer for drug-target interaction prediction. Bioinformatics **37**(6), 830–836 (2021)

38. Chen, L., Tan, X., Wang, D., et al.: TransformerCPI: improving compound-protein interaction prediction by sequence-based deep learning with self-attention mechanism and label reversal experiments. Bioinformatics **36**(16), 4406–4414 (2020)

39. Zixuan, E., Qiao, G., Wang, G., et al.: GSL-DTI: graph structure learning network for drug-target interaction prediction. Methods **223**, 136–145 (2024)

40. Jiang, M., Li, Z., Zhang, S., et al.: Drug-target affinity prediction using graph neural network and contact maps. RSC Adv. **10**(35), 20701–20712 (2020)

41. Guo, B., Zheng, H., Jiang, H., et al. Enhanced compound-protein binding affinity prediction by representing protein multimodal information via a coevolutionary strategy. Briefings Bioinform. **24**(2): bbac628 (2023)

42. Li, Y., Rezaei, M.A., Li, C., et al.: DeepAtom: A framework for protein-ligand binding affinity prediction. In: 2019 IEEE International Conference on Bioinformatics and Biomedicine (BIBM). ie,pp. 303–310 (2019)

43. Zeng ,Y., Chen, X., Luo, Y., et al.: Deep drug-target binding affinity prediction with multiple attention blocks. Briefings Bioinform. **22**(5), bbab117 (2021)

44. Zheng, L., Fan, J., Mu, Y.: Onionnet: a multiple-layer intermolecular-contact-based convolutional neural network for protein-ligand binding affinity prediction. ACS Omega **4**(14), 15956–15965 (2019)

45. Nguyen, T., Le, H., Quinn, T.P., et al.: GraphDTA: predicting drug-target binding affinity with graph neural networks. Bioinformatics **37**(8), 1140–1147 (2021)

46. Wu, Z., Ramsundar, B., Feinberg, E.N., et al.: MoleculeNet: a benchmark for molecular machine learning. Chem. Sci. **9**(2), 513–530 (2018)

47. Zhang, L., Wang, C.C., Zhang, Y., et al.: GPCNDTA: prediction of drug-target binding affinity through cross-attention networks augmented with graph features and pharmacophores. Comput. Biol. Med. **166**, 107512 (2023)

48. Wishart D S, Knox C, Guo A C, et al. DrugBank: a knowledgebase of drugs, drug actions, and drug targets. Nucleic acids research, 2008, 36(suppl_1): D901-D906

49. Kuhn, M., Letunic, I., Jensen, L.J., et al.: The SIDER database of drugs and side effects. Nucleic Acids Res. **44**(D1), D1075–D1079 (2016)

50. Wang, Y., Xiao, J., Suzek, T.O., et al.: PubChem: a public information system for analyzing bioactivities of small molecules. Nucleic Acids Res. **37**(suppl_2), W623-W633 (2009)

51. Gaulton, A., Bellis, L.J., Bento, A.P., et al.: ChEMBL: a large-scale bioactivity database for drug discovery. Nucleic Acids Res. **40**(D1), D1100–D1107 (2012)

52. Kanehisa, M., Furumichi, M., Tanabe, M., et al.: KEGG: new perspectives on genomes, pathways, diseases, and drugs. Nucleic Acids Res. **45**(D1), D353–D361 (2017)

53. Günther, S., Kuhn, M., Dunkel, M., et al.: SuperTarget and Matador: resources for exploring drug-target relationships. Nucleic Acids Res. **36**(suppl_1), D919-D922 (2007)

54. Keshava Prasad, T.S., Goel, R., Kandasamy, K., et al.: Human protein reference database-2009 update. Nucleic Acids Res. **37**(suppl_1): D767-D772 (2009)

55. UniProt: the universal protein knowledgebase in 2021. Nucleic Acids Res. **49**(D1), D480-D489 (2021)

56. Burley, S.K., Berman, H.M., Kleywegt, G.J., et al.: Protein Data Bank (PDB): the single global macromolecular structure archive. Protein Crystallography: Methods Protocols, 627–641 (2017)

57. Chen, X., Ji, Z.L., Chen, Y.Z.: TTD: therapeutic target database[J]. Nucleic Acids Res. **30**(1), 412–415 (2002)

58. Finn, R.D., Bateman, A., Clements, J., et al.: Pfam: the protein families database. Nucleic Acids Res. **42**(D1), D222–D230 (2014)

59. Liu, T., Lin, Y., Wen, X., et al:. BindingDB: a web-accessible database of experimentally determined protein-ligand binding affinities. Nucleic Acids Res. **35**(suppl_1), D198-D201 (2007)

60. Li, Z., Han, P., You, Z.H., et al.: In silico prediction of drug-target interaction networks based on drug chemical structure and protein sequences. Sci. Rep. **7**(1), 11174 (2017)

61. Rifaioglu, A.S., Cetin Atalay, R., Cansen Kahraman, D., et al.: MDeePred: novel multi-channel protein featurization for deep learning-based binding affinity prediction in drug discovery. Bioinformatics **37**(5), 693–704 (2021)

62. Song, T., Zhang, X., Ding, M., et al.: DeepFusion: a deep learning-based multi-scale feature fusion method for predicting drug-target interactions. Methods **204**, 269–277 (2022)

63. Zhao Q, Xiao F, Yang M, et al. AttentionDTA: prediction of drug-target binding affinity using attention model. In: IEEE International Conference on Bioinformatics and Biomedicine (BIBM), ,pp. 64–69. San Diego: IEEE (2019)

64. Su, X., Hu, P., Yi, H., et al.: Predicting drug-target interactions over heterogeneous information network. IEEE J. Biomed. Health Inform. **27**(1), 562–572 (2022)

65. Mahmud, S.M.H., Chen, W., Liu, Y., et al.: PreDTIs: prediction of drug-target interactions based on multiple feature information using gradient boosting framework with data balancing and feature selection techniques. Briefings Bioinform. **22**(5), bbab046 (2021)

66. Zhang, Y., Jiang, Z., Chen, C., et al.: DeepStack-DTIs: predicting drug-target interactions using LightGBM feature selection and deep-stacked ensemble classifier. Interdisciplinary Sci. Comput. Life Sci., 1–20 (2022)

67. Cheng, Z., Zhao, Q., Li, Y., et al.: IIFDTI: predicting drug-target interactions through interactive and independent features based on attention mechanism. Bioinformatics **38**(17), 4153–4161 (2022)

68. Pu, Y., Li, J., Tang, J., et al.: DeepFusionDTA: drug-target binding affinity prediction with information fusion and hybrid deep-learning ensemble model. IEEE/ACM Trans. Comput. Biol. Bioinf. **19**(5), 2760–2769 (2021)

69. Mei, S., Zhang, K.: A machine learning framework for predicting drug-drug interactions. Sci. Rep. **11**(1), 17619 (2021)

70. Lin , X.: DeepGS: Deep Representation Learning of graphs and sequences for drug-target binding affinity prediction. arXiv, 2003.13902v2 (2020)

71. Zeng, X., Chen, W., Lei, B.: CAT-DTI: cross-attention and Transformer network with domain adaptation for drug-target interaction prediction. BMC Bioinform. **25**(1), 141 (2024)

72. Yang, Z., Zhong, W., Zhao, L., et al.: MGraphDTA: deep multiscale graph neural network for explainable drug-target binding affinity prediction. Chem. Sci. **13**(3), 816–833 (2022)

73. Zhang, J., Liu, Z., Pan, Y., et al.: IMAEN: An interpretable molecular augmentation model for drug-target interaction prediction. Expert Syst. Appl. **238**, 121882 (2024)

74. Landrum, G.: RDKit: a software suite for cheminformatics, computational chemistry, and predictive modeling. Greg Landrum, , **8**(31.10), 5281 (2013)

75. Steinbeck, C., Hoppe, C., Kuhn, S., et al.: Recent developments of the chemistry development kit (CDK)-an open-source java library for chemo- and bioinformatics. Curr. Pharm. Des. **12**(17), 2111–2120 (2006)

76. Yap, C.W.: PaDEL-descriptor: an open source software to calculate molecular descriptors and fingerprints. J. Comput. Chem. **32**(7), 1466–1474 (2011)

77. Dong, J., Cao, D.S., Miao, H.Y., et al.: ChemDes: an integrated web-based platform for molecular descriptor and fingerprint computation. J. Cheminform. **7**, 1–10 (2015)

78. Cao D S, Liang Y Z, Yan J, et al. PyDPI: freely available Python package for chemoinformatics, bioinformatics, and chemogenomics studies (2013)

79. Cao, D.S., Xiao, N., Xu, Q.S., et al.: Rcpi: R/Bioconductor package to generate various descriptors of proteins, compounds, and their interactions. Bioinformatics **31**(2), 279–281 (2015)

80. Waterhouse, A., Bertoni, M., Bienert, S., et al.: SWISS-MODEL: homology modeling of protein structures and complexes. Nucleic Acids Res. **46**(W1), W296–W303 (2018)

81. Kelley, L.A., Mezulis, S., Yates, C.M., et al.: The Phyre2 web portal for protein modeling, prediction and analysis. Nat. Protoc. **10**(6), 845–858 (2015)

82. Jumper, J., Evans, R., Pritzel, A., et al.: Highly accurate protein structure prediction with AlphaFold. Nat. **596**(7873), 583–589 (2021)

83. DeLano, W.L.: Pymol: an open-source molecular graphics tool. CCP4 Newsl. Protein Crystallogr, **40**(1), 82–92 (2002)

84. Teufel, F., Almagro Armenteros, J.J., Johansen, A.R., et al.: SignalP 6.0 predicts all five types of signal peptides using protein language models. Nat. Biotechnol. **40**(7), 1023–1025 (2022)

85. Briesemeister, S., Rahnenfï¿½hrer J., Kohlbacher, O.: YLoc-an interpretable web server for predicting subcellular localization. Nucleic Acids Res. **38**(suppl_2), W497-W502 (2010)

86. Chou, K.C., Shen, H.B.: Cell-PLoc: a package of Web servers for predicting subcellular localization of proteins in various organisms. Nat. Protoc. **3**(2), 153–162 (2008)

87. Gouet, P., Robert, X., Courcelle, E.: ESPript/ENDscript: extracting and rendering sequence and 3D information from atomic structures of proteins. Nucleic Acids Res. **31**(13), 3320–3323 (2003)

88. Liu, W., Xie, Y., Ma, J., et al.: IBS: an illustrator for the presentation and visualization of biological sequences. Bioinformatics **31**(20), 3359–3361 (2015)

89. Waterhouse, A.M., Procter, J.B., Martin, D.M.A., et al.: Jalview Version 2-a multiple sequence alignment editor and analysis workbench. Bioinformatics **25**(9), 1189–1191 (2009)

90. Bai, P., Miljković, F., John, B., et al.: Interpretable bilinear attention network with domain adaptation improves drug-target prediction. Nat. Mach. Intell. **5**(2), 126–136 (2023)

91. Zhang, W., Jing, K., Huang, F., et al.: SFLLN: a sparse feature learning ensemble method with linear neighborhood regularization for predicting drug-drug interactions. Inf. Sci. **497**, 189–201 (2019)

92. Nguyen, D.A., Nguyen, C.H., Petschner, P., et al.: SPARSE: a sparse hypergraph neural network for learning multiple types of latent combinations to accurately predict drug-drug interactions. Bioinformatics, **38**(Supplement_1), i333-i341 (2022)

93. Liang, X., Zhang, P., Yan, L., et al.: LRSSL: predict and interpret drug-disease associations based on data integration using sparse subspace learning. Bioinformatics **33**(8), 1187–1196 (2017)

94. Abbas ,S., Sampedro, G.A., Abisado, M., et al.: A novel drug-drug indicator dataset and ensemble stacking model for detection and classification of drug-drug interaction indicators. IEEE Access (2023)

95. Rayhan, F., Ahmed, S., Shatabda, S., et al.: iDTI-ESBoost: identification of drug target interaction using evolutionary and structural features with boosting. Sci. Rep. **7**(1), 17731 (2017)
96. Wan, F., Zhu, Y., Hu, H., et al.: DeepCPI: a deep learning-based framework for large-scale in silico drug screening. Genomics Proteomics Bioinform. **17**(5), 478–495 (2019)
97. Nguyen, T.M., Nguyen, T., Tran, T.: Mitigating cold-start problems in drug-target affinity prediction with interaction knowledge transferring. Briefings Bioinform. **23**(4), bbac269 (2022)
98. Chen, J., Zhang, L., Cheng, K., et al.: Predicting drug-target interaction via self-supervised learning. IEEE/ACM Trans. Comput. Biol. Bioinform. (2022)
99. Li, F., Zhang, Z., Guan, J., et al.: Effective drug–target interaction prediction with mutual interaction neural network. Bioinformatics **38**(14), 3582–3589 (2022)
100. Ma, X.: Research on drug-target interaction prediction method based on generative adversarial network. Henan University, Henan (2023)
101. Zeng, X., Xiang, H., Yu, L., et al.: Accurate prediction of molecular properties and drug targets using a self-supervised image representation learning framework. Nat. Mach. Intell. **4**(11), 1004–1016 (2022)
102. Singh, R., Sledzieski, S., Bryson, B., et al.: Contrastive learning in protein language space predicts interactions between drugs and protein targets. Proc. Natl. Acad. Sci. **120**(24), e2220778120 (2023)

The Joint Entity-Relation Extraction Model Based on Span and Interactive Fusion Representation for Chinese Medical Texts with Complex Semantics

Danni Feng[1], Runzhi Li[2(⊠)], Jing Wang[1], Siyu Yan[3], Lihong Ma[3], and Yunli Xing[4]

[1] School of Zhengzhou University, Zhengzhou, China
[2] Cooperative Innovation Center of Internet Healthcare, Zhengzhou University, Zhengzhou, China
fdn@gs.zzu.edu.cn
[3] National Center for Cardiovascular Diseases, Fuwai Hospital, Chinese Academy of Medical Sciences and Peking Union Medical College, Beijing, China
[4] Department of Geriatrics, Beijing Friendship Hospital, Capital Medical University, Beijing, China

Abstract. Joint entity-relation extraction is a critical task in transforming unstructured or semi-structured text into triplets, facilitating the construction of large-scale knowledge graphs, and supporting various downstream applications. Despite its importance, research on Chinese text, particularly with complex semantics in specialized domains like medicine, remains limited. To address this gap, we introduce the CH-DDI, a Chinese drug-drug interactions dataset designed to capture the intricacies of medical text. Leveraging the strengths of attention mechanisms in capturing long-range dependencies, we propose the SEA module, which enhances the extraction of complex contextual semantic information, thereby improving entity recognition and relation extraction. Additionally, to address the inefficiencies of existing methods in facilitating information exchange between entity recognition and relation extraction, we present an interactive fusion representation module. This module employs Cross Attention for bidirectional information exchange between the tasks and further refines feature extraction through BiLSTM. Experimental results on both our CH-DDI dataset and public CoNLL04 dataset demonstrate that our model exhibits strong generalization capabilities. On the CH-DDI dataset, our model achieves an F1-score of 96.73% for entity recognition and 78.43% for relation extraction. On the CoNLL04 dataset, it attains an entity recognition precision of 89.54% and a relation extraction accuracy of 71.64%.

Keyword: joint entity-relation extraction·interactive fusion·semantic enhancement

© The Author(s), under exclusive license to Springer Nature Singapore Pte Ltd. 2025
Y. Zhang et al. (Eds.): CHIP 2024, CCIS 2433, pp. 196–216, 2025.
https://doi.org/10.1007/978-981-96-3752-2_12

1   Introduction

Entity recognition and relation extraction are pivotal components in the establishment of large-scale knowledge graphs (KG). Lots of researches focus on them. One is two-stage pipeline method that trains two tasks independently [1–3]. However, this approach encounters some significant challenges. Firstly, it tends to overlook the interplay between entity recognition and relation extraction. Secondly, it encounters error propagation.

To solve the above problems, various joint entity relation extraction methods have been proposed. In which, traditional methods rely on labor-intensive and time-consuming feature engineering [4,5]. Neural network-based joint entity relation extraction methods [6–8] demonstrate the capability to extract triplets in a single step. Nevertheless, lacking constraints on entity types, makes it difficult to guide relation prediction. Conversely, methods that leverage shared parameters offer flexibility, typically prioritizing entity recognition before relation extraction. However, they may overlook semantic information, which is particularly important for joint extraction of entities and relations, especially for Chinese texts. For instance, Zeng et al. [9] employ Convolutional Neural Networks (CNN) to extract contextual information. Miwa et al. [10] and Zheng et al. [11] utilize Long Short-Term Memory (LSTM) networks to extract semantic information. However, These approaches struggle to effectively capture intricate details within sentences and grapple with capturing long-term dependencies. Subsequently, Eberts et al. [12] leverage the CLS token as a semantic indicator for entity recognition purposes. However, the CLS representation derived from BERT [13] may be susceptible to information loss or inadequate comprehension of the broader context. JI B et al. [14] improved this work, achieving sentence-level semantic acquisition and span-level semantic acquisition through four different attention variants, but this also requires storing a large number of attention parameters.

Our research focuses on extracting structured knowledge from Chinese medical texts, which often contain complex semantics. To facilitate this, we constructed the CH-DDI, a drug-drug interactions dataset. When performing entity recognition, we integrate the advantages of existing models, maximize potential entity spans through span partitioning, and introduce attention-based SEA modules to effectively extract long-range contextual information. In addition, during the creation process of CH-DDI, we identified an important issue of relation overlap, where one drug may have the same or different interactions with multiple other drugs. Therefore, accurate semantic understanding during relation extraction is also crucial. To address this issue, we introduce local contextual semantics between span pairs through max-pooling during relation extraction.

Moreover, facilitating information exchange between the two tasks is deemed advantageous for enhancing model performance. Specifically, entity recognition by having awareness of the potential relations within a sentence can lead to more precise recognition of entities, and vice versa. For instance, given two potential location entities, the semantic relation in the sentence may be "Located_in" rather than "Promotion". Xiong et al. [15] demonstrated the usefulness of information exchange between tasks by implementing the gating mechanism for task interaction. Based on the idea that implementing information exchange between tasks can improve model performance, we propose an interactive fusion representation module to achieve bidirectional information exchange between entity recognition and relation extraction.

In this work, we propose a joint entity-relation extraction model based on span and interactive fusion representation for Chinese medical texts with complex semantics. In which, the interactive fusion representation module facilitates information exchange between entity recognition and relation extraction by Cross Attention and BiLSTM. And we use the span feature extraction module to obtain segmented spans and various features for spans. It should be noted that we treat the contextual semantics used in entity recognition as sentence-level semantics and use SEA for processing while treating the local context between span pairs used in relation extraction as spans. Similar to the extraction of internal features within spans, we use max-pooling to preserve the important features of the local context. The final entity recognition and relation extraction are the implementation of traditional classification.

Overall, our contributions are as follows:

1. We propose a joint entity-relation extraction model based on span and interactive fusion representation for Chinese medical texts with complex semantics, which captures long sentence dependencies through attention mechanism and extracts features again using BiLSTM, ultimately obtaining contextual semantics that consider both sentence importance and sentence sequence order.
2. We propose an interactive fusion representation module based on Cross Attention. The encoder in the model includes feedforward neural networks, which can obtain specific representations for entity recognition and relation extraction. The interactive fusion representation module can perform dual Cross Attention on these two representations and further use BiGRU for feature fusion.
3. We establish a Chinese drug-drug interactions dataset CH-DDI and conduct experiments on both CH-DDI and the public dataset CoNLL04. Compared with the baseline models, the best results are achieved on both Chinese and English datasets.

2   Related Work

Entity recognition and relation extraction stand as pivotal sub-tasks within the realm of natural language processing(NLP). The initial two-stage model was gradually abandoned due to the difficulty in achieving interaction between two sub-tasks and the problem of error propagation. Currently, the joint extraction model for unified modeling the two tasks is used, and the extracted structured triplets are convenient for constructing large-scale knowledge graphs(KG) or completing other downstream tasks.

Parameter Sharing-Based Methods. The shared-parameter joint extraction framework has been shown to enhance the performance of relation extraction through the synergistic optimization of entity recognition processes. Wei et al. [16] utilizes the binary taggers to predict all potential head entities, and subsequently utilizes these predictions to infer their corresponding tail entities and relations. Fu et al. [17] innovatively constructs entities and relations as graphs, where entities are nodes and relations are edges. The method Bekoulis et al. [18] proposed is similar to the work Huang et al. [19] proposed, they both use BIO annotation combined with CRF for entity recognition and allow for the prediction of multiple potential relations between a word and other words during relation extraction. The only difference lies in the selection of the basic encoder. However, the multi-head selection method lacks the use of semantic information for judgment. STER [20] is a model that uses knowledge distill, it has two teachers that study the information for entity recognition and relation extraction respectively. Our work, similar to SpERT [12] and SPAN [14], utilizes spans for overlapping entity recognition. However, neither of these methods can effectively achieve task interaction, and SpERT lacks effective acquisition of complex semantics. On the other hand, SPAN achieves sentence-level semantic supplementation through multiple attention mechanisms, which often require more storage of attention parameters.

Joint Decoding Algorithm-Based Methods. The methods based on the decoding algorithm often blur the distinction between entity recognition and relation extraction, enabling the direct extraction of triplets in a single step. Common approaches that use joint decoders include tag-based and table-based. Zheng et al. [6] proposed a method that involves assigning a tag to each input token to denote the head or tail entities along with the relations, and subsequently inferring the triplet through tag prediction and parsing. However, the method based on tables often generates one table for each relation. Feiliang Ren et al. [7] introduces a global feature-oriented relational triple extraction model, Wang et al. [21] proposed a method that formulates joint extraction as a token pair linking problem and introduces a novel handshaking tagging scheme that aligns the boundary tokens of entity pairs under each relation type. Shang Y M et al. [8] introduce a novel scoring based classifier to parallel tag and a Rel-Spec Horns Tagging strategy to ensure efficient decoding. Nevertheless, these methods often rely on predefined encoding and decoding strategies, and these methods often lack entity type constraints.

Generative Models-Based Methods. With the widespread application of generative models such as Transformer [22] in multiple fields, some researchers have also attempted to use generative models for entity relation extraction. Dianbo Sui et al. [23] used generative models to generate sets, where the elements in the set are the desired triplets. However, the output produced by the generative model is more stochastic, and this model often relies on richer training data. LinkNER [24] is the first work exploring how to fine-tune models synergistically with LLMs for NER tasks. Asada M et al. [25] Proposed a novel relation extraction method enhanced by large language models (LLMs).

3   Method

3.1   Overview

In this work, we propose a novel span-based joint entity-relation extraction model named ISER. It is illustrated in Fig. 1. It primarily comprises five components that consist of the encoder module, the interactive fusion representation module, the span-based feature extraction module, the entity recognition module, and the relation extraction module. The encoder is a pre-trained BERT followed by two feedforward layers. The interactive fusion representation module carries out Cross Attention first and then executes BiLSTM to achieve representation fusion of entity and relation. The span-based feature extraction module implements span partition strategy, in which span width is embedded and span context is concated. The entity recognize module and relation extract module are traditional classification modules.

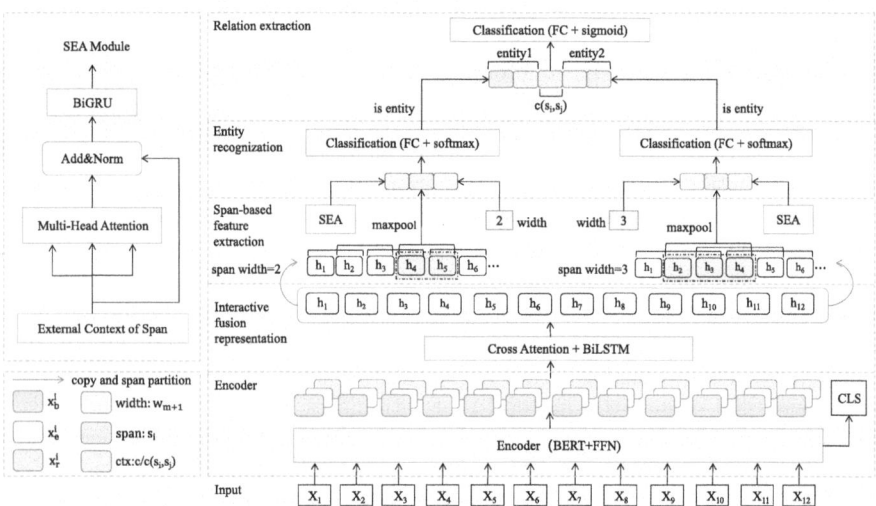

Fig. 1. The overall architecture of our model. The encoder can convert input sequences into three embedding representations: the embeddings obtained by BERT, representations for entity recognition and representations for relation extraction; the interactive fusion representation module can realize the information exchange between entity recognition and relation extraction; the span-based feature extraction module obtains three types features of spans: the internal features of spans, the width embedding and the external context; the entity recognition and relation extraction modules composed of traditional classifiers

3.2   Encoder

The encoder module is composed of a pre-trained BERT model and two feedforward neural networks (FFNs). The input sentence X is tokenized, obtaining a sequence of n tokens and passed through the encoder, obtaining an embedding sequence $(x_b^1, x_b^2, x_b^3 \ldots, \text{CLS})$ of length n+1, along with specific embedding representations $X_e(x_e^1, x_e^2, \ldots x_e^n)$ and $X_r(x_r^1, x_r^2, \ldots x_r^n)$ of length n, which are derived through the FFN layers(Eq. 1,2) and respectively for entity recognition and relation extraction. In order to facilitate the completion of subsequent tasks, we map all features generated by the encoder to the same dimension as the BERT output and denote it as d.

$$\text{FFN}(x_b^i) = \left(\text{ReLU}(x_b^i W_e^1 + b_e^1)\right) W_e^2 + b_e^2 \tag{1}$$

$$\text{FFN}(x_b^i) = \left(\text{ReLU}(x_b^i W_r^1 + b_r^1)\right) W_r^2 + b_r^2 \tag{2}$$

Both W and b are trainable weights and biases.

3.3 Interactive Fusion Representation

The employment of the attention mechanism facilitates the selective focus on critical information within input sequences, and Cross Attention allows for the exchange of information across disparate data, thereby enhancing the model's capacity to comprehend semantic context. As outlined in the introduction, we are supposed to consider the impact of entity recognition on relation extraction and vice versa. Consequently, the integration of Cross Attention is proposed to promote mutual interaction between entity recognition and relation extraction. After the interactive information is concatenated, it is further fused through BiLSTM. The architecture of the interactive fusion representation is depicted in Fig. 2.

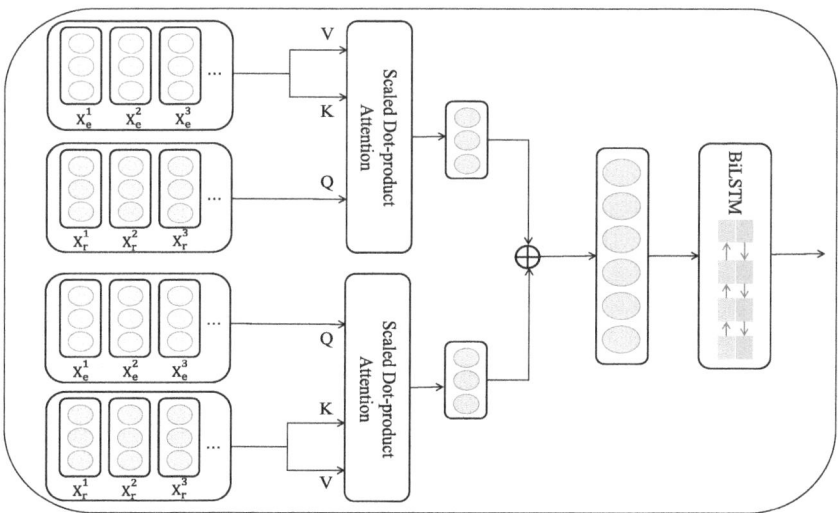

Fig. 2. The overall architecture of the interactive fusion representation

In this work, we use the scaled dot-product attention mechanism to implement Cross Attention. Specifically, using one of the representations obtained by the encoder for entity recognition(X_e) and relation extraction(X_r) as Query and the other as Key and Value. Through the computation of the scaled dot-product operation (Eq. 3, 4), revised representations for both entity recognition and relation extraction are derived. Subsequently, these revised representations $\widetilde{X}_e$ and $\widetilde{X}_r$ undergo concatenation via a Bidirectional Long Short-Term Memory (BiLSTM) architecture (Eq. 5), resulting in a novel embedding sequence $H = (h_1, h_2, ... h_n)$. This newly formed representation, reflecting the latest state post bilateral information exchange, is harnessed for the execution of subsequent tasks.

$$\widetilde{X}_e = \text{softmax}\left(\frac{X_r X_e^T}{\sqrt{d}}\right) X_e \tag{3}$$

$$\widetilde{X}_r = \text{softmax}\left(\frac{X_e X_r^T}{\sqrt{d}}\right) X_r \tag{4}$$

$$H = BiLSTM(\widetilde{X}_e \oplus \widetilde{X}_r) \tag{5}$$

H is the final result obtained by the interactive fusion representation module, and each token h_i in it is a d-dimensional vector.

3.4   Span-Based Feature Extraction

In our span-based feature extraction module, a slide window strategy is employed to facilitate effective span partition from input sequences. Consider an input sequence of length n, where the sliding window is configured with a size k. This approach systematically traverses the sequence, extracting all candidate spans of size k, illustrated in Fig 3(a). We constrain the window size because named entities tend not to span excessively long sequences, thereby enhancing computational efficiency. For each candidate span generated, a dual mask technique is applied to encode both the span and its contextual information. The encoding of span is that positions occupied by span tokens are assigned 1 while assigning 0 to all non-span positions; Inversely, the context mask assigns span token positions with 0 and all other context positions with 1, as depicted in Fig 3(b).

After partitioning the span, we extract three types of span features separately. For the existing sequence $H = (h_1, h_2, ... h_n)$ obtained through interactive fusion representation module and the span s $= (h_i, h_{i+1}, h_{i+2})$ with width of 3 to be predicted, we use max-pooling to extract internal features across spans(Eq. 6); We then use word embedding to map the discrete span width to a fixed dimensional continuous vector, and this feature is denoted as w_3 for span s and is used to clarify the boundary information of the span. Finally, We use the proposed SEA module for context feature extraction, which consists of Multi-Head Attention and BiGRU, as shown in Fig. 4. The input of the SEA module is the sequence with the span has been masked $H_{mask} = (h_1, ... h_{i-1}, [mask], [mask], [mask], h_{i+3}, .. h_n)$. Then the Multi-head Self-attention is used to capture contextual semantic information. To ensure the

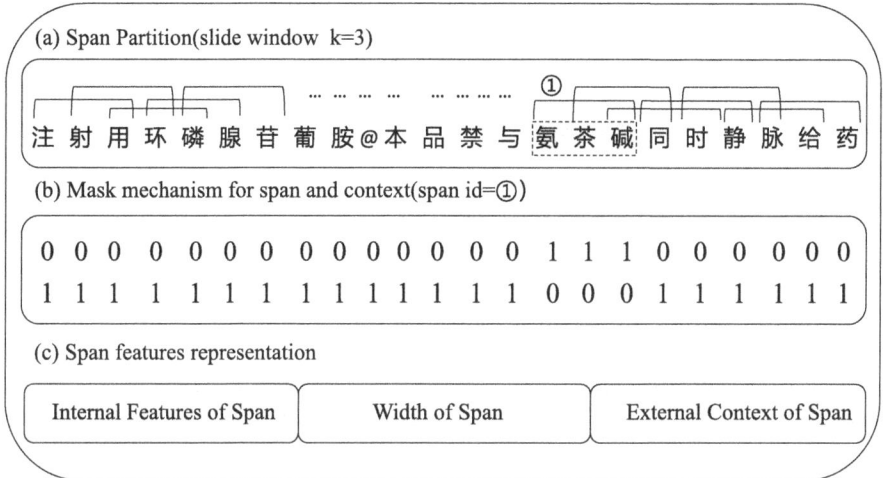

Fig. 3. The overall process of feature extraction based on span

integrity of the original information, residual structures are introduced. Meanwhile, due to the temporal insensitivity of the attention mechanism, a Bidirectional Gated Recurrent Unit (BiGRU) network is integrated into the SEA architecture. The final output of the SEA module is denoted as c. For inputs with dimension d, the calculation formulas of the SEA module are as follows (Eq. 7,8,9).

$$s = \text{maxpool}(h_i, h_{i+1}, h_{i+2}) \tag{6}$$

$$K/Q/V = H_{mask}W_{K/Q/V} \tag{7}$$

$$\text{Attention(K,Q,V)} = \text{softmax}\left(\frac{QK^T}{\sqrt{d}}\right)V \tag{8}$$

$$c = \text{BiGRU(Attention(K, Q, V))} \tag{9}$$

W_K, W_Q, W_V are trainable weights.

In Fig. 3(c), the three types of span features are concatenated and then used for entity recognition.

3.5 Entity Recognition

Our entity recognition classifier is a multi-class classifier and it uses any candidate spans as input. For example, let span $=(h_i, h_{i+1}, ... h_{i+m})$ represent a span whose width is m+1. We let ε represent the set of entity types included in the dataset, the classifier can map the span to an entity class. During the entity recognition phase, the representations we use are the concatenated representations obtained from the span-based feature extraction module z_e.

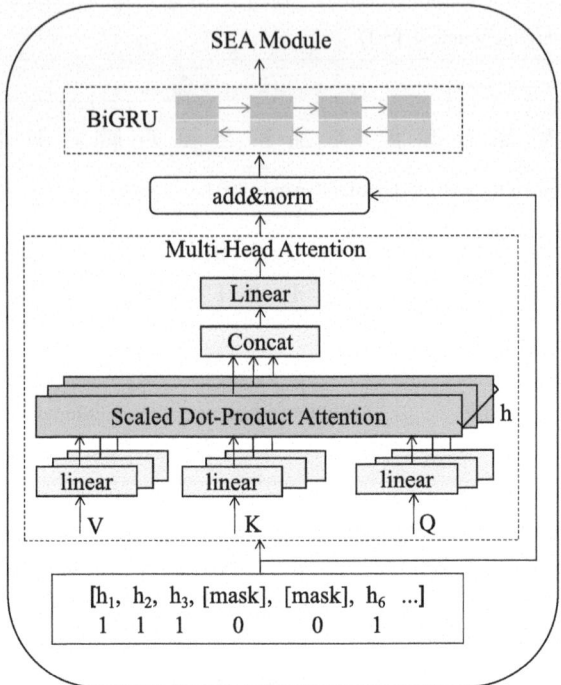

Fig. 4. The architecture of the SEA module

$$z_e = s \oplus w_{m+1} \oplus c \tag{10}$$

$$\tilde{y}_e = softmax(W'_e \cdot z_e + b'_e) \tag{11}$$

3.6   Relation Extraction

The relation extraction classifier uses candidate span pairs and the local context between them as input to predict whether there is a relation. For the given span pair (s_1, s_2) whose widths are p,q respectively, the span pair (s_1, s_2) are represented by their internal features and width features, and we can easily obtain contextual information between span pairs because we save mask records of spans when partitioning them, and we defined the context between the span pairs as $c(s_1, s_2)$. As relations are often asymmetric, we will predict whether there is a relation both in (s_1, s_2) and (s_2, s_1). It should be noted that we also consider the local context between span pairs as "spans", and like obtaining internal features of spans, we use max-pooling to obtain contextual information.

$$z_r^1 = (s_1 \oplus w_p) \oplus c(s_1, s_2) \oplus (s_2 \oplus w_q) \tag{12}$$

$$z_r^2 = (s_2 \oplus w_q) \oplus c(s_2, s_1) \oplus (s_1 \oplus w_p) \tag{13}$$

$$\tilde{y}_r^{1/2} = \sigma \left(W'_r \cdot z_r^{1/2} + b'_r \right) \tag{14}$$

3.7   Training

We use text annotated with entities and relations for training. By training, the fine-tuning BERT, a width embedding matrix for spans, and classifiers for entity recognition and relation extraction can be obtained. The loss of our model we defined is as follows (Eq. 15).

$$L = L_e + L_r \tag{15}$$

The L_e is the entity recognition loss and the L_r is the relation extraction loss. In the context of entity recognition, the model's output necessitates processing through a softmax activation function to yield the entity type with the maximum probability. The cross-entropy loss function (Eq. 16) is employed to compute the discrepancy between the predicted and actual categorical distributions for entity labels. Conversely, for relation extraction, the task reduces to determining whether a specific relation exists or not, which can be framed as a binary classification problem. Thus, the sigmoid function is utilized to map the model's output to a probabilistic representation confined between 0 and 1, and subsequently, the binary cross-entropy loss function is applied to measure the loss incurred during this binary classification process (Eq. 17). (y_e and y_r are the Ground Truth)

$$L_e = CrossEntropyLoss(\widetilde{y}_e, y_e) \tag{16}$$
$$L_r = BCEWithLogits(\widetilde{y}_r, y_r) \tag{17}$$

4   Experiments

4.1   Datasets

CoNLL04: The CoNLL04 dataset [26] is a widely-used public benchmark for joint entity and relation extraction, it comprises four primary entity types (Location, Organization, Person, and Other) and five distinct relation types (Work_for, Kill, Live_in, Organized_in, and Located_in). In this paper, We conducted experiments using the dataset provided by SpERT, which includes 922 training datasets and 231 testing datasets.

CH-DDI: This is a self-built Chinese drug-drug interactions dataset, which uses drug information from the website Yimaitong. Specifically, the steps for constructing the dataset are as follows: (1) Crawl drug-drug interactions in drug instrcutions related to five chronic diseases (coronary heart disease, COPD (Chronic Obstructive Pulmonary Disease), diabetes, hypertension, and osteoporosis), remove useless information, and obtain the original data after preliminary processing. Taking the treatment of hypertension with bumetanib tablets as an example, the raw data obtained is"<布美他尼片><药物相互作用><1.与多巴胺合用，利尿作用加强。2.肾上腺糖、盐皮质激素，促肾上腺皮质激素及雌激素能降低本药的利尿作用。3.与拟交感神经药物及抗惊厥药物合用，利尿

作用减弱>". (2) Perform sentence segmentation to obtain sentences containing complete drug interactions. After this processing, the above example will obtain "布美他尼片@与多巴胺合用，利尿作用加强—— 布美他尼片@肾上腺糖、盐皮质激素，促肾上腺皮质激素及雌激素能降低本药的利尿作用—— 布美他尼片@与拟交感神经药物及抗惊厥药物合用，利尿作用减弱" (3) Refer to the annotation of CoNLL04 to achieve annotation of our dataset. Taking the first sentence after sentence segmentation as an example, the annotated data obtained is "{"text": "布美他尼片@与多巴胺合用，利尿作用加强", "spo_list": ["predicate": "协同", "object_type": "@value": "药物", "subject_type": "药物", "object": "@value": "布美他尼片", "subject": "多巴胺"]}". In summary, under the guidance of clinical doctors, drug interactions are defined as seven types (antagonism, inhibition, synergy, taboo, irrelevance, promotion, addition), and we only marked drug entities with significant interactions. The processing flow of the entire dataset follows the above process and has been checked by three people.

The statistical results of the two datasets introduced above are shown in Table 1, And the statistical of the relations in the CH-DDI are presented in Table 2.

Table 1. The statistic of CoNLL04 and CH-DDI

	CoNLL04			CH-DDI		
	sentence	entity	relation	sentence	entity	relation
train	922	3377	1283	585	1830	1276
test	231	893	343	147	527	386

Table 2. The Statistic of Relations in CH-DDI

Relation types	Training dataset	Testing dataset
Antagonism	252	76
Inihibition	120	22
Synergy	319	118
Taboo	279	91
Irrelevance	187	31
Promotion	95	42
Addition	24	6

4.2 Evaluation Metrics and Experiment Settings

Evaluation Metrics: This article assesses the performance of the model in entity recognition and relation extraction. For entity recognition, a prediction is considered correct when a span is identified as an entity and its boundaries and types exactly match the ground truth. As for relation extraction, it is deemed accurate if both spans are correctly recognized as entities and the relation between these spans is accurately predicted. In particular, we compute the precision (Eq. 18), recall(Eq. 19), and F1-score (Eq. 20) on both macro and micro indicators for both entity recognition and relation extraction.

$$\text{Precision} = \frac{\text{TP}}{\text{TP} + \text{FP}} \tag{18}$$

$$\text{Recall} = \frac{\text{TP}}{\text{TP} + \text{FN}} \tag{19}$$

$$\text{F1} = \frac{2 * \text{Precision} * \text{Recall}}{\text{Precision} + \text{Recall}} \tag{20}$$

Experiment Settings: The model architecture incorporates BERT*base* as the underlying encoder for the CoNLL04 dataset, while Bio-BERT, specifically pre-trained on medical text, is utilized for the CH-DDI dataset. Both BERT models undergo fine-tuning during the training process to adapt to the respective tasks. Training involves the implementation of the Adam optimizer with a learning rate decay schedule, commencing with a peak learning rate of 2e-5. To optimize computational efficiency and convergence properties, the batch size for training iterations is empirically determined to be 2 following extensive experimental validations. Subsequently, the batch size is adjusted to 1 during the testing phase. Through meticulous experimentation, a relation threshold of 0.4 is established for the relation extraction. Based on Fig. 5, we set the dropout for the CoNLL04 to 0.1 and for the CH-DDI, it is 0.75. The epoch for training we set is 70. The same method as Eberts was used to generate negative samples, 100 negative entity and relation samples were generated during the training for each sentence in CoNLL04 and 50 negative entity and relation samples for each sentence in CH-DDI.

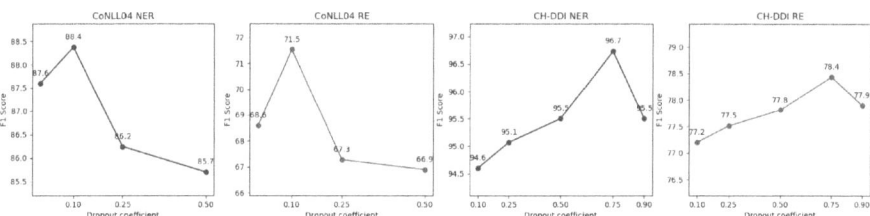

Fig. 5. Effect of dropout coefficient on CoNLL04 and CH-DDI

4.3   Comparison with Baseline Models

Table 3 and Table 4 shows the comparison results between our model and other models on two datasets. To ensure the reliability of our comparison, we reproduced all the benchmark models and conducted experiments on the two datasets introduced above to obtain and compare the best results.

GraphRel [17]: It is an end-to-end relation extraction model that uses graph convolutional networks (GCNs) to jointly learn named entities and relations.

CasRel [16]: This model utilizes binary taggers to extract entities and relations. It needs to pre-define the relation patterns (subject_type, relation, object_type).

SPN4RE [23]: SPN4RE is a prediction model designed for triple sets, which does not require consideration of the sequential output of traditional seq2seq models.

Multi-head [18]: It uses the CRF layer for entity recognition and then uses a Multi-head selection mechanism in the relation extraction.

SpERT [12]: This model is a span-based joint extraction method, which uses an entity classifier and a relation classifier to obtain entities and relations.

OneRel [8]: It is based on decoding algorithms and obtains relation triplets in one step.

STER [20]: It is a joint extraction model with knowledge distill framework and it has two teacher models for entity recognition and relation extraction respectively.

W2NER [27]: This model is based on tables, which generates a table for each input sequence and decodes the table to obtain the predicted entity and entity type.

ISER $_{GRU}$: It refers to remove the Semantic Enhancement Attention(SEA) module and only uses GRU to extract context information.

ISER $_{ChineseBERT}$: It refers to uses Chinese_BERT for CH-DDI rather than the Bio-BERT which has trained on large biomedical materials.

Table 3. Compares our model with other models on the CH-DDI

Methods	NER			RE		
	P	R	F	P	R	F
GraphRel$_{1p}$ [17]	51.98	68.85	59.23	31.76	49.48	38.69
GraphRel$_{2p}$ [17]	53.19	63.35	57.83	36.42	47.64	41.31
SPN4RE [23]	85.54	81.61	83.53	**84.04**	80.17	**82.06**
Multi-head [18]	89.03	91.67	90.33	69.21	70.83	70.01
SpERT [12]	92.63	97.72	95.11	75.38	76.96	76.17
OneRel [8]	–	–	–	**78.89**	78.27	**78.58**
STER [20]	94.09	96.64	95.35	74.27	80.10	77.08
W2NER [27]	95.05	96.04	95.54	–	–	–
ISER$_{GRU}$	94.11	97.53	95.79	74.87	78.01	76.41
ISER$_{ChineseBERT}$	94.01	98.29	96.10	75.25	79.58	77.35
ISER(micro)	**95.22**	**98.17**	**96.73**	**76.11**	**80.89**	**78.43**
ISER(macro)	**98.40**	**99.43**	**98.90**	**77.24**	**83.09**	**79.30**

Table 4. Compares our model with other models on the CoNLL04

Methods	NER			RE		
	P	R	F	P	R	F
GraphRel$_{1p}$ [17]	41.28	48.98	44.80	36.90	47.23	41.43
GraphRel$_{2p}$ [17]	44.39	48.40	46.30	40.78	45.77	43.13
CasRel [16]	–	–	–	58.95	43.83	50.28
SPN4RE [23]	63.67	57.73	60.55	63.02	57.14	59.94
Multi-head [18]	83.75	84.06	83.90	63.75	60.43	62.04
SpERT [12]	86.69	86.79	86.74	72.31	64.72	68.31
OneRel [8]	–	–	–	68.62	70.64	69.62
STER [20]	88.88	86.79	87.82	**75.00**	64.72	69.48
W2NER [27]	84.86	85.18	85.02	–	–	–
ISER$_{GRU}$	86.99	87.57	87.28	71.47	66.47	68.88
ISER(micro)	**89.54**	**87.23**	**88.37**	71.64	71.43	71.53
IESR(macro)	**86.66**	**82.44**	**84.32**	72.92	73.42	72.77

Comparative analysis of evaluation metrics reveals the necessity of leveraging domain-specific pre-training models such as the use of Bio-BERT for the medical field, because the Bio-BERT can provide some potential knowledge. As shown in Sect. 4.1, the annotation data our self-built dataset is:"{"text": "布美他尼片@与多巴胺合用，利尿作用加强", "spo_list": ["predicate": "协同", "object_type": "@value": "药物", "subject_type": "药物", "object": "@value": "布美他尼片", "subject": "多巴胺"]}. Before the "@" symble, it is an entity involved in drug interactions, which can be seen as entity prompting. And the dataset only contains one entity type Therefore, the performance of entity recognition on this dataset is excellent. Moreover, from the statistical situation of various relation types in Table 2, there is a data imbalance problem in the CH-DDI dataset, which may have a certain impact on relation extraction.

Our model demonstrates superior performance in joint extraction tasks. Experiments with the Graphrel [17] and Casrel [16] models indicate their reliance on substantial training data, the small-sized dataset we use leading to subpar performance. SPN4RE [23] is a seq2seq model designed for end-to-end task, simultaneously generating labels for entities and their corresponding triples. As a result, the model maintains consistent performance across both entity recognition and relation extraction. Our approach resembles a pipeline model, it concentrates on the two tasks for entities and relations, including improving performance in both tasks to ensure broad applicability. The multi-head selection [18] model excels in entity recognition but falls short in relation extraction due to limited semantic information. Shang et al. [8] proposed the one-stage triplet extraction model OneRel. It can effectively address the problem of relation overlap and has shown good performance on both datasets we use. STER is a model that uses knowledge distill to joint extract entities and relations which has excellent performance. In contrast to the span-based SpERT [12] model, our model achieves superior performance in both entity recognition and relation extraction. On the CH-DDI dataset, the F1-score of our model for both tasks increases by 1.62% and 2.26%. On the CoNLL04 dataset, our model exhibits improvements of 1.63% and 3.22% in the F1-score for entity recognition and relation extraction, respectively. The W2NER [27] achieves comprehensive entity recognition across domains and languages, showcasing superior performance. However, from Table 3 and Table 4, it can be seen that our model performs better than W2NER on both the CH-DDI dataset and the CoNLL04 dataset, with F1-score improved by 1.19% and 3.35% respectively.

Table 5. The results of the ablation study on CH-DDI

	NER			RE		
	P	R	F	P	R	F
-interactive fusion	94.03	98.67	96.30	74.88	79.58	77.16
SEA->CLS	94.11	96.96	95.51	74.62	77.75	76.15
LC->LC$_{att}$	94.98	97.83	96.38	76.92	79.11	78.00
LC->LC$_{BERT}$	94.81	97.15	95.97	76.84	78.13	77.48
LC->CLS	94.83	97.53	96.16	75.14	78.80	76.93
LC->GC$_{BERT}$	94.68	97.91	96.27	76.08	78.27	77.16
LC->GC	95.18	97.34	96.25	77.00	78.01	77.50
ISER	**95.22**	**97.72**	**96.73**	**76.11**	**80.89**	**78.43**

Table 6. The results of the ablation study on CoNLL04

	NER			RE		
	P	R	F	P	R	F
-interactive fusion	87.40	87.01	87.21	70.59	66.47	68.47
SEA->CLS	87.77	87.75	87.67	68.19	69.39	68.79
LC->LC$_{att}$	88.55	88.02	88.28	70.78	69.93	70.35
LC->LC$_{BERT}$	88.46	87.57	88.01	73.62	65.89	69.54
LC->CLS	88.98	87.68	88.32	60.44	71.72	65.60
LC->GC$_{BERT}$	87.90	86.23	87.05	61.52	66.18	63.76
LC->GC	88.94	86.45	87.67	66.28	66.47	66.38
ISER	**89.54**	**87.32**	**88.37**	**71.64**	**71.43**	**71.53**

4.4   Ablation Study

We performed seven ablation experiments, the results are presented in Table 5 and Table 6. In these experiments, "-interactive fusion" refers to the removal of the interactive fusion representation module; "SEA -> CLS" denotes the elimination of the proposed SEA module and the utilization of the CLS token generated by BERT; "LC -> LC_{att}" means we use self-attention to obtain the local context; "LC ->LC_{BERT}" refers to using the local context in the original BERT output; "LC -> CLS" signifies the utilization of the CLS token output by BERT; "LC -> GC_{BERT}" refers to using the whole output generated by BERT and "LC -> GC" denotes utilizing the whole output obtained through interactive fusion representation module.

Based on the experimental results presented in Table 5 and Table 6, it can be observed that our proposed interactive fusion representation module effectively enhances model performance, particularly in relation extraction, with an increase of 1.27% and 3.06% in F1-score on the CH-DDI and CoNLL04 datasets, respectively. After removing the Semantic Enhancement Attention (SEA) module we proposed and replacing it with the token CLS, the performance of entity recognition on both datasets decreased, which in turn affected subsequent relation extraction.

In addition, we focused on discussing the semantic information used in the relation extraction, the Fig 6 illustrates the comparison of F1-score for the replacement of the local context we use. It can be seen that whether using global or local context, the results obtained by using the representations through the interactive fusion representation module are better than using the original representations generated by BERT. On the CoNLL04 dataset, using the interactive global context increased the F1-Score for relation extraction by 2.62% compared to using the original BERT global context, and the results using the original BERT local context decreased the F1-Score by 1.99%. The same pattern was observed on the CH-DDI dataset. This once again proves the effectiveness of our proposed interactive fusion representation module. We also processed the local context using self-attention mechanism and compared the results. From Table 5 and Table 6, it can be seen that the results of using attention mechanism are not significantly improved from those of using max-pooling. Considering the efficiency of the model, we ultimately decide to use max-pooling. In addition, we can observe that on the CoNLL04 dataset, the performance of relation extraction fluctuates greatly after not using the local context. For example, when using global context obtained by BERT and the token CLS respectively, the F1-score decreases by 7.77% and 5.93%. On the dataset CH-DDI, there is not much change in performance, which is determined by the language characteristics. English often determines relations based on certain keywords, so the introduction of complete semantic information is equivalent to introducing too much redundant information, while some complex Chinese relations need to be judged based on complete semantics.

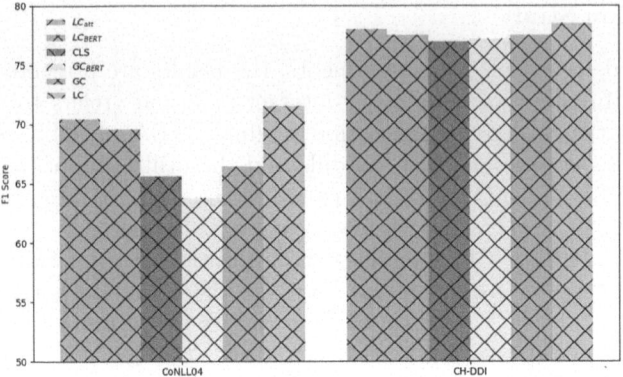

Fig. 6. The comparison of F1-Score for the ablation study

5   Interpretability Analysis

In this section, we visualized and analyzed the Cross Attention we use. Specifically, we aggregate the weight matrices obtained through scaled dot-product attention at the token level and normalize them. Figure 7 and Fig. 8 are specific visualization examples for ConLL04 and CH-DDI. From the figures, we can see that when using the relation representations as the query, the updated representations pay more attention to the overall semantics, especially the potential entities. The example in CoNLL04 dataset shows that the model assigns higher attention to "*WilkesBooth*" and "*Lincion*" and in the CH-DDI dataset, "注射用环磷腺苷葡胺" has high weight. While using entity representations as the query, Words related to relations are given higher weight. For example, in Fig. 7, "*assassinate*" is given the highest weight and it often implies a "*kill*" relation

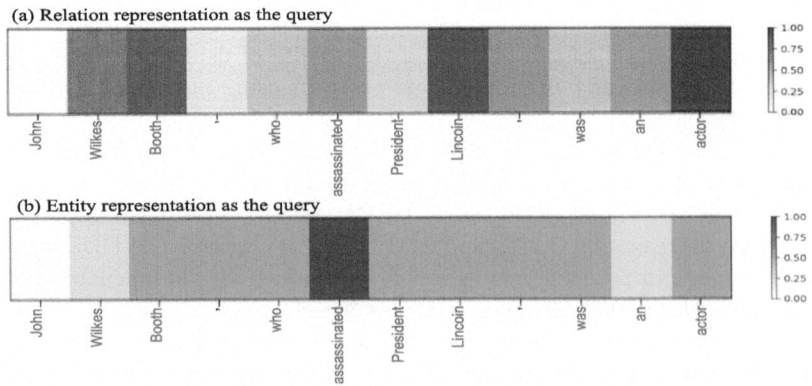

Fig. 7. Visualization of Cross Attention (CoNLL04)

in the sentence. In Fig. 8, the "禁与" has the highest weight and it means that there may be a "*taboo*" relation.

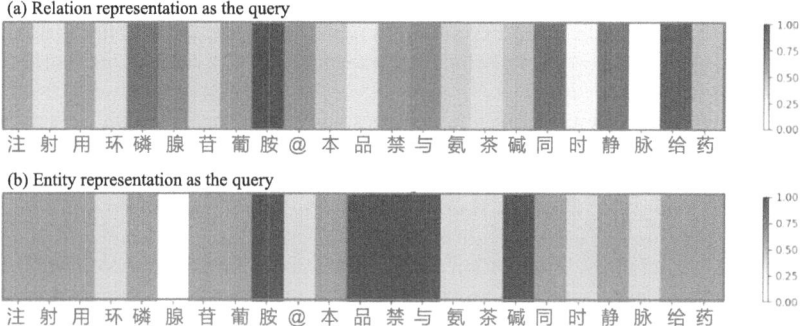

Fig. 8. Visualization of Cross Attention (CH-DDI)

6   Conclusion

This paper proposes a joint entity-relation extraction model based on span and Interactive fusion representation for Chinese medical texts with complex semantics, which achieves bidirectional information interaction between entity recognition and relation extraction. When performing entity recognition, the proposed SEA module can effectively obtain contextual semantics for partitioned spans, thereby improving the performance. The local context is used to supplement semantics in relation extraction to help circumvent potential confusion within the relation classifier caused by relation overlap issues. Our model performs well on the public dataset CoNLL04 and the self-bulit CH-DDI dataset.

In the future, we will do our best to improve our dataset CH-DDI to address the issue of data imbalance, and we will also explore more methods for information exchange in entity recognition and relation extraction.

Acknowledgment. This work was funded by the National Science and Technology Major Project (2021ZD0111000) and Henan Province Science and Technology Research Project (232102311232).

References

1. Mintz, M., Bills, S., Snow, R., Jurafsky, D.: Distant supervision for relation extraction without labeled data. In: Proceedings of the Joint Conference of the 47th Annual Meeting of the ACL and the 4th International Joint Conference on Natural Language Processing of the AFNLP, pp. 1003–1011 (2009)

2. Zhong, Z., Chen, D.: A frustratingly easy approach for entity and relation extraction. arXiv preprint arXiv:2010.12812 (2020)

3. Liu, Z., Li, H., Wang, H., Liao, Y., Liu, X., Gaojie, W.: A novel pipelined end-to-end relation extraction framework with entity mentions and contextual semantic representation. Expert Syst. Appl. **228**, 120435 (2023)

4. Ren, X., et al.: Cotype: Joint extraction of typed entities and relations with knowledge bases. In: Proceedings of the 26th International Conference on World Wide Web, pp. 1015–1024 (2017)

5. Yu, X., Lam, W.: Jointly identifying entities and extracting relations in encyclopedia text via a graphical model approach. In: Coling 2010: Posters, pp. 1399–1407 (2010)

6. Zheng, S., Wang, F., Bao, H., Hao, Y., Zhou, P., Xu, B.: Joint extraction of entities and relations based on a novel tagging scheme. In: Proceedings of the 55th Annual Meeting of the Association for Computational Linguistics (Volume 1: Long Papers), Vancouver, Canada, pp. 1227–1236. Association for Computational Linguistics (July 2017)

7. Ren, F., et al.: A novel global feature-oriented relational triple extraction model based on table filling. In Proceedings of the 2021 Conference on Empirical Methods in Natural Language Processing, Online and Punta Cana, Dominican Republic, pp. 2646–2656. Association for Computational Linguistics (November 2021)

8. Shang, Y.-M., Huang, H., Mao, X.: Onerel: Joint entity and relation extraction with one module in one step. In: Proceedings of the AAAI Conference on Artificial Intelligence, vol. 36, pp. 11285–11293 (2022)

9. Zeng, D., Liu, K., Lai, S., Zhou, G., Zhao, J.: Relation classification via convolutional deep neural network. In: Proceedings of COLING 2014, the 25th International Conference on Computational Linguistics: Technical Papers, pp. 2335–2344 (2014)

10. Miwa, M., Bansal, M.: End-to-end relation extraction using lstms on sequences and tree structures. arXiv preprint arXiv:1601.00770 (2016)

11. Zheng, S., et al.: Joint entity and relation extraction based on a hybrid neural network. Neurocomputing **257**, 59–66 (2017)

12. Eberts, M., Ulges, A.: Span-based joint entity and relation extraction with transformer pre-training. In: European Conference on Artificial Intelligence (2019)

13. Devlin, J., Chang, M.-W., Lee, K., Toutanova, K.: BERT: Pre-training of deep bidirectional transformers for language understanding. In: Proceedings of the 2019 Conference of the North American Chapter of the Association for Computational Linguistics: Human Language Technologies, Volume 1 (Long and Short Papers), Minneapolis, Minnesota, pp. 4171–4186. Association for Computational Linguistics (June 2019)

14. Ji, B., et al.: Span-based joint entity and relation extraction with attention-based span-specific and contextual semantic representations. In: Proceedings of the 28th International Conference on Computational Linguistics, pp. 88–99 (2020)

15. Xiong, X., Liu, Y., Liu, A., Gong, S., Li, S.: A multi-gate encoder for joint entity and relation extraction. In: China National Conference on Chinese Computational Linguistics, pages 163–179. Springer (2022). https://doi.org/10.1007/978-3-031-18315-7_11

16. Wei, Z., Su, J., Wang, Y., Tian, Y., Chang, Y.: A novel cascade binary tagging framework for relational triple extraction. In Proceedings of the 58th Annual Meeting of the Association for Computational Linguistics, pp. 1476–1488. Association for Computational Linguistics (July 2020)

17. Fu, T.-J., Li, P.-H., Ma, W.-Y.: Graphrel: modeling text as relational graphs for joint entity and relation extraction. In: Proceedings of the 57th Annual Meeting of the Association for Computational Linguistics, pp. 1409–1418 (2019)
18. Bekoulis, G., Deleu, J., Demeester, T., Develder, C.: Joint entity recognition and relation extraction as a multi-head selection problem. Expert Syst. Appl. **114**, 34–45 (2018)
19. Huang, W., Cheng, X., Wang, T., Chu, W.: BERT-based multi-head selection for joint entity-relation extraction. In: Tang, J., Kan, M.-Y., Zhao, D., Li, S., Zan, H. (eds.) NLPCC 2019. LNCS (LNAI), vol. 11839, pp. 713–723. Springer, Cham (2019). https://doi.org/10.1007/978-3-030-32236-6_65
20. Zhao, X., Yang, M., Qu, Q., Xu, R., Li, J.: Exploring privileged features for relation extraction with contrastive student-teacher learning. IEEE Trans. Knowl. Data Eng. (2022)
21. Wang, Y., Yu, B., Zhang, Y., Liu, T., Zhu, H., Sun, L.: TPLinker: single-stage joint extraction of entities and relations through token pair linking. In: Scott, D., Bel, N., Zong, C. (eds.) Proceedings of the 28th International Conference on Computational Linguistics, pp. 1572–1582, Barcelona, Spain. International Committee on Computational Linguistics (December 2020)
22. Vaswani, A., et al.: Attention is all you need. Adv. Neural Inform. Process. Systems **30** (2017)
23. Sui, D., Zeng, X., Chen, Y., Liu, K., Zhao, J.: Joint entity and relation extraction with set prediction networks. IEEE Trans. Neural Netw. Learn. Syst. (2023)
24. Zhang, Z., Zhao, Y., Gao, H., Mengting, H.: Linkner: linking local named entity recognition models to large language models using uncertainty. In: Proceedings of the ACM on Web Conference 2024, pp. 4047–4058 (2024)
25. Asada, M., Fukuda, K.: Enhancing relation extraction from biomedical texts by large language models. In: International Conference on Human-Computer Interaction, pp. 3–14. Springer (2024). https://doi.org/10.1007/978-3-031-60615-1_1
26. Carreras, X., Màrquez, L.:Introduction to the CoNLL-2004 shared task: Semantic role labeling. In: Proceedings of the Eighth Conference on Computational Natural Language Learning (CoNLL-2004) at HLT-NAACL 2004, 6 May - 7 May, Boston, Massachusetts, USA, pp. 89–97. Association for Computational Linguistics (2004)
27. Lu, Y., et al.: Unified structure generation for universal information extraction. arXiv preprint arXiv:2203.12277 (2022)
28. Nasar, Z., Jaffry, S.W., Malik, M.K.: Named entity recognition and relation extraction: State-of-the-art. ACM Comput. Surv. (CSUR) **54**(1), 1–39 (2021)
29. Li, J., et al.: Unified named entity recognition as word-word relation classification. In: Proceedings of the AAAI Conference on Artificial Intelligence, vol. 36, pp. 10965–10973 (2022)
30. Zelenko, D., Aone, C., Richardella, A.: Kernel methods for relation extraction. J. Mach. Learn. Res. **3**, 1083–1106 (2003)
31. Miwa, M., Sasaki, Y.: Modeling joint entity and relation extraction with table representation. In: Proceedings of the 2014 Conference on Empirical Methods in Natural Language Processing (EMNLP), pp. 1858–1869 (2014)
32. Su, J., et al.: Global pointer: Novel efficient span-based approach for named entity recognition. arXiv preprint arXiv:2208.03054 (2022)
33. Wang, H., et al.: Extracting multiple-relations in one-pass with pre-trained transformers. arXiv preprint arXiv:1902.01030 (2019)
34. Cao, J., Ananiadou, S.: Generativere: incorporating a novel copy mechanism and pretrained model for joint entity and relation extraction. In: Findings of the Association for Computational Linguistics: EMNLP 2021, pp. 2119–2126 (2021)

35. Kipf, T.N., Welling, M.: Semi-supervised classification with graph convolutional networks. arXiv preprint arXiv:1609.02907 (2016)
36. Dixit, K., Al-Onaizan, Y.: Span-level model for relation extraction. In: Proceedings of the 57th Annual Meeting of the Association for Computational Linguistics, pp. 5308–5314 (2019)
37. Wang, S., et al.: Gpt-ner: Named entity recognition via large language models. arXiv preprint arXiv:2304.10428 (2023)
38. Chan, Y.S., Roth, D.: Exploiting syntactico-semantic structures for relation extraction. In: Proceedings of the 49th Annual Meeting of the Association for Computational Linguistics: Human Language Technologies, pp. 551–560 (2011)
39. Tang, R., Chen, Y., Qin, Y., Huang, R., Zheng, Q.: Boundary regression model for joint entity and relation extraction. Expert Syst. Appl. **229**, 120441 (2023)

Multi-task Learning-Based Knowledge Graph Question Answering for Pediatric Epilepsy

Yingjie Han, Mengyuan Wang, Kunli Zhang[(⊠)], Jinzhao Zhang, Tengfei Chen, and Zhongtian Hua

College of Computer and Artificial Intelligence, Zhengzhou University, Zhengzhou, China
{ieyjhan,ieklzhang}@zzu.edu.cn

Abstract. In the field of Knowledge graph Question Answering (KGQA), Semantic Parsing-based (SP) methods have become increasingly prominent. These methods, particularly those translating natural language into logical forms via generative models, have shown promising results. However, a key challenge in SP-based KGQA is the potential for noise introduction when incorrect or irrelevant information is used during the learning process. This noise can significantly degrade the performance of logical form generation, a critical aspect of KGQA. To tackle this issue, we propose a framework named the Multi-task with Loss Optimization for KGQA (MLO-KGQA), which significantly employs the balanced uncertainty weight loss approach to optimize the loss function in multi-task learning. MLO-KGQA takes logical form generation as the primary task, with entity disambiguation and subgraph selection as subtasks. The critical innovation of our framework is the application of balanced uncertainty weighting, which optimizes loss weights during multi-task learning, effectively reducing the noise problem. Experimental results on Pediatric Epilepsy Knowledge Graph Question Answer (PEKGQA) and CCKS2023-CKBQA show that the MLO-KGQA demonstrates a significant improvement in performance.

Keywords: Knowledge Graph · Question answering · Multi-task Learning · Logical Form Generation

1 Introduction

Knowledge Graph Question Answering (KGQA) aims to answer natural language questions using facts extracted from large-scale Knowledge Graphs (KGs). Examples of prominent KGs include Freebase [1], DBpedia [2], Wikidata [3], KQApro [4], Zhishi.me [5], and PKUbase [6], which provide a solid data foundation for the development of KGQA systems. Mainstream KGQA methods are roughly categorized as either Information Retrieval (IR) [7–9] or Semantic Parsing (SP) [10–12]. The first method directly scores the relevance between the question and query path, making it challenging to address intricate questions. Using the SP-based approach, natural language is converted into logical forms (λ-DCS [13], SPARQL [14], S-expressions [15]) and executed against the knowledge base to produce answers. These logical forms are generated by fine-tuning a pre-trained encoder-decoder model.

© The Author(s), under exclusive license to Springer Nature Singapore Pte Ltd. 2025
Y. Zhang et al. (Eds.): CHIP 2024, CCIS 2433, pp. 217–233, 2025.
https://doi.org/10.1007/978-981-96-3752-2_13

However, the basic model cannot generate entities and relations that have not been learned during training. To address this problem, Das et al. [16] augmented logical form generation with question-query pairs as auxiliary information. Ye et al. [17] ranked the candidate logical forms, then enhanced the generation process with the top-ranked candidates. However, these two methods did not effectively use fine-grained auxiliary information. Although they introduced auxiliary information, noise is also introduced into the generated model, which makes it difficult to generate accurate logical form.

To reduce the impact of noise and improve the generalization of logical forms, Zhang et al. [18] extracted relevant fine-grained auxiliary information from a knowledge base and reconstructed this information into medium-grained knowledge pairs. This approach aimed to generate final logical expressions that can be executed after transformation. However, it did not consider the linkages between individual tasks. Hu et al. [19] introduced a multitask learning approach to jointly learn entity disambiguation, relationship classification, and logical form generation, to mitigate the impact of noise in auxiliary information. Multi-task learning can effectively use auxiliary information and reduces the noise, but the method cannot guarantee that the classified relations are related to the subject entity, and does not consider the issue of balancing loss weights across tasks, which results in the model not getting effective learning from the entity disambiguation and relation classification tasks, and introduces noisy entities or relations, and reduces the overall performance of the model.

To address loss weight imbalance in multitask learning, Kendall et al. [20] introduced a Bayesian correlation framework. This approach considers prediction uncertainty in semantic and instance segmentation tasks in computer vision. It automatically adjusts task weights based on their current magnitudes. However, in tasks involving both regression and classification, the model may exhibit bias towards the regression task, negatively impacting the learning of the classification task.

In summary, we propose a KGQA framework called MLO-KGQA, which treats entity disambiguation and subgraph filtering as classification tasks and logical form generation as a regression task. The framework uses multi-task learning to jointly train each task and incorporates a balanced uncertainty-weighted approach to auto-tuning the loss weights of each subtask in the multi-task learning process.

2   Method

This section offers a comprehensive introduction to the MLO-KGQA framework. The preprocessing module is utilized to extract candidate entities and subgraphs that are relevant to the given question. The multi-task learning module enhances the generation of the logical form of questions through entity disambiguation and subgraph filtering, focusing on disambiguation, subgraph filtering, and logical generation. During this process, we use a method that balances uncertainty to optimize the loss in training. After obtaining the logical form of the question, the logical form is converted to obtain SPARQL, and SPARQL is executed in the knowledge base to obtain the answer (Fig. 1).

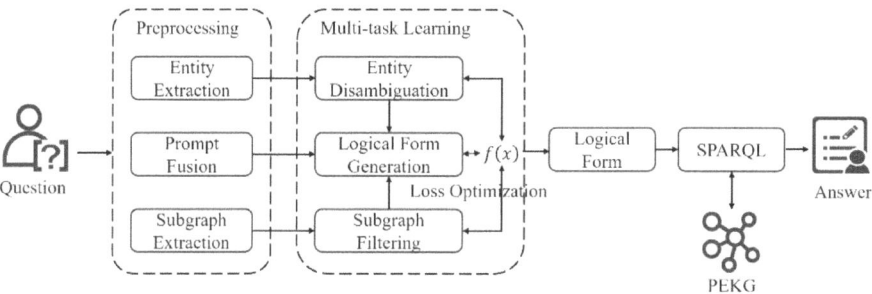

Fig. 1. MLO-KGQA framework.

2.1 Preprocessing

The KGQA requires understanding and answering questions, which requires preprocessing steps such as entity identification and relation extraction [21]. Entity extraction, prompt combination, and subgraph extraction are realized by the question q preprocessing module, with the goal of obtaining candidate entities e and candidate subgraphs g, and designing a reasonable prompt for the logical form generation task to prepare for subsequent tasks.

Entity Extraction. Entity extraction is a necessary pre-processing step in KGQA that aims to identify key entities from user-provided queries to better understand questions. As illustrated in Fig. 2, this process comprises three main modules—Named Entity Recognition (NER), Entity Linking, and Entity Ranking—to generate candidate entities. NER combines deep learning models [22] and rule-based entity recognition methods to improve the accuracy and recall of entity recognition. The Entity Linking module processes entity mentions using an inverted index table and an alias dictionary. This step retrieves all related entities in the knowledge graph that correspond to the entity mentioned in the question. The Entity Ranking considers two primary features—the similarity between candidate entities and the query, and entity weight—to rank these entities. The top 10 entities in the ranking are retained as candidate entities for further processing in the next stage.

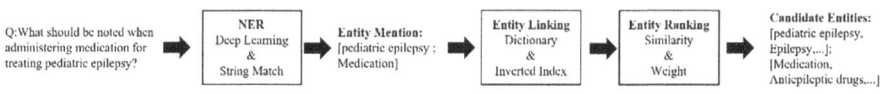

Fig. 2. Entity Processing Flow.

Prompt Combination. In the fine-tuning of downstream tasks, the T5-Pegasus [23] model relies significantly on prompts. These prompts serve as essential guides, equipping the model with relevant information for effectively executing specific tasks. To assist the model in understanding and generating the logical form corresponding to a given question, a specific prompt is designed: 'Transform the question into an S-expression: question. | {entity} | {subgraph}.' For instance, the prompt for the question 'What should be noted when administering medication for treating pediatric epilepsy?' would be: 'Transform the question into an S-expression: What should be noted when administering medication for treating pediatric epilepsy? | {entity} | {subgraph}.' Here, {entity} and {subgraph} serve as markers for different auxiliary information.

Subgraph Extraction. The subgraph is formed by combining triple query paths. To control the size of candidate subgraphs and ensure that all questions are covered as much as possible, paths within 3-hop of the candidate entities are extracted to construct the set of candidate subgraphs. The number of subgraphs linked to an entity grows exponentially with the increase in number of path hops. Addressing this issue involves the application of cluster search to regulate the expansion of retrieval paths. As shown in Fig. 3, using the question "What should be noted when administering medication for treating pediatric epilepsy?" as an example, only the three most relevant paths to this question are preserved at each hop during the retrieval process. Relevance is determined based on the similarity between the question and the subgraph.

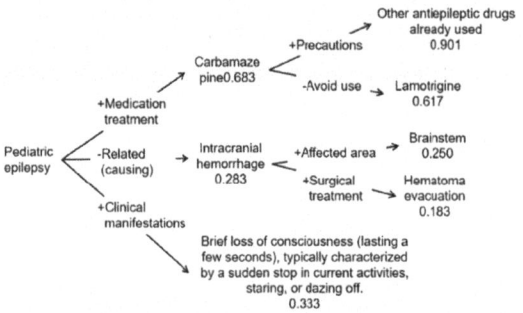

Fig. 3. Beam search with integrated direction.

2.2 The Logical Form Generation Model Based on Multi-Task Learning

In order to effectively utilize auxiliary information for the generation of logical forms, a multi-task learning model was designed, as shown in Fig. 4. Serving as the core of the MLO-KGQA framework, this model employs T5-Pegasus as its base model, utilizing its encoder as a shared encoder to obtain vector representations of queries, entities, and subgraphs. These vectors are then fed into corresponding neural networks, facilitating entity disambiguation, subgraph filtering, and logical form generation. The aim of this model is to fully exploit the shared encoder, thereby achieving efficient use of information from queries, entities, and subgraphs.

Entity Disambiguation. The task of entity disambiguation is treated as a text-matching task, where the relevance between the question and an entity is assessed and ranked to identify the most pertinent entity. Recognizing the limitations of the semantic information inherent in a single entity for effective semantic computation, the relationships within one hop of the entity are considered as supplementary semantic information.

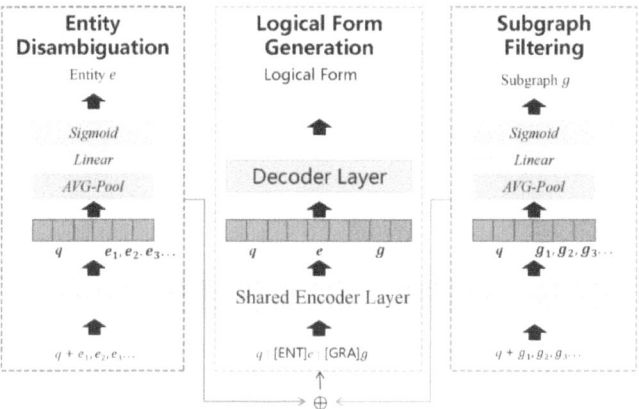

Fig. 4. Multi-task learning model.

The BM25 [24] algorithm is employed to rank relationships within one hop of an entity, and the three most relevant groups of relationships are selected as its supplementary semantic information. Upon obtaining this supplementary information, it is concatenated with the entity e to form an "entity- relationship" combination. By integrating relationships within one hop of the entity, the model can more comprehensively consider the relationship between the candidate entity and the question.

The formal description of entity filtering is shown in Eqs. (1)–(4). The question q is concatenated with the entity-relationship combination e_i and input into the T5-Pegasus encoder. The resulting vector is then averaged using pooling, and the average pooled result is fed into a fully connected layer to calculate the relevance score $s(\cdot)$ between the entity-relationship combination and the question. The entity disambiguation loss function $\mathcal{L}^{ENT}$ is the binary cross-entropy loss. Here, $FC(\cdot)$ represents the fully connected layer, e_i denotes the entity to be filtered, i is the entity's classification label, and k is the number of candidate entities.

$$Encoder\_output = T5\_encoder(q + E) \tag{1}$$

$$Avg\_polling = \frac{1}{N} \sum_{i=1}^{N} Encoder\_output_i \tag{2}$$

$$s(q, e_i) = Sigmoid(FC(Avg\_poling)) \tag{3}$$

$$\mathcal{L}^{ENT} = -\frac{1}{k} \sum_{1}^{k} \left[v_i \cdot log(s(q, e_i)) + (1 - v_i) \cdot log(1 - s(q, e_i)) \right] \tag{4}$$

Subgraph Filtering. Subgraph filtering is achieved by calculating the semantic similarity between the subgraph and the question. The question q is concatenated with the subgraph, and then passed through the T5-Pegasus encoder for average pooling, followed by a fully connected layer. The Sigmoid function is used to calculate the similarity between the question q and the subgraph g. This computational process is illustrated in Eqs. (5) and (6). Binary cross-entropy loss is employed as the loss function for subgraph filtering.

$$s(q, g_i) = Sigmoid(FC(Avg\_polling(T5\_encoder(q + g)))) \tag{5}$$

$$\mathcal{L}^{GRA} = -\frac{1}{k} \sum_{1}^{k} [v_i \cdot log(s(q, e_i)) + (1 - v_i) \cdot log(1 - s(q, e_i))] \tag{6}$$

Logical Form Generation. The objective of the logical form generation task is to generate the logical form of a given question. The filtered entity and subgraph are utilized as auxiliary information to enhance the generation of the logical form. Specifically, the question q, entity e, and subgraph g are concatenated using special symbols. Moreover, to explicitly inform the model of the type of each element, the labels "[ENT]" and "[GRA]" are added before each entity and subgraph, respectively. This representation, which incorporates the query and auxiliary information, is denoted as shown in (7), Q_{all} represents the representation of the question with auxiliary information, where i denotes the number of entities and j denotes the number of subgraphs.

$$Q_{all} = question|[ENT]e_1, e_2|[GRA]g_1, g_2 \tag{7}$$

The calculation of the probability of the target logical form generated by T5-Pegasus is depicted in (8)–(10). This involves obtaining a vector through the T5-Pegasus encoder, where x_i represents the i-th token of the input, and n is the number of tokens. y_i denotes the i-th token of the target logical form. Subsequently, the T5-Pegasus decoder decodes this representation token by token into the logical form.

$$[h_1, h_2 \ldots h_n] = T5\_encoder(Q_{all}) \tag{8}$$

$$p_j = T5\_decoder(a_1, a_2 \ldots a_n, h_1, h_2 \ldots h_n) \tag{9}$$

$$\mathcal{L}^{LOG} = -\frac{1}{m} \sum_{j=1}^{m} logp_j, a_j \tag{10}$$

2.3   Balanced Uncertainty Weight Loss

The MLO-KGQA framework is divided into three subtasks: entity disambiguation, subgraph filtering and logical form generation. The training objective of the multitask learning model is formulated as a loss function as shown in (11), where ω_i is the task-specific weight and $\mathcal{L}_i$ is the task-specific loss function.

$$\mathcal{L} = \sum_i \omega_i \cdot \mathcal{L}_i \tag{11}$$

Model performance is affected by the weights w_i. As shown in Fig. 5, when w_i is equal, the model is dominated by the logical form generation task.Entity disambiguation and subgraph filtering are not converged.The case study shows that logical form generation is wrong when the entities and sub-diagrams of the auxiliary information are incorrect.The results were shown experimentally that the probability of logical form generation can be improved by correct auxiliary information.Important steps for generating correct logical form are taken by entity disambiguation and subgraph filtering. It is required to balance the loss weights of the three tasks. Weights can be adjusted manually, and it can be a tedious and time-consuming process.

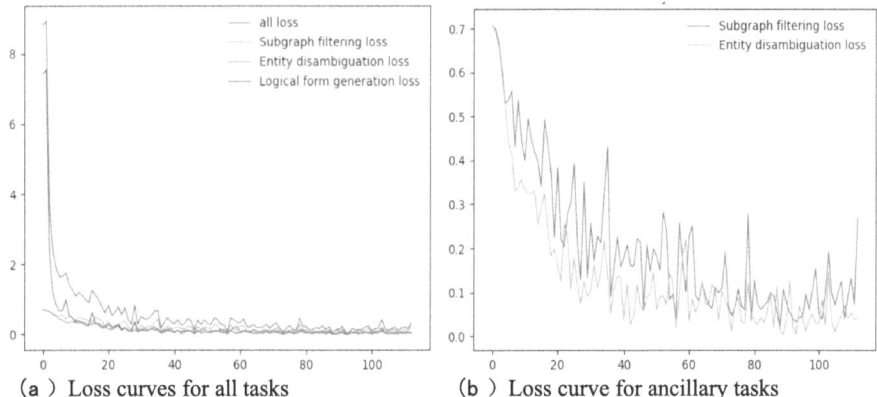

(a) Loss curves for all tasks   (b) Loss curve for ancillary tasks

Fig. 5. Loss curves for each task on PEKGQA.

In order to solve unbalanced loss weights, a method is designed to automatically balance the loss weights, as shown in (12), (13). The simultaneous occurrence of a generation task and a regression task in loss computation cannot be handled by the method of uncertainty weighting [25]. To solve this problem, losses from entity disambiguation and subgraph filtering are deflated by balanced uncertainty weight loss to the same order of magnitude as the logical form generation task. Finally, balanced uncertainty weight loss is used to balance the loss weights of multiple tasks.

$$\mathcal{L} = \frac{1}{2\sigma_1^2}\mathcal{L}^{LOG} + \frac{c_1}{2\sigma_2^2}\mathcal{L}^{ENT} + \frac{c_2}{2\sigma_3^2}\mathcal{L}^{GRA} + log\sigma_1\sigma_2\sigma_3 \qquad (12)$$

$$c_1 = \frac{\mathcal{L}^{LOG}}{\mathcal{L}^{ENT}} \; c_2 = \frac{\mathcal{L}^{LOG}}{\mathcal{L}^{GRA}} \qquad (13)$$

For the loss functions of entity disambiguation and subgraph screening, the ratios $\mathcal{L}^{LOG}/\mathcal{L}^{ENT}$ and $\mathcal{L}^{LOG}/\mathcal{L}^{GRA}$ are calculated in the computational graph and used to separate these tasks from the graph before computation. The uncertain parameter σ_i is a learnable parameter designed to represent task-specific uncertainty. It is initialized during training and updated through gradient descent based on the loss functions, enabling it to adapt to the inherent uncertainty of each task.

By introducing uncertainty as a loss weight for each task, the model is added the ability to dynamically adjust the loss. By introducing an optimization strategy that balances uncertainty weighting, entity disambiguation and subgraph screening tasks are accommodated by the model while completing the logical form generation task. The performance effect on the sub-tasks is improved by this optimization strategy. The reduction of noise introduced by erroneous auxiliary information is enhanced by this optimization strategy.

3 Experiment

3.1 Datasets and Evaluation Metrics

Datasets. The PEKGQA dataset is constructed based on PEKG [26] (**P**ediatric **E**pilepsy **K**nowledge **G**raph) and PEQAC (**P**ediatric **E**pilepsy **Q**uestion **A**nswering **C**orpus), aiming to provide a high-quality data source for pediatric epilepsy question answering systems. This dataset supports intelligent question answering systems in clinical decision support, patient education, and medical inquiry applications. The construction of PEKG follows medical standards and guidelines, and after discussions with medical experts, the conceptual layers of the knowledge graph in the pediatric epilepsy domain were established. The knowledge graph was built through four key steps: data collection and processing, knowledge extraction, manual-checking, and knowledge fusion. In the end, PEKG includes 25 entity types, 53 relationship types, totaling 38,634 entities, and 176,577 triples. PEQAC, on the other hand, was formed through data collection, processing, manual verification, and clustering analysis, resulting in 11,141 high-quality question-answer pairs. The PEKGQA dataset is generated by combining the entities and relational triples from PEKG with the question intent distributions and query templates from PEQAC. It employs both rule-based and contextual learning methods to construct the questions. According to the statistics, The PEKGQA dataset contains 5,400 data entries, of which 28.7% are simple questions, while 72.2% are complex questions. An example is provided in Table 1.

Table 1. Example of PEKGQA.

Data type	example
Question	What precautions should be taken when administering medication for the treatment of West syndrome?
SPARQL	Select ? y where { <West syndrome > < Medication treatment > ? y. ?y < Precautions > ?x}
Answer	This product may affect the results of certain laboratory tests…

The CCKS2023-CKBQA [27] (**C**hinese **K**nowledge **B**ase **Q**uestion **A**nswering) serves as a comprehensive Open Domain Knowledge Graph Q&A dataset, encompassing questions from diverse fields such as culture, sports, history, finance, and healthcare.

The dataset comprises a total of 7,625 entries, with an equal distribution of 1,292 entries each in the validation and test sets. The knowledge base was derived from PKU-base, a large-scale Chinese knowledge base developed by Peking University, which boasts 41,009,141 triples involving 13,930,117 entities. Training data and validation data are presented in the form of "question-SPARQL query-answer", as shown in Table 2.

Table 2. Example of CCKS2023-CKBQA.

Data type	example
Question	What are the recommended 5-km hotels near Ningbo Nanyuan Global Hotel
SPARQL	select ?y where { <Nanyuan Universe Deluxe Hotel > < distance > ?cvt. ?cvt < entity name > ?y. ?cvt < distance > ?distance. Filter(?distance < = 5).?y < type > < hotel >.}
Answer	< Ningbo Kaiyuan Mingdu Hotel > < Ningbo Nanyuan Hotel >

To investigate the performance of MLO-KGQA on different types of questions, an analysis was conducted based on the question classification system proposed in papers [28, 29], focusing on common questions in pediatric epilepsy. The questions were categorized into three main types and nine subtypes based on SPARQL query characteristics. The specific categories and their associated SPARQL features are summarized in Table 3. Single-hop questions are classified as simple, while the remaining types are considered complex.

In the PEKGQA dataset, 28.7% of the questions are simple, while 72.2% are complex. Among the complex questions, 22.2% are multi-hop, 33.3% are constraint-based, and 16.7% involve logical reasoning. In the CCKS2023-CKBQA dataset, 56% of the questions are simple, 27% are multi-hop, 12% are constraint-based, and 5% are logical operation questions. Additionally, 1% of the questions in the CCKS2023-CKBQA dataset fall into 'other' categories, which include those that don't fit into the aforementioned classifications.

Evaluation Metrics. The goal of KGQA is to use entities in the knowledge base to answer natural language questions. The validity of their methods in KGQA was averaged using Precision, R(Recall) and F1 values and the formulae are shown in (14)–(16). Q denotes the set of questions, A_i denotes the set of answers given by the system for the i-th question, and G_i denotes the standard answer for the i-th question.

$$P_i = \frac{|A_i \cap G_i|}{|A_i|} \qquad (14)$$

$$R_i = \frac{|A_i \cap G_i|}{|G_i|} \qquad (15)$$

$$F1 = \frac{1}{|Q|} \sum_{i=1}^{|Q|} \frac{2P_i R_i}{P_i + R_i} \qquad (16)$$

Table 3. Question types and Features

Question Type	Subtype	SPARQL Features
Chain Questions	Single-Hop Questions Multi-Hop Questions	One topic entity, variable types equal to the number of triples
Constraint Restrictions	Entity Constraint Relation Constraint Conditional Constraint	Multiple topic entities, one type of variable, one relation Multiple topic entities, one type of variable, multiple relations Multiple topic entities, multiple variables, fewer relations than triples
Logical Operations	Statistical Operations Comparison Operations Aggregation Operations Composite Operations	One topic entity, contains "COUNT" keyword One topic entity, contains "FILTER" keyword One topic entity, contains "ORDER BY" keyword Multiple topic entities, composite questions, containing multiple operators

3.2 Implementation Detail

Hyperparameters. The model is generated using T5-Pegasus [23]. The number of candidates for entities and subgraphs was set to 10, and the learning rate was initialized to 0.0001. Adam was used as the optimizer, and the model was trained for 30 rounds with a batch size of 16. Generating 50 sets of S-expressions is used to ensure that the decoded generated S-expressions are executable, converted to SPARQL queries and executed sequentially until a non-empty query result is returned.

3.3 Experimental Results and Analysis

Main Results. In order to validate the effectiveness, we compare the performances of our model with a wide range of state-of-the-art models, which include image captioning Yang et al. [30], ChatKBQA [31], KB-BINDER [32], RNG-KBQA [17], FC-KBQA [18],GMT-KBQA [19].

As shown in Table 4., the F1 score of MLO-KGQA on the PEKGQA dataset reaches 83.2%. Although this is 3.4% and 2.6% lower than the methods proposed by Yang et al. and KB-BINDER, respectively, the parameter size of the generative model used is 0.2 B, which is significantly smaller than the base models of Yang et al. and KB-BINDER, leading to more resource efficiency. Furthermore, the semantic understanding capability of T5-Pegasus is inherently weaker compared to Chat GLM and LLAMA, which somewhat affects the model's overall semantic comprehension ability. But MLO-KGQA can achieve more noticeable results when using the same number of parameters. Upon further analysis, RNG-KBQA constructs logical forms from all 2-hop subgraphs of the topic entity, introducing excessive auxiliary information, which cause difficult in semantic

Table 4. Comparison in PEKGQA datasets.

Models	Size	Methods	F1(%)
ChatGLM	6B	Yang	**86.6**
LLAMA	7B	ChatKBQA	82.2
		KB-BINDER	85.8
T5-Pegasus	0.2B	RNG-KBQA	79.7
		GMT-KBQA	73.3
		FC-KBQA	67.7
		MLO-KGQA	83.2

understanding. In contrast, GMT-KBQA does not consider the convergence trends of loss weights between multiple tasks during multi-task learning, which negatively impacts the accuracy of auxiliary tasks and thus degrades overall performance. Although FC-KBQA reduces the amount of auxiliary information, the multiple inferences, from fine-grained to coarse-grained reasoning, result in noise accumulation.

To validate the generalizability of MLO-KGQA on public test datasets, we conducted comparative experiments on the CCKS2023-KBQA dataset. Table 5 presents the evaluation results of MLO-KGQA on the CCKS2023-CKBQA dataset. The top-ranked method achieved a score of 75.63%, while the second-ranked method scored 74.34%. These results were sourced from the evaluation leaderboard [27].

Table 5. Comparison on CCKS2023-CKBQA datasets.

Model	F1(%)
Yang	**75.63**
USTC	74.34
GMT-KBQA	51.82
FC-KBQA	48.97
MLO-KGQA	74.33

The results show that the F1 score of the MLO-KGQA method on the CCKS2023-CKBQA task test set reached 74.33%, closely approaching the scores of the first and second-ranked models. Upon analysis, it was observed that both the FC-KBQA and GMT-KBQA methods rely on directly extracting relations from the question and then ranking them. However, in this dataset, the relations in the questions are often difficult to directly map to the knowledge base. Incorrectly identified relations introduce noisy data, leading to suboptimal overall performance. In contrast, the subgraph extraction and filtering steps effectively handle the retrieval of relations. Although the overall performance of MLO-KGQA on the public test did not meet initial expectations, it demonstrated promising results in handling complex relations, validating the potential effectiveness of the proposed approach. Future improvements in relation mapping strategies and noise control mechanisms are expected to yield better performance on public datasets.

Ablation Studies. To validate that the introduction of the multi-task learning approach can more effectively extract auxiliary information, we conducted an ablation study by removing both the multi-task learning and loss optimization methods to assess the impact on the auxiliary information extraction task. The ablation experiments were carried out on the CCKS2023-CKBQA dataset, which is more diverse and challenging compared to the PEKGQA dataset. As a result, this dataset was selected to perform the ablation study. The experimental results are presented in Table 6.

Table 6. Effect of multi-task learning on entity disambiguation and subgraph screening in CCKS2023-CKBQA.

Model	Entity Disambiguation			Subgraph filtering		
	P(%)	R(%)	F1(%)	P(%)	R(%)	F1(%)
MLO-KGQA	**79.00**	72.35	**75.52**	**96.47**	94.51	**95.47**
w/o LO	76.37	69.52	72.48	94.58	**95.49**	95.03
w/o MTL	70.03	**74.39**	72.14	85.73	86.17	85.94

Multi-task learning approach is more effective in extracting auxiliary information is proved experimentally. Experiments are used to verify the effectiveness of the auxiliary information extraction task after removing the multi-task learning with loss optimization approach. The experimental results are shown in Table 5. Without using a multi-task learning strategy: in the entity disambiguation task, both precision and F1 are degraded and recall is improved; in the subgraph screening task, all three metrics are degraded. Multi-task learning and loss optimization strategies can be used to improve model performance on sub-tasks.

In order to explore the impact of the sub-tasks and their combinations in depth for the ablation analysis, different frameworks were combined and used for comparison. w/o Entity denotes that the entity linking task was removed from the framework. w/o Graph denotes that the subgraph screening task was removed from the framework.

Table 7. Ablation experiment on CCKS2023- CKBQA.

Framework	F1(%)	Δ (%)
MLO-KGQA	**74.33**	–
w/o Entity	72.56	−1.77
w/o Graph	72.30	−2.03
w/o Entity, Graph	70.48	−3.85

The data is displayed in Table 7. And the MLO-KGQA performance is considered significantly better than the others. With the removal of subgraph information, the overall performance of the model was degraded. The overall performance was affected by the subgraph information. Entities, relationships, and path directions are included in the subgraphs, providing rich auxiliary information for generating the model. Meanwhile, the importance of auxiliary tasks is further demonstrated by the fact that model performance is generally degraded as more tasks are removed.

Loss Weight Optimization Results.   In order to verify the necessity of loss weight optimization method based on balanced uncertainty weighting for multitask learning strategy, BART, T5, and T5-Pegasus are used as the base generating models, respectively. Different loss weight optimization strategies are selected for experiments on the base generation models. The experimental results are shown in Table 8.

Table 8. Optimization results of loss weight of different basic models (F1(%))

Base Model	T5-Pegasus	T5	BART
Uncertainty [25]	73.97	72.59	60.11
Balance	73.63	72.30	59.24
Not optimized [19]	70.30	69.33	55.82
Balance Uncertainty	**74.33**	**73.12**	**61.37**

As can be seen from the experimental results, the performance of the loss weighting optimization strategy is boosted on different models. The order of magnitude of the loss between tasks was not taken into account by the uncertainty weighting. This strategy leads to the overall performance of the task, balancing the uncertainty weighting effect is boosted. Multi-task learning is experimentally verified to be effective. Due to the lack of consideration for the magnitude of losses among various tasks in uncertainty weighting, there is a resultant decline in overall task performance. Conversely, balancing uncertainty weighting yields the most pronounced improvement in effectiveness.

Experimental Results on Different Question Types.   To assess the performance of MLO-KGQA in handling different types of complex questions, experiments were conducted, and the results are presented in Table 9.

The experimental results show that on the PEKGQA dataset, MLO-KGQA achieves F1 scores of 97.6% for simple questions and 95.7% for entity constraint-based questions. On the CCKS2023-CKBQA dataset, the F1 score for chain questions is 75.9%, while it is 97.3% for entity constraint-based questions. The experimental results of MLO-KGQA on logical operation questions are generally lower. To investigate the reasons for its poor performance on conditional constraint and logical operation type questions, we will conduct a case study below.

Table 9. Experimental results of MLO-KGQA on different question types.

Question Type	Subtype	F1(%)	
		PEKGQA	CCKS2023-CKBQA
Chain Questions	Single-Hop Questions	97.6	75.9
	Multi-Hop Questions	83.4	
Constraint Restrictions	Entity Constraint	95.7	97.3
	Relation Constraint	92.6	59.3
	Conditional Constraint	77.0	26.9
Logical Operations	Statistical Operations	45.9	6.8
	Aggregation Operations	49.5	11.0
	Composite Operations	54.8	15.8
	Composite Operations	44.9	5.0
Other	Relationship Query	–	79.2
	No entity	–	5.7
Average	–	83.2	74.3

Case Study. To evaluate the strengths and weaknesses of the MLO-KGQA method, this paper presents a case study on two questions, analyzing the intermediate results generated during the SPARQL query process in MLO-KGQA, as shown in Table 10.

Table 10. Case study of MLO-KGQA on the PEKGQA dataset.

Query	Intermediate Output	Ground Truth	Predicted Result
What diseases can cognitive epilepsy induce?	Entity	Cognitive epilepsy	Cognitive epilepsy
	Subgraph	Cognitive epilepsy + Related (causing)	Cognitive epilepsy + Related (causing)
	S-expression	(AND (R Related (causing)) cognitive epilepsy)	(AND (R Related (causing)) cognitive epilepsy)
What are the drugs that cost less than 50 yuan to treat epilepsy?	Entity	Epilepsy; "50"	Epilepsy; "50"
	Subgraph	Epilepsy + Drug Treatment + Price	Epilepsy + Drug Treatment; 50 – Price
	S-expression	(AND (LT Price 50)) (JOIN (R Drug Treatment) Epilepsy)	(AND (JOIN Price 50)) (JOIN (R Drug Treatment) Epilepsy)

Taking the question "What diseases can cognitive epilepsy induce?" as an example, the entities were correctly extracted, and the corresponding query subgraph was successfully identified, leading to the correct generation of the S-expression. However, for the question "What are the drugs that cost less than 50 yuan to treat epilepsy?", although the entities were correctly extracted, the optimal query subgraph was not identified, resulting in an incorrect S-expression. Analysis shows that when the question involves logical operations, semantic parsing becomes more challenging, making it harder to identify the optimal subgraph, and thus leading to errors in generating the logical form.

4 Conclusion

This paper addresses the issue of noise introduced by the improper inclusion of auxiliary information in Knowledge Graph Question Answering for Pediatric Epilepsy. We propose a multi-task learning approach for KGQA that incorporates balanced uncertainty weight loss optimization. Multi-task learning reduces model parameters and memory footprint by sharing underlying structures, leading to more efficient task processing. It also leverages inter-task relationships to improve overall performance. Balanced uncertainty loss optimization dynamically adjusts the loss weights of individual tasks, effectively addressing the issue of divergent convergence behaviors during multi-task training. Experimental results demonstrate that, even under resource-constrained conditions, the proposed method achieves performance comparable to large-scale models on the PEKGQA dataset. MLO-KGQA no restrictions on the syntax of logical forms or the representation of entities and relationships. Therefore, it is applicable to new knowledge graphs. The CCKS2023-CKBQA results further validate the method's generalization ability. Future work will focus on enhancing the performance of logical operation-based complex questions through advanced techniques in semantic parsing and subgraph identification.

Acknowledgments. The work was partially supported by the National Science and Technology Major Project – "New Generation of Artificial Intelligence" (No. 2021ZD0111000), the Science and Technology Tackling Project of the Henan Provincial Science and Technology Department (No. 232102211039), and the Key Research and Development Program of Henan Province (No. 241111212700). We sincerely thank the anonymous reviewers for their insightful comments and constructive suggestions, which greatly contributed to improving this paper.

References

1. Bollacker, K., Evans, C., Paritosh, P., et al.: Freebase: a collaboratively created graph database for structuring human knowledge. In: Proceedings of the 2008 ACM SIGMOD International Conference on Management of Data, pp. 1247–1250 (2008)
2. Lehmann, J., Isele, R., Jakob, M., et al.: Dbpedia–a large-scale, multilingual knowledge base extracted from Wikipedia. Semantic web 6(2), 167–195 (2015)
3. Vrandečić, D., Krötzsch, M.: Wikidata: a free collaborative knowledgebase. Commun. ACM 57(10), 78–85 (2014)
4. Cao, S., Shi, J., Pan, L., et al.: KQA pro: A dataset with explicit compositional programs for complex question answering over knowledge base. arXiv preprint arXiv:2007.03875, (2020)
5. Niu, X., Sun, X., Wang, H., et al.: Zhishi. me-weaving Chinese linking open data. In: The Semantic Web–ISWC 2011: 10th International Semantic Web Conference, Bonn, Germany, October 23–27, 2011, Proceedings, Part II 10, pp. 205–220. Springer, Berlin (2011). https://doi.org/10.1007/978-3-642-25093-4_14

6. http://pkubase.gstore.cn/
7. Bordes, A., Usunier, N., Chopra, S., et al.: Large-scale simple question answering with memory networks. arXiv preprint arXiv:1506.02075, (2015)
8. Wang, Z., Zhang, J., Feng, J., et al.: Knowledge graph embedding by translating on hyperplanes. In: Proceedings of the AAAI Conference on Artificial Intelligence, vol. 28(1) (2014)
9. Lin, Y., Liu, Z., Sun, M., et al.: Learning entity and relation embeddings for knowledge graph completion. In: Proceedings of the AAAI Conference on Artificial Intelligence, vol. 29(1) (2015)
10. Berant, J., Chou, A., Frostig, R., et al.: Semantic parsing on freebase from question-answer pairs. In: Proceedings of the 2013 Conference on Empirical Methods in Natural Language Processing, pp. 1533–1544 (2013)
11. ;Ye, X., Yavuz, S., Hashimoto, K., et al. RNG-KBQA: generation augmented iterative ranking for knowledge base question answering. In: Proceedings of the 60th Annual Meeting of the Association for Computational Linguistics (Volume 1: Long Papers), pp. 6032–6043 (2022)
12. Zhang, L., Zhang, J., Wang, Y., et al.: FC-KBQA: a fine-to-coarse composition framework for knowledge base question answering. In: Proceedings of the 61st Annual Meeting of the Association for Computational Linguistics (Volume 1: Long Papers), pp. 1002–1017 (2023)
13. Liang, P.: Lambda dependency-based compositional semantics. arXiv preprint arXiv:1309.4408, (2013)
14. Pérez, J., Arenas, M., Gutierrez, C.: Semantics and complexity of SPARQL. ACM Transactions on Database Systems (TODS) **34**(3), 1–45 (2009)
15. Gu, Y., Kase, S., Vanni, M., et al.: Beyond IID: three levels of generalization for question answering on knowledge bases. In: Proceedings of the Web Conference 2021, pp. 3477–3488 (2021)
16. Das, R., Zaheer, M., Thai, D., et al.: Case-based reasoning for natural language queries over knowledge bases. In: Proceedings of the 2021 Conference on Empirical Methods in Natural Language Processing, pp. 9594–9611 (2021)
17. Ye, X., Yavuz, S., Hashimoto, K., et al.: RNG-KBQA: generation augmented iterative ranking for knowledge base question answering. In: Proceedings of the 60th Annual Meeting of the Association for Computational Linguistics (Volume 1: Long Papers), pp. 6032–6043 (2022)
18. Zhang, L., Zhang, J., Wang, Y., et al.: FC-KBQA: a fine-to-coarse composition framework for knowledge base question answering. In: Proceedings of the 61st Annual Meeting of the Association for Computational Linguistics (Volume 1: Long Papers), pp. 1002–1017 (2023)
19. Hu, X., Wu, X., Shu, Y., et al.: Logical form generation via multi-task learning for complex question answering over knowledge bases. In: Proceedings of the 29th International Conference on Computational Linguistics, pp. 1687–1696 (2022)
20. Kendall, A., Gal, Y., Cipolla, R.: Multi-task learning using uncertainty to weigh losses for scene geometry and semantics. In: Proceedings of the IEEE Conference on Computer Vision and Pattern Recognition, pp. 7482–7491 (2018)
21. Han, X., Wang, Z., Zhang, J., et al.: Overview of the CCKS 2019 knowledge graph evaluation track: entity, relation, event and QA. arXiv preprint arXiv:2003.03875, (2020)
22. Zhang, K., Zhang, C., Ye, Y., et al.: Named entity recognition in electronic medical records based on transfer learning. In: Proceedings of the 2022 International Conference on Intelligent Medicine and Health, pp. 91–98 (2022)
23. Su, J.: T5 PEGASUS - ZhuiyiAI.2021.https://github.com/ZhuiyiTechnology/t5-pegasus
24. Gomaa, W.H., Fahmy, A.A.: A survey of text similarity approaches. International Journal of Computer Applications **68**(13), 13–18 (2013)
25. Robertson, S., Zaragoza, H.: The probabilistic relevance framework: BM25 and beyond. Foundations and Trends® in Information Retrieval, vol. 3(4), pp. 333–389 (2009)

26. Zhang, K., Gao, Q., Zhang, J., et al.: Construction of Chinese pediatric epilepsy Knowledge Graph. In: 2023 IEEE 36th International Symposium on Computer-Based Medical Systems(CBMS), pp. 241–244. IEEE (2023)
27. https://tianchi.aliyun.com/competition/entrance/532100/rankingList
28. Bao, J., Duan, N., Yan, Z., et al.: Constraint-based question answering with knowledge graph. In: Proceedings of COLING 2016, the 26th International Conference on Computational Linguistics: Technical Papers, pp. 2503–2514 (2016)
29. Jia, Y.: Research on Knowledge Base Question Answering Based on Query Graph. Soochow University (2022). https://doi.org/10.27351/d.cnki.gszhu.2022.001585
30. Yang, S., Teng, M., Dong, X., et al.: LLM-Based SPARQL generation with selected schema from large scale knowledge base. In: China Conference on Knowledge Graph and Semantic Computing. Singapore: Springer Nature Singapore, pp. 304–316 (2023)
31. Luo, H., Tang, Z., Peng, S., et al.: Chatkbqa: a generate-then-retrieve framework for knowledge base question answering with fine-tuned large language models. arXiv preprint arXiv:2310.08975, (2023)
32. Li, T., Ma, X., Zhuang, A., et al.: Few-shot In-context Learning for Knowledge Base Question Answering. arXiv preprint arXiv:2305.01750, (2023)

Hypertension Medication Recommendation Based on Synergy and Selectivity of Heterogeneous Medical Entities

Ke Zhang[1] , Zhichang Zhang[1(✉)] , Yali Liang[1] , Wei Wang[1] , and Xia Wang[2]

[1] College of Computer Science and Engineering, Northwest Normal University, Lanzhou 730070, Gansu, China
zzc@nwnu.edu.cn
[2] Gansu Provincial Hospital, Lanzhou 730070, Gansu, China

Abstract. Electronic health records (EHR) store rich data of medical entities, such as diagnoses, procedures, and medications, which are invaluable in the development of automated systems for hypertension medication recommendations. These entities within EHR demonstrate significant synergies during the treatment process. However, existing medication recommendation methods predominantly focus on homogeneous graphs, thus overlooking the crucial synergistic relationships among heterogeneous medical entities. Moreover, accurately modeling the progression of hypertension using EHR is essential for precise medication recommendations, but current approaches often lack comprehensive temporal modeling and do not fully meet clinical requirements. To overcome these challenges, this paper introduces a novel model for hypertension medication recommendation that leverages the synergy and selectivity of heterogeneous medical entities. Initially, patient EHRs are utilized to construct both heterogeneous and homogeneous graphs. The inter-entity synergies are then captured using a multi-head graph attention mechanism, which enhances the entity-level representations. Subsequently, a dual-layer temporal selection mechanism calculates selective coefficients between current and historical visit records, thereby aggregating these to form refined visit-level representations. Ultimately, medication recommendation probabilities are determined based on these comprehensive patient representations, yielding practical and actionable recommendations. Experimental evaluations conducted on the real-world dataset MIMIC-IV v2.2 demonstrate that our model significantly outperforms baseline models. It achieves a Jaccard similarity coefficient of 55.82%, a precision-recall AUC of 80.69%, and an F1 score of 64.83%, thereby demonstrating its superior efficacy in medication recommendation. These results underscore the potential of our model to enhance clinical decision-making in the management of hypertension.

Keywords: Hypertension Medication Recommendation · Electronic Health Records · Heterogeneous Graph · Multi-head Graph Attention Mechanism · Time Series Selective Mechanism

© The Author(s), under exclusive license to Springer Nature Singapore Pte Ltd. 2025
Y. Zhang et al. (Eds.): CHIP 2024, CCIS 2433, pp. 234–250, 2025.
https://doi.org/10.1007/978-981-96-3752-2_14

1 Introduction

Hypertension is a common chronic disease and a major risk factor for cardiovascular mortality, making timely pharmacological intervention for blood pressure management crucial [1]. With the increasing trend of an aging population, the rising number of hypertension patients has placed a significant burden on healthcare systems [2]. Consequently, automated medication recommendation systems for hypertension have been developed.

Early hypertension medication recommendation methods are primarily rule-based. For example, Wu et al. developed a hypertension ontology and reasoning rules to recommend appropriate antihypertensive medications to patients [3]. However, these methods relied only on predefined rules and a limited set of case data, neglecting other critical patient information, which resulted in recommendations that lacked flexibility and personalization. In recent years, numerous neural network models for recommending hypertension medications based on Electronic Health Records (EHR) have been proposed [4, 5]. These models have shown improved outcomes and effectively address many limitations inherent in earlier algorithms.

Nevertheless, the complexity of EHR data continues to present significant challenges for medication recommendation tasks, particularly in two critical areas:

Insufficient Synergy Among Heterogeneous Medical Entities: EHR generated during medical visits include diverse medical entities such as diagnoses, treatment procedures, and medications, which have a significant synergistic effect during patient treatment. For example, diagnostic results often inform a patient's health status, which in turn guides the formulation of treatment plans. The selected treatment procedures and medications within these plans are expected to work synergistically to optimize treatment efficacy. Capturing this synergy between diverse medical entities is essential for effective medication recommendations. Current methods primarily use graph structures to address this issue, with models like MiME [6] and GCT [7] exploring potential causal relationships among different medical codes. Based on this assumption, MiME learns multilevel representations in a hierarchical sequence, while GCT concurrently learns the hidden causal structures of entities during prediction. However, these studies focus only on homogeneous graphs and overlook the heterogeneity of medical entities in original health records.

Neglect of Temporal Dynamics in Patient Condition: As a chronic disease, hypertension evolves over time. In clinical practice, physicians often synthesize both current and historical medical visit data to fully capture the progression of a patient's condition and tailor treatment plans accordingly. Therefore, effectively integrating visit information for temporal modeling of disease progression is another key issue in medication recommendation. Yang et al. modeled the time dependency of medications through two medical sequences but did not consider the correlation between these sequences [8]. Similarly, Liu and colleagues used three heterogeneous LSTM models to simulate the correlation between different medical sequences while ignoring the impact of the patient's current condition on treatment decisions [9]. These methods have not fully modeled the development process of a patient's condition.

To address the issues mentioned above, this paper introduces CSRec, a hypertension medication recommendation model that leverages the integration of heterogeneous medical entities and selective temporal modeling. The model comprises two key modules: the Heterogeneous Synergy Module and the Temporal Selectivity Module. In the Heterogeneous Synergy Module, to capture the synergistic effects between different medical entities, the model first extracts data from individual medical visits to construct both heterogeneous and homogeneous graphs, then employs a Multi-Head Graph Attention Mechanism (GAT) to update nodes and obtain entity-level representations of medical entities. In the Temporal Selectivity Module, to effectively simulate the progression of hypertension, the model calculates selection coefficients for the current health status against historical medical visits for the same patient, selectively aggregating historical visit data to achieve visit-level medical entity representations. Finally, various types of medical entities are concatenated to form a comprehensive patient representation, which is utilized for personalized hypertension medication recommendations. Additionally, to ensure the safety of recommended medications, the model integrates knowledge about Drug-Drug Interactions (DDI).

The main contributions of this paper are as follows:

- We present CSRec, a model that constructs a graph from EHR integrating diverse medical entities. Utilizing graph attention, CSRec learns enhanced collaborative entity representations. It also employs a temporal selection mechanism to model hypertension progression, achieving comprehensive patient representation for hypertension medication recommendations.
- To fully capture the synergistic effects between medical entities, we innovatively modify the traditional GAT to focus more on neighboring node information, thus obtaining a more aggregated representation of the principal nodes.
- Extensive experiments are conducted on the public dataset MIMIC-IV [10] to demonstrate the advanced nature and effectiveness of the proposed model.

2 Related Work

2.1 Graph Neural Network-Based Medication Recommendation

Graph Neural Networks (GNN) are capable of learning node embeddings in a graph and effectively aggregating information from neighboring nodes. Therefore, researchers often utilize GNN to model EHR in medication recommendations. For instance, Shang et al. proposed the GAMENet model, which used a graph convolutional network to integrate medical knowledge from EHR graphs and Drug-Drug Interaction (DDI) graphs, addressing the issue of potential side effects caused by medication interactions [11]. However, this model did not integrate knowledge from other medical entities such as diagnoses and procedures. To more comprehensively learn information from different medical entities, Shang et al. further employed pre-training techniques to propose the G-BERT model, but it overlooked the medication safety issue [12]. Subsequently, Wang et al. introduced the CompNet model, which modeled medications in a graph in an unordered manner. However, this model incurred high learning costs and poor stability when dealing with large numbers of patients and a vast medication space [13]. Yang et al. attempted to model the molecular structures of medications as graphs to simulate interactions between medication molecules and their effects on diseases, thereby facilitating medication recommendations [14]. Meanwhile, Li et al. used graph contrastive learning to model differences between current and historical medical visits [15]. However, existing graph-based studies struggled to ensure both the effectiveness and safety of medication recommendations simultaneously.

Therefore, this paper proposes modeling EHR as complete heterogeneous graphs and extending the conventional Graph Attention Network (GAT) to learn within this framework.

2.2 Temporal Modeling-Based Medication Recommendation

Research on temporal modeling of EHR for medication recommendations has been extensive. For example, the RETAIN model proposed by Choi et al. utilized an attention mechanism to precisely identify historical medical visits and key clinical variables that have significant impacts on the treatment process [16]. An et al. employed an interactive Long Short-Term Memory network to model time dependencies and capture hierarchical relationships between different sequences to simulate the decision-making process of physicians [17]. Hung et al. utilized a memory-enhanced neural network model to simulate complex interactions and long-term dependencies between two asynchronous sequential views [18]. Yang et al. focused on the prescription medications from the most recent visit and captured changes in patient health status between two adjacent visits through a residual mechanism [19]. Wu et al. used the Transformer architecture to model the temporal relationships among a patient's historical diagnoses, medications, and current diagnosis, and introduced a copying mechanism to determine whether to replicate previous medications or generate new ones [20].

Inspired by previous research, this paper designs a Temporal Selectivity Module to effectively simulate the progression of diseases.

3 Problem Formulation

3.1 Electronic Health Records

Electronic Health Records (EHR) encompass a variety of medical visit information collected from patients. For a specific patient, EHR can be represented as a collection of multiple medical visit records, denoted as $V = \left[V^1, V^2, \cdots, V^T\right]$, where V^t represents the t-th visit and T is the total number of visits for the patient. Specifically, the t-th visit can be represented as $V^t = \left[V_d^t, V_p^t, V_m^t\right]$, where $V_d^t \in \{0,1\}^{|D|}$, $V_p^t \in \{0,1\}^{|P|}$, and $V_m^t \in \{0,1\}^{|M|}$ are the multi-hot encoded vectors for diagnosis, procedures, and medications, respectively. Here, $|*|$ denotes the total number of categories for the respective medical entities.

3.2 Heterogeneous Medical Entities

In this paper, different types of medications are defined as medication entities within the model. Any medication appearing in the EHR has its corresponding medication entity, where each entity corresponds to a unique identifier, denoted as $\{m_1, m_2, \cdots\}$, and is embedded independently in the model with the same dimension. Similarly, diagnoses and procedures are classified into diagnostic entities and procedural entities, respectively. These three types of entities are collectively referred to as heterogeneous medical entities.

3.3 Hypertension Medication Recommendation

Using the patient's current visit diagnosis information V_d^t, procedure information V_p^t, historical visit sequence $V = [V^1, V^2, \cdots, V^{T-1}]$, and the heterogeneous medical entity graph G, the model recommends appropriate antihypertensive medications $\hat{y}_t \in \{0,1\}^{|M|}$ to the patient.

4 Hypertension Medication Recommendation Based on the Collaborative and Selective Properties of Heterogeneous Medical Entities

In this section, we will detail the architecture of the CSRec model. As illustrated in Fig. 1, the model consists of three modules: (1) In the Heterogeneous Collaborative Module, we designed both heterogeneous and homogeneous graph networks, focusing on aggregating the collaboration between different entities to update the entity-level representations. (2) In the Temporal Selectivity Module, we calculate the selection coefficients of the current visit against previous visit records through a bidirectional selection mechanism, and then integrate these into a visit-level representation. (3) The Interaction Prediction Module is used for integration and output. We concatenate the visit-level representations of heterogeneous medical entities into the final patient representation, which is then transformed into probabilities of medication recommendation. Medications exceeding the threshold are outputted as results.

4.1 Heterogeneous Collaborative Module

For a specific patient, we initially construct a complete medication graph $G_{mm}(t-1) = \{M(t-1), A^{mm}\}$, where $M(t-1)$ represents the set of all medications from the patient's historical visits, and A^{mm} denotes the med-med collaborative interaction adjacency matrix. Each element in the matrix represents the initial collaboration coefficient between the corresponding nodes. The process of constructing the matrix is shown in Fig. 2. Initially, A^{mm} is set as a zero matrix. If medication i and medication j co-occur during a specific visit, $A[i,j] = 1$; if medication i and j co-occur across multiple visits, the corresponding value in A^{mm} is incremented, with higher values indicating stronger collaboration between the medications.

Each medication node $m \in M(t-1)$ in the graph corresponds to its initial embedding vector.

$$e_m = V_m^{t-1} E_m \tag{1}$$

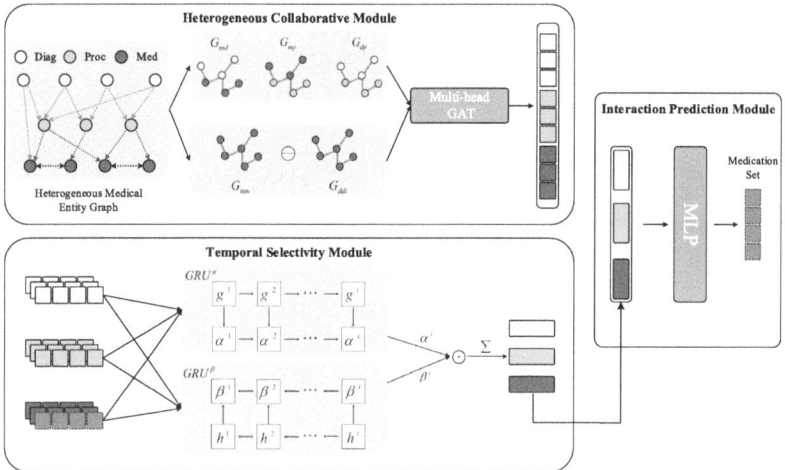

Fig. 1. The framework of CSRec.

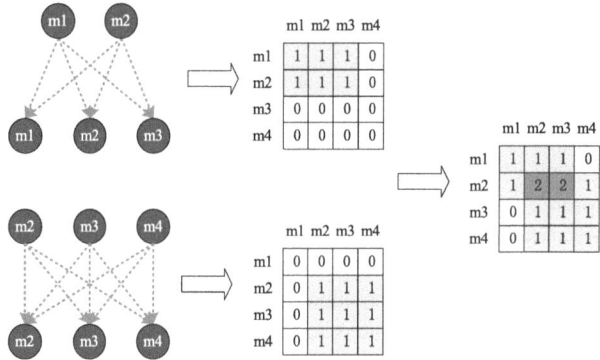

Fig. 2. The med-med synergy matrix construction process.

Moreover, some medications may have harmful interactions (DDI) and should be avoided when used together. To address this, we integrate the medication collaboration graph G_{mm} with the medication safety graph G_{ddi}, enhancing the comprehensive representation of the medication nodes.

$$G_m = G_{mm} - \lambda G_{ddi} \qquad (2)$$

Subsequently, we use a GAT-based graph neural approach to learn the representations of medication nodes in the graph G_m:

- Utilize the attention mechanism to calculate the attention coefficients between a node and its neighbors, followed by normalization

$$\alpha_{ij}^{(m)} = \frac{exp\left(g_{ij}^{(m)}\right)}{\sum_{k \in N_i^{(m)}} exp\left(g_{ik}^{(m)}\right)} \tag{3}$$

Specially, $g_{ij}^{(m)} = LeakyReLU\left(\beta^{(m)^T}\left(h_i^{(m)} \| h_j^{(m)}\right)\right); N_i^{(m)}$ represents the set of neighbor nodes of node m_i in the graph G_m, $\beta^{(m)}$ is the learnable attention vector, and $\|$ denotes the concatenation operation.

- Employ the calculated attention coefficients to perform weighted aggregation of neighbor nodes, thereby obtaining the representation of node m_i:

$$e_i^{(m)} = \sigma\left(\sum_{j \in N_i^{(m)}} \gamma_{ij}^{(m)} h_j^{(m)}\right) \tag{4}$$

- To overcome the limitations of a single perspective, we employ a multi-head attention mechanism, using a linear layer to map node representations into multiple subspaces, and then aggregate representations under each subspace. This can be represented as:

$$e_i^{(m)} = \|_{h=1}^{H} \sigma\left(\sum_{j \in N_i^{(m)(h)}} \gamma_{ij}^{(m)(h)} h_j^{(m)(h)}\right) \tag{5}$$

In this equation, H is the number of attention heads, the superscript (h) indicates the current attention head index, and $\|$ represents concatenating outputs from different heads. This method captures unique node information in respective dimensions, integrating features from various subspaces to significantly enhance the accuracy and robustness of the model's node representations.

During the training process, each medication entity is updated according to the above steps, resulting in an aggregated representation of the medication set $V_m = \{v_m^1, v_m^2, \cdots v_m^{t-1}\}$.

Similarly, we define three heterogeneous complete graphs: the diag-pro graph $G_{dp}(t) = \{D(t), P(t), A^{dp}\}$, the med-diag graph $G_{md}(t) = \{M(t-1), D(t), A^{md}\}$, and the med-pro graph $G_{mp}(t) = \{M(t-1), P(t), A^{mp}\}$. Following a similar learning approach to the medication graph G_m, we first initialize the diagnosis and procedure nodes in the three heterogeneous graphs.

$$e_d = V_d^t E_d, e_p = V_p^t E_p \tag{6}$$

Then, we learn from the diag-pro graph according to steps (3)–(5) to obtain aggregated sets of diagnosis codes $V_d = \{v_d^1, v_d^2, \cdots v_d^t\}$ and procedure nodes $V_p = \{v_p^1, v_p^2, \cdots v_p^t\}$.

Finally, based on the aggregated medication nodes from the medication graph G_m and the learned diagnosis and procedure nodes from the diag-pro graph G_{dp}, we learn from the med-diag graph G_{md} and the medication-procedure graph G_{mp}, updating to obtain entity-level representations of the medication, diagnosis, and procedure sets:

$$V_D = \left\{ V_d^1, V_d^2, \cdots V_d^t \right\}$$
$$V_P = \left\{ V_p^1, V_p^2, \cdots V_p^t \right\} \tag{7}$$
$$V_M = \left\{ V_m^1, V_m^2, \cdots V_m^{t-1} \right\}$$

It is important to highlight that this paper employs a multi-head Graph Attention Network (GAT) mechanism to learn and update nodes within the graph. While traditional GAT models consider intrinsic features and aggregate neighboring features, our approach with the heterogeneous graph network prioritizes enhancing the representations of medications, diagnoses, and procedures through the relationships between heterogeneous medical entities. Consequently, our model focuses more intensively on neighboring nodes to prevent excessive node information merging. Thus, we have adapted the traditional GAT to concentrate exclusively on the information from neighboring nodes in the learning process of the heterogeneous graph.

4.2 Temporal Selectivity Module

To accurately capture the temporal dynamics of a patient's condition progression, this paper introduces a dual-layer temporal selection mechanism utilizing Gated Recurrent Units (GRU). Compared to traditional Recurrent Neural Networks (RNN), GRU exhibits enhanced modelling capabilities and is capable of effectively capturing temporal dependencies in time series data. It mitigate common issues such as gradient vanishing and the extensive parameterization typical of Long Short-Term Memory networks (LSTM). The relatively streamlined architecture of GRU, coupled with the faster training speed, renders it particularly suitable for medication recommendation tasks.

Specifically, we first utilize GRU^α to learn the diagnostic sequence, generating forward diagnostic selection coefficients.

$$g^1, g^2, \cdots, g^t = GRU_d^\alpha \left(V_d^1, V_d^2, \cdots, V_d^t \right) \tag{8}$$

$$\alpha^j = tanh \left(W^\alpha g^j + b^\alpha \right), j = 1, \cdots, t \tag{9}$$

Concurrently, GRU^β is employed in the reverse temporal order to learn the diagnostic sequence, thereby ensuring that the backward selection coefficients are generated at different time steps, which enhances the computational stability.

$$h^t, h^{t-1}, \cdots, h^1 = GRU_d^\beta \left(V_d^t, V_d^{t-1}, \cdots, V_d^1 \right) \tag{10}$$

$$\beta^j = tanh\,shrink \left(W^\beta h^j + b^\beta \right), j = t, \cdots, 1 \tag{11}$$

Based on the generated dual-layer diagnostic selection coefficients, we can capture key visit information and entity information within the visit sequence, thereby obtaining a diagnostic representation that integrates historical visit information.

$$d^t = \sum_{j=1}^{t} \alpha^j \beta^j \odot V_d^j \qquad (12)$$

After a series of similar processing steps, we obtain the patient's final procedural and medication representations.

$$p^t = \sum_{j=1}^{t} \alpha^j \beta^j \odot V_p^j, m^{t-1} = \sum_{j=1}^{t-1} \alpha^j \beta^j \odot V_m^j \qquad (13)$$

4.3   Interaction Prediction Module

Based on the output of the above modules, for the patient's t -th visit, we concatenate the medical entity sequence to make medication recommendations:

$$\hat{y}^t = \sigma\left(\left[d^t; p^t; m^{t-1}\right]\right) \qquad (14)$$

In this paper, medication recommendation is defined as a multi-label classification task [21, 22]. During the model training process, the binary cross-entropy loss function is optimized using the Adam optimizer [23].

$$L = -\sum_{t=1}^{T} \sum_{i=1}^{|M|} y_i^t \log \hat{y}_i^t + (1 - y_i^t) \log\left(1 - \hat{y}_i^t\right) \qquad (15)$$

5   Experiments and Analysis

5.1   Dataset Description

In this study, we utilized the MIMIC-IV v2.2 dataset[1] [10] for our experiments. This dataset originates from the Massachusetts Institute of Technology and encompasses medical records of patients admitted to intensive care units between 2008 and 2019. The experiments primarily utilized the HOSP module of the dataset, which includes data on diagnoses, procedures, and medications. The diagnosis and procedure data employ the ICD-9 coding system,[2] while the medication data use the NDC (National Drug Code) system in the United States.[3] To study medication recommendations for patients with hypertension, this paper extracted corresponding data based on the ICD-9 codes for hypertension from the dataset and selected patients who had at least two visits, following previous studies [4, 19, 20], while filtering out medications that appeared less than 2000 times. Subsequently, the dataset was divided into training, validation, and test sets in a ratio of 4:1:1. Detailed information about the dataset used in the final experiments and examples of patient data are shown in Table 1 and Table 2.

---

[1] https://physionet.org/content/mimiciv/2.2/
[2] https://en.wikipedia.org/wiki/List_of_ICD9_codes.
[3] http://www.whocc.no/atc/structure_and_principles.

Table 1. The detailed information of experimental dataset.

Item	Number
# patients	19,609
# visits	55,239
# diagnosis	2,000
# procedure	5,488
# medication	14
avg # of visits	2.8169
avg # of diagnosis	9.3666
avg # of procedure	2.5492
avg # of medication	1.0804

Table 2. The samples of Electronic Health Records.

Sub_ID	Hadm_ID	Diagnoses	Procedures	Medications
10001217	24597018	3240,3484,3485,5180, 340,04109,3051,4019, V168,V161	139,331,3897	HydrALAzine, LeVETiracetam, Vancomycin, Bisacodyl, Meropenem,...
10001217	27703517	3240,3485,340,04102, 04184,4019,3051	139	HydrALAzine, Vancomycin, Meropenem, Bisacodyl, Lidocaine...

5.2 Evaluation Metrics

To validate the effectiveness of CSRec, the following evaluation metrics are used:

- **Jaccard Similarity Coefficient (Jaccard).** A high Jaccard coefficient indicates a high degree of similarity between the predicted and target sets of medications.

$$Jaccard = \frac{1}{T}\sum_{t=1}^{T}\frac{\left|y^t \cap \hat{y}^t\right|}{\left|y^t \cup \hat{y}^t\right|} \tag{16}$$

- **Precision-Recall AUC (PRAUC).** A high PRAUC indicates that the model recommends appropriate medications while keeping a low error rate.

$$\Delta Recall(i)^t = Recall(i)^t - Recall(i-1)^t \tag{17}$$

$$PRAUC = \frac{1}{T}\sum_{t=1}^{T}\sum_{i=1}^{|M|}Precision(i)^t \Delta Recall(i)^t \tag{18}$$

- **F1 Score (F1).** A high F1 score in medication recommendations indicates that the model balances accuracy and recall effectively.

$$Precision^t = \frac{\left|y^t \cap \hat{y}^t\right|}{\left|\hat{y}^t\right|}, Recall^t = \frac{\left|y^t \cap \hat{y}^t\right|}{\left|y^t\right|} \tag{19}$$

$$F1 = \frac{1}{T}\sum_{t=1}^{T} \frac{2 \times Precision^t \times Recall^t}{Precision^t + Recall^t} \tag{20}$$

- **Drug-Drug Interaction Rate (DDI).** A lower DDI rate ensures that the recommended combination of medications is safer in clinical practice.

$$DDI = \frac{1}{T}\sum_{t=1}^{T} \frac{\sum_{i=1}^{\left|\hat{y}^t\right|}\sum_{j=i+1}^{\left|\hat{y}^t\right|} 1\left\{A_d\left[\hat{y}_i^t, \hat{y}_j^t\right]\right\}}{\sum_{i=1}^{\left|\hat{y}^t\right|}\sum_{j=i+1}^{\left|\hat{y}^t\right|} 1} \tag{21}$$

5.3   Comparative Models

The following baseline models are selected for comparison with proposed CSRec:

- **LR**: Logistic Regression with L2 regularization.
- **ECC** [24]: Enhances predictions by connecting multiple classifiers, commonly used in multi-label classification tasks to improve model performance.
- **RETAIN** [16]: Constructs a hierarchical attention model that uses a two-level reverse time attention mechanism for predicting diagnoses, suitable for sequential prediction tasks such as medication recommendation.
- **LEAP** [25]: Utilizes Recurrent Neural Networks (RNNs) to extract meaningful representations during current medical visits and generate medication sequences.
- **DMNC** [18]: Employs a memory-augmented network to simulate the interaction between two asynchronous sequences in therapeutic prediction tasks.
- **GAMENet** [11]: Uses a graph-enhanced dynamic memory network that integrates medication interaction knowledge and views temporal patient records as queries to retrieve medications from the memory.
- **MICRON** [19]: Focuses on changes in patients' electronic health records, updating historical medication combinations when new symptoms appear to maximize therapeutic effects and minimize adverse reactions.
- **SafeDrug** [8]: Concentrates on the chemical and biological information between medications and patient health status to recommend safer medication combinations.
- **COGNet** [20]: Introduces a copy-predict mechanism that incorporates useful medications from previous combinations into the current recommendation sequence.

5.4   Performance Comparison

In this section, we comprehensively compare CSRec with the aforementioned medication recommendation baseline models to assess its performance. Experimental results on the MIMIC-IV 2.2 dataset are shown in Table 3 (bold indicates optimal data, ↑ indicates a preference for larger values, ↓ indicates a preference for smaller values).

Table 3. The comparison experimental results.

Model	Jaccard↑	PRAUC↑	F1↑	DDI↓
LR	0.4248	0.7426	0.5125	0.2821
ECC	0.4389	0.7498	0.5305	0.3064
RETAIN	0.5349	0.7964	0.6356	0.3431
LEAP	0.4186	0.5047	0.5326	**0.0104**
DMNC	0.5139	0.7678	0.5392	0.2801
GAMENet	0.5151	0.7781	0.6069	0.2884
MICRON	0.4297	0.7543	0.5151	0.2866
SafeDrug	0.5173	0.7770	0.6109	0.3084
COGNet	0.5087	0.7448	0.5948	0.3261
CSRec	**0.5582**	**0.8069**	**0.6483**	0.2760

After detailed analysis, we can observe several key findings:

- The CSRec model proposed in this paper outperforms most comparative models across multiple evaluation metrics, fully demonstrating its significant effectiveness in hypertension medication recommendation.
- LR and ECC performed poorly, primarily because these methods focus only on the patient's current medical state and overlook the impact of historical medical information on the current state. In contrast, the model presented in this paper, along with RETAIN, GAMENet, and other models integrating longitudinal medical histories, performed better, highlighting the importance of capturing historical medical information in hypertension medication recommendations.
- Compared with longitudinal models like RETAIN, GAMENet, and COGNet, CSRec still outperforms other methods, thanks to the model's accurate simulation of patient disease progression and effective capture of the relationships between heterogeneous medical entities.
- Although the CSRec model proposed in this paper is not the best in the DDI metric, it still ranks as suboptimal. This is mainly because the best-performing LEAP model only considers the patient's current health condition, thus recommending the fewest medications, leading to the lowest DDI values.

5.5   Ablation Study

To evaluate the effectiveness and rationality of each component of the CSRec, ablation experiments were conducted by comparing CSRec with its variants.

- **WO_S**: Removes the selection module based on the cyclic mechanism.
- **WO_C**: Removes the collaborative module based on the heterogeneous graph.
- **GAT_GCN**: Replaces the multi-head GAT in the collaborative module with a GCN.

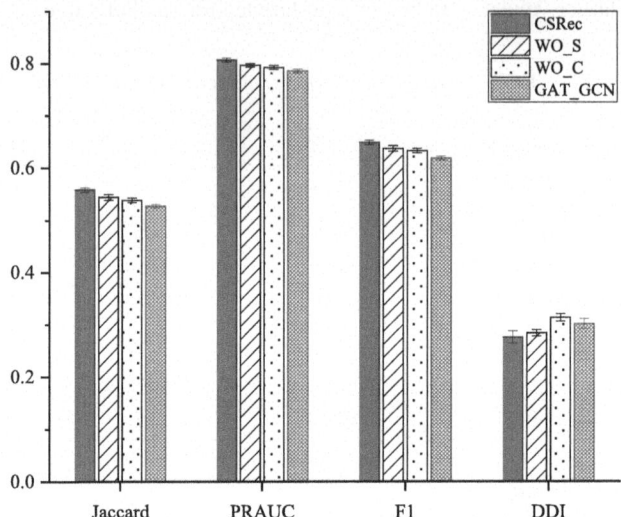

Fig. 3. The ablation study of different components.

The results displayed in Fig. 3 indicate that the performance of CSRec declines when any module is removed or replaced, demonstrating that each component of CSRec is indispensable. The collaborative module effectively models the correlations between different medical events during each visit, enhancing the representation of medical entities; the selective module globally models the patient's medical history, focusing on the impact of each point in time on the current health condition, thereby accurately simulating the progression of hypertension in patients; and the multi-head attention mechanism aggregates richer information in the heterogeneous graph compared to the convolutional network, accurately representing the nodes and edges of medical entities.

The paper also explores the impact of different types of medical entity information (diagnosis, procedure, and medication DDI information) on hypertension medication recommendation, as shown in Fig. 4. Experimental results show that the performance of CSRec declines when any type of medical entity is removed (WO_DM, WO_PM, WO_DP), indicating that different types of medical entities are highly relevant to medication recommendation. Moreover, removing medication co-occurrence and interaction information (WO_MM) significantly reduces the safety of the recommended medications, indicating that DDI information is also essential.

5.6 Parameter Sensitivity

To explore the effect of the number of heads in the multi-head graph attention mechanism within the heterogeneous collaborative module on model performance, a series

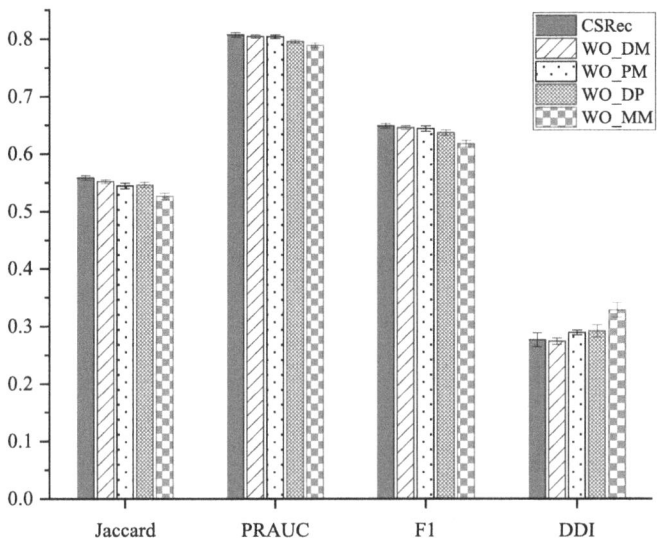

Fig. 4. The ablation study of different medical entities.

of experiments were conducted comparing different numbers of attention heads, with specific results shown in Fig. 5.

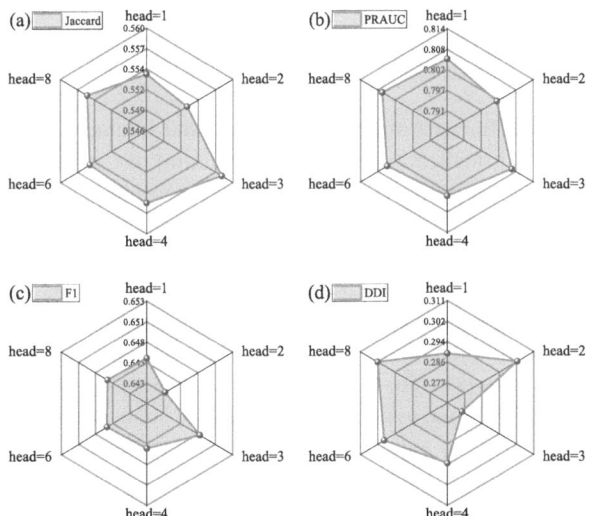

Fig. 5. The effect of different number of heads in the multi-head GAT.

It was found that a setting of three attention heads (head = 3) achieves optimal performance, and thus, in other experiments in this paper, the number of attention heads is set to three. Additionally, the data shows that even if the number of heads changes, the resulting performance fluctuations are relatively small, further demonstrating the robustness and reliability of the model presented in this paper.

5.7 Case Study

To visualize the learning process of the model presented in this paper, a patient was randomly selected from the test set for a case study. Taking diagnosis and medication entities as examples, the entire learning process is shown in Fig. 6.

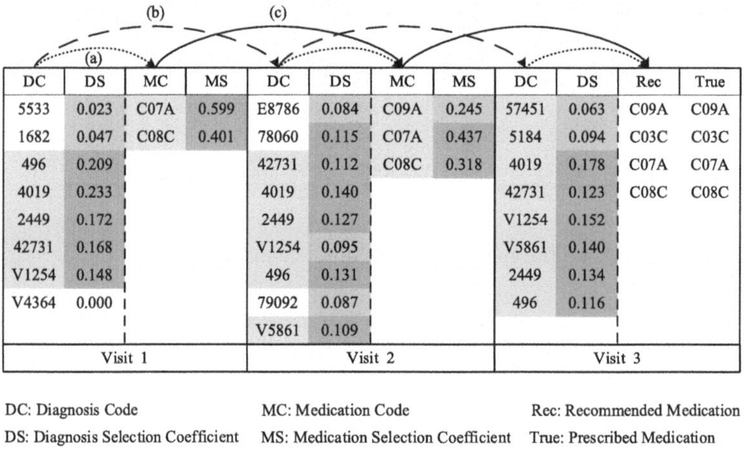

DC	DS	MC	MS	DC	DS	MC	MS	DC	DS	Rec	True
5533	0.023	C07A	0.599	E8786	0.084	C09A	0.245	57451	0.063	C09A	C09A
1682	0.047	C08C	0.401	78060	0.115	C07A	0.437	5184	0.094	C03C	C03C
496	0.209			42731	0.112	C08C	0.318	4019	0.178	C07A	C07A
4019	0.233			4019	0.140			42731	0.123	C08C	C08C
2449	0.172			2449	0.127			V1254	0.152		
42731	0.168			V1254	0.095			V5861	0.140		
V1254	0.148			496	0.131			2449	0.134		
V4364	0.000			79092	0.087			496	0.116		
				V5861	0.109						
Visit 1				Visit 2				Visit 3			

DC: Diagnosis Code   MC: Medication Code   Rec: Recommended Medication
DS: Diagnosis Selection Coefficient   MS: Medication Selection Coefficient   True: Prescribed Medication

Fig. 6. Case Study.

Initially, in the collaborative process (a), the model interacts between diagnostic codes (DC column) and medication codes (MC column) at the visit level, enhancing the effect of diagnostic information on medication information. Furthermore, due to the temporal dependency of EHR data, the recommended medications not only depend on the diseases diagnosed in the third visit DC column but are also closely related to past prescription medications and disease progression. Therefore, as shown in process (c), medication codes from historical visits are assigned higher selection coefficients, emphasizing their importance in the recommendation process. Similarly, in process (b), diagnostic codes from previous visits receive more attention, with higher selection coefficients. In each DC column, hypertension diseases are consistently assigned a higher selection coefficient, aligning with the data characteristics of hypertension treatment records.

6 Conclusion

This paper presents the CSRec model for hypertension medication recommendation, which is based on the collaboration and selection of heterogeneous medical entities. By learning the correlations between different types of medical entities and combining the temporal evolution characteristics of clinical entities, the model provides more precise and effective medication guidance for hypertension treatment. Future research will focus on three main areas: 1) further investigating the model's performance on the cold start problem; 2) attempting to use other methods to comprehensively model the correlations and collaboration between medical entities; 3) exploring recommendations for medication dosages alongside medication types.

Acknowledgments. This paper is supported by the National Natural Science Foundation of China (No. 62163033), the Talent Innovation and Entrepreneurship Project of Lanzhou, China (No. 2021-RC-49), the Natural Science Foundation of Gansu Province, China (No. 22JR5RA145, No. 21JR7RA781, No. 21JR7RA116), the Major Research Project Incubation Program of Northwest Normal University, China (No. NWNU-LKZD2021–06). The funding body had no role in study design, data collection and analysis, decision to publish, or preparation of the manuscript.

Disclosure of Interests. The authors declare that they have no known competing financial interests or personal relationships that could influence the work reported in this paper.

References

1. Hypertension Branch of Chinese Geriatrics Society, Beijing Hypertension Association, National Clinical Research Center of the Geriatric Diseases.: 2023 Guidelines for the management of hypertension in the elderly population in China. Chin. J. Hypertension **31**(06), 508–538 (2023)

2. The Writing Committee of the Report on Cardiovascular Health and Diseases in China.: Interpretation of report on cardiovascular health and diseases in China 2022. Chin. J. Cardiovascular Med. **28**(04), 297–312 (2023)

3. Wu, H., Xie, H.: Research on hypertension diagnosis and treatment system based on ontology and CBR. Comput. Appli. Softw. **30**(12), 155–159+206 (2013)

4. Li, X., Liang, S., Hou, Y., Ma, T.: StratMed: Relevance stratification between biomedical entities for sparsity on medication recommendation. Knowl.-Based Syst. **284**, 111239 (2024)

5. Zhang, H., Yang, X., Bai, L.: Enhancing drug recommendations via heterogeneous graph representation learning in EHR networks. IEEE Trans. Knowl. Data Eng. **36**(07), 3024–3035 (2024)

6. Choi, E., Xiao, C., Stewart, W.: Mime: Multilevel medical embedding of electronic health records for predictive healthcare. Adv. Neural. Inf. Process. Syst. **31**, 4552–4562 (2018)

7. Choi, E., Xu, Z., Li, Y.: Learning the graphical structure of electronic health records with graph convolutional transformer. In: Proceedings of the AAAI Conference on Artificial Intelligence 2020, vol. 34, pp. 606–613. AAAI Press, Palo Alto (2020)

8. Yang, C., Xiao, C., Ma, F.: Safedrug: dual molecular graph encoders for recommending effective and safe drug combinations. In: Zhou, Z. (ed.) Proceedings of the Thirtieth International Joint Conference on Artificial Intelligence 2021, pp. 3735–3741. IJCAI Press, Montreal (2021)

9. Liu, S., Wang, X., Xiang, Y.: Multi-channel fusion LSTM for medical event prediction using EHRs. J. Biomed. Inform. **127**, 104011 (2022)

10. Johnson, A.E., Bulgarelli, L., Shen, L.: MIMIC-IV, a freely accessible electronic health record dataset. Scientific data **10**(1), 1 (2023)

11. Shang, J., Xiao, C., Ma, T.: Gamenet: graph augmented memory networks for recommending medication combination. In: Proceedings of the AAAI Conference on Artificial Intelligence 2019, vol. 33, pp. 1126–1133. AAAI Press, Honolulu (2019)

12. Shang, J., Ma T., Xiao, C.: Pre-training of graph augmented transformers for medication recommendation. In: Proceedings of the Twenty-Eighth International Joint Conference on Artificial Intelligence 2019, pp. 5953–5959. IJCAI Press, Macao (2019)

13. Liang, X., Yang, J., Lu, G.: Compnet: Competitive neural network for palmprint recognition using learnable gabor kernels. IEEE Signal Process. Lett. **28**, 1739–1743 (2021)

14. Yang, N., Zeng, K., Wu, Q.: Molerec: combinatorial drug recommendation with substructure-aware molecular representation learning. In: Ding, Y., Tang, J., Sequeda, J. (eds.) Proceedings of the ACM Web Conference 2023, pp.4075–4085. ACM Press, New York (2023)

15. Li, X., Zhang, Y., Li, X.: DGCL: distance-wise and graph contrastive learning for medication recommendation. J. Biomed. Inform. **139**, 104301 (2023)

16. Choi, E., Bahadori, M.T., Sun, J.: RETAIN: an interpretable predictive model for healthcare using reverse time attention mechanism. In: Proceedings of the 30th International Conference on Neural Information Processing Systems 2016, vol. 29, pp. 3512–3520. ACM Press, Red Hook (2016)

17. An, Y., Zhang, L., You, M.: MeSIN: Multilevel selective and interactive network for medication recommendation. Knowl.-Based Syst. **233**, 107534 (2021)

18. Le, H., Tran, T., Venkatesh, S.: Dual memory neural computer for asynchronous two-view sequential learning. In: Guo, Y., Farooq, F. (eds) Proceedings of the 24th ACM SIGKDD international conference on knowledge discovery & data mining 2018, pp. 1637–1645. ACM Press, New York (2018)

19. Yang, C., Xiao, C., Glass, L.: Change matters: medication change prediction with recurrent residual networks. In: Proceedings of the Thirtieth International Joint Conference on Artificial Intelligence 2021, pp. 3728–3734. IJCAI Press, Montreal (2021)

20. Wu, R., Qiu, Z., Jiang, J.: Conditional generation net for medication recommendation. In: Proceedings of the ACM Web Conference 2022, pp. 935–945. ACM Press, New York (2022)

21. Zhao, D., Shi, Y., Cheng, L.: Time interval uncertainty-aware and text-enhanced based disease prediction. J. Biomed. Inform. **139**, 104239 (2023)

22. Nguyen, M.V., Nguyen, D.T., Trinh, Q.H.: ALGNet: attention Light Graph Memory Network for Medical Recommendation System. In: Proceedings of the 12th International Symposium on Information and Communication Technology 2023, pp. 570–577. ACM Press, New York (2023)

23. Kingma, D.P.: Adam: A method for stochastic optimization. arXiv preprint arXiv:1412.6980 (2014)

24. Read, J., Pfahringer, B., Holmes, G.: Classifier chains for multi-label classification. Mach. Learn. **85**, 333–359 (2011)

25. Zhang, Y., Chen, R., Tang, J.: LEAP: learning to prescribe effective and safe treatment combinations for multimorbidity. In: Proceedings of the 23rd ACM SIGKDD international conference on knowledge Discovery and data Mining 2017, pp. 1315–1324. ACM Press, New York (2017)

Integrating TCM's "One Root of Medicine and Food" Principle Into Dietary Recommendations with Retrieval-Augmented LLMs

Fan Gong[1], Hangyu Sha[2], Runfeng Liu[2], Tianxing Wu[2,3], Bo Liu[4(✉)], and Haofen Wang[5]

[1] Department of Endocrinology, Shuguang Hospital, Affiliated to Shanghai University of Traditional Chinese Medicine, Shanghai, China
[2] Southeast University, Nanjing, China
{hysha,runfengliu,tianxingwu}@seu.edu.cn
[3] Key Laboratory of New Generation Artificial Intelligence Technology and Its Interdisciplinary Applications (Southeast University), Ministry of Education, Nanjing, China
[4] Informatization Office, Shanghai University of Traditional Chinese Medicine, Shanghai, China
liubo@shutcm.edu.cn
[5] Tongji University, Shanghai, China

Abstract. This paper addresses the challenge of integrating Traditional Chinese Medicine (TCM) principles with contemporary artificial intelligence to generate accurate and personalized dietary recommendations. Focusing on the TCM concept of "One Root of Medicine and Food," we develop a novel method that employs Retrieval-Augmented Generation (RAG) techniques based on Large Language Models (LLMs). We confront the difficulties of translating nuanced TCM wisdom into actionable advice compatible with AI systems, ensuring high accuracy and relevance in personalized recommendations, and maintaining scientific rigor while preserving traditional knowledge. To overcome these obstacles, we design a unified set of prompt engineering instructions tailored for TCM dietary guidance and evaluate several mainstream LLMs, ultimately selecting Qwen as the optimal base model. By integrating RAG with a specialized TCM knowledge base, we enhance the model's accuracy and professionalism; experimental results show significant improvements, with the ROUGE-L score increasing from 0.294 to 0.427 and the Accuracy score rising from 0.315 to 0.439. Case studies further demonstrate that our method enhances the rationality and customization of recommendations, ensuring they are scientifically sound and tailored to individual needs. This approach significantly improves the relevance and fidelity of TCM-based dietary recommendations, bridging traditional wisdom and modern technology for personalized healthcare.

© The Author(s), under exclusive license to Springer Nature Singapore Pte Ltd. 2025
Y. Zhang et al. (Eds.): CHIP 2024, CCIS 2433, pp. 251–267, 2025.
https://doi.org/10.1007/978-981-96-3752-2_15

Keywords: Dietary recommendations · Traditional chinese medicine ·
One root of medicine and food · Large language models ·
Retrieval-augmented generation

1   Introduction

The concept of "One Root of Medicine and Food" in Traditional Chinese Medicine (TCM) has a long history, and is deeply rooted in China's rich cultural heritage. Through extensive practice, practitioners have explored and summarized the relationship between food and medicine, concluding that food shares similar properties with medicine. This includes theories of nature and flavor, such as the Four Natures (Cold, Hot, Warm, Cool) and Five Flavors (Sour, Bitter, Sweet, Pungent, Salty), meridian tropism, and the principles of rising, descending, floating, and sinking [1]. These valuable insights have been documented in numerous ancient pharmacopoeias. The Huangdi Neijing Taisu [2] states: "When used to satisfy hunger, it is called food; when used to treat illness, it is called medicine." This highlights that diet not only meets basic physiological needs but also plays a crucial role in maintaining health and preventing diseases.

In modern health management, the "One Root of Medicine and Food" theory has been widely applied, notably in the prevention and management of chronic diseases [3]. By considering an individual's constitution and health condition, and adhering to TCM dietary principles, a well-designed dietary plan can significantly improve health levels. However, providing personalized dietary recommendations based on this concept faces several challenges. Firstly, such recommendations heavily rely on professional knowledge, often requiring the involvement of experienced specialists, which increases the cost and complexity of service delivery. Secondly, significant differences in individuals' physical conditions, lifestyles, and personal preferences, make it challenging to meet users' personalized needs while ensuring scientific accuracy and avoiding homogenization [4].

To address these challenges, we propose leveraging modern artificial intelligence technologies, specifically Large Language Models (LLMs) enhanced with Retrieval-Augmented Generation (RAG), to generate accurate and personalized dietary recommendations. LLMs like ChatGPT [5], after training on large-scale datasets, have demonstrated strong capabilities in language understanding and generation, making them suitable for producing relevant and coherent advice [6]. The RAG technique further enhances these models by retrieving and integrating information from specialized domain knowledge bases during generation [7], compensating for the lack of specific domain knowledge in LLMs and improving the reasoning ability and accuracy of recommendations.

In this paper, we systematically evaluate the performance of several mainstream LLMs in generating personalized dietary recommendations based on the "One Root of Medicine and Food" concept. We also explore how the integration of RAG can further enhance these models in providing personalized and professional dietary guidance tailored to users with different constitutions and health conditions. The key contributions of this paper are as follows:

- *Construction of a Comprehensive Knowledge Base:* We develop a RAG knowledge base containing a wide range of documents related to TCM's "One Root of Medicine and Food" principles, providing a rich source of domain-specific information.
- *Evaluation of Mainstream LLMs:* We design tailored prompt engineering instructions and systematically evaluate the performance of mainstream LLMs, ultimately selecting Qwen as the optimal base model for our application.
- *Enhancement through RAG Integration:* By introducing external TCM knowledge through RAG, our method enhances the richness, relevance, customization, and medical soundness of generated dietary recommendations.
- *Demonstration of Effectiveness:* Experimental results and case studies demonstrate that our approach significantly improves the scientific accuracy and individualization of TCM-based dietary recommendations.

This approach provides a practical tool for personalized healthcare, harmonizing traditional wisdom with modern technology, and addresses the urgent need for cost-effective, accurate, and personalized dietary guidance based on TCM principles.

2   Related Work

Dietary recommendation generation involves utilizing computational algorithms and data analysis techniques to automatically produce personalized dietary suggestions based on individual needs, health status, dietary preferences, and nutritional information. The goal is not only to provide scientifically sound dietary guidance but also to consider users' lifestyles and cultural backgrounds, thereby achieving higher acceptance and practical effectiveness.

Traditional dietary recommendation methods are predominantly rule-based, relying on expert knowledge and predefined guidelines to generate suggestions. While straightforward, they often lack flexibility and personalization, failing to meet the diverse needs of users effectively. This limitation has propelled researchers to explore more intelligent and personalized recommendation systems.

In recent years, the application of deep learning models and knowledge graphs has significantly advanced dietary recommendation systems. Manoharan [8] introduced a recommendation system based on K-clique embedded deep learning classifiers (K-DLRS), which automatically tailors diets to patients' specific health conditions, such as blood pressure and cholesterol levels. This system demonstrated superior precision and accuracy compared to traditional machine learning methods. Chen et al. [9] developed a personalized food recommendation framework utilizing Knowledge Graph Question Answering (KBQA). By incorporating user preferences and health guidelines as constraints, they optimized food recommendations to better suit individual needs. Tang et al. [10] proposed an anticancer recipe recommendation system that integrates a cancer dietary knowledge graph with Knowledge Graph Attention Networks (KGAT) and Long Short-Term Memory (LSTM) networks. This approach significantly improved the accuracy of personalized recommendations by dynamically adjusting to users' evolving taste preferences. Similarly, Chen et al. [11] introduced a health-aware food recommendation system that employs a collaborative recipe knowledge graph and multi-task learning to balance health requirements with dietary preferences. Their model outperformed baseline models in providing suitable recommendations. Ma et al. [12] proposed a nutrition-related knowledge graph neural network (NRKG) using graph convolutional networks. By integrating nutritional data with user preferences, their approach enhances food recommendations, promoting healthier and more diverse eating habits. Furthermore, Xu et al. [13] developed *ElCombo*, a personalized meal recommendation system for older adults. Leveraging a food knowledge graph, *ElCombo* improves dietary diversity and quality, demonstrating superior performance in simulation tests compared to users' autonomous choices.

With the rapid development of LLMs, researchers have increasingly explored their applications in dietary recommendations. Jin et al. [14] utilized Generative Pre-trained Transformers (GPT) to develop a dietary recommendation system aimed at managing potassium intake in hemodialysis patients, effectively reducing hyperkalemia rates compared to traditional methods. Sun et al. [15] created an AI-based nutritionist program that integrates LLMs with image recognition technology to manage type 2 diabetes. Their system provides accurate, personalized dietary recommendations and achieves food ingredient recognition accuracy comparable to that of professional dietitians. Hannon et al. [16] introduced *Chef Dalle*, a multimodal recipe recommendation system that leverages voice, text, and image interactions for personalized cooking guidance. By employing advanced models such as GPT-Vision and DALL-E 3, this system enhances accessibility and promotes healthier eating habits. Similarly, Kopitar et al. [17] proposed a generative AI system for personalized meal planning in inpatient clinical dietetics. By integrating patient data from electronic health records with clinical guidelines, they created adaptable meal plans and visual representations, thereby enhancing patient engagement and adherence to dietary recommendations. Collectively, these studies highlight the potential of LLMs to generate more personalized and effective dietary recommendations.

The TCM concept of "one root of medicine and food" posits that many foods possess therapeutic properties extending beyond mere nutritional value. Current studies [18–20] indicate that certain foods can not only fulfill dietary requirements but also support and enhance various physiological functions, aiding in the prevention and management of diseases. By recognizing the medicinal qualities of food, TCM advocates for a diet that aligns with an individual's specific health conditions, promoting a proactive approach to health and wellness.

Despite these advancements, a significant gap exists in integrating TCM principles, especially the "one root of medicine and food" concept, with modern AI for dietary recommendations. Most existing systems focus on Western dietary principles, overlooking the potential benefits of combining traditional wisdom with cutting-edge technology. Our work addresses this gap by uniquely integrating TCM principles with LLMs enhanced by RAG, offering personalized guidance that considers both nutritional and medicinal aspects of food.

3 Methodology

An overview of the proposed method is illustrated in Fig. 1. The system comprises two main phases: **knowledge retrieval** and **answer generation**.

In the knowledge retrieval phase, the process begins with *prompt engineering* [27]. Carefully designed prompts guide the LLM to accurately extract key information from the user's query. This information typically includes the user's dietary preferences, current health conditions, and specific nutritional needs. For example, if a user states, "I have a cold constitution and often feel fatigued," the system extracts keywords such as *cold constitution* and *fatigue*.

Using these extracted keywords, the system employs a retriever to search the pre-constructed TCM knowledge base for relevant document blocks. The retrieved documents are then ranked based on their relevance, ensuring that the most pertinent information is prioritized for the subsequent answer generation phase. This ensures that the LLM has access to authoritative TCM knowledge aligned with the user's specific condition.

In the answer generation phase, the system combines the top-k document blocks from the knowledge retrieval phase with the user's original query. Through further prompt engineering, this integrated information is provided as input to the LLM. The model then generates personalized dietary recommendations that consider the user's unique circumstances, while referencing the retrieved professional TCM theoretical knowledge and practical experience.

Continuing the earlier example, the LLM might suggest warming foods that invigorate energy, such as ginger tea or dishes with lamb, which are recommended in TCM for individuals with a cold constitution and fatigue. The final recommendation is directly presented to the user, offering tailored advice that merges modern AI capabilities with traditional TCM wisdom.

3.1 Construction of the Knowledge Base

The construction of our knowledge base for RAG is built upon a rich tapestry of TCM literature, ranging from ancient texts to modern research. Unlike typical knowledge bases that often rely on structured datasets, our approach captures the nuanced insights of TCM literature in document form. This comprehensive, document-centric methodology provides a robust foundation for our dietary recommendation system, integrating the time-honored "One Root of Medicine and Food" concept with contemporary scientific understanding.

Ancient and Classical Sources. Our knowledge base incorporates seminal works that have shaped TCM dietary theory:

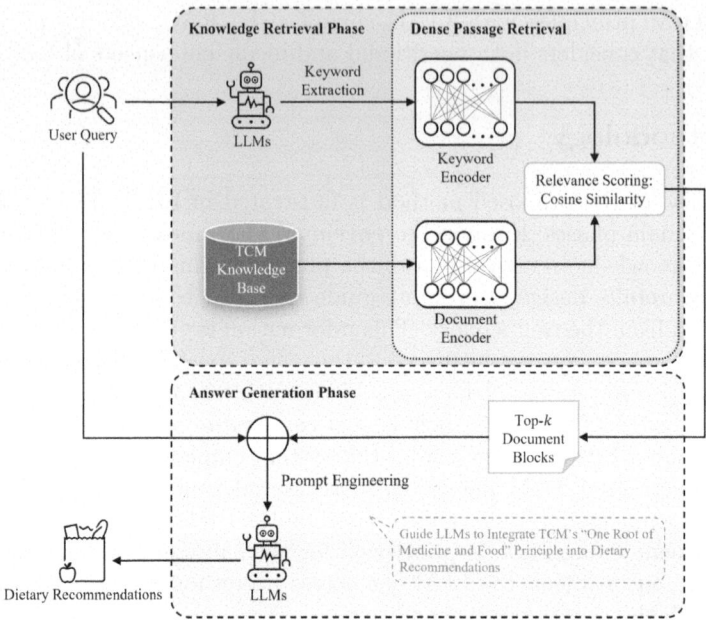

Fig. 1. Framework for Generating Dietary Recommendations Based on TCM's "One Root of Medicine and Food" Principles Using Retrieval-Augmented Large Language Models.

- *Huangdi Neijing Suwen* [21]: This foundational text eloquently articulates the interconnectedness of food and medicine, stating: "Toxic drugs attack pathogens, while grains provide nourishment, fruits assist, livestock benefit, and vegetables satisfy, all taken in harmony of flavor to replenish essence and invigorate qi."
- *The Shiliao Bencao(Dietetic Materia Medica)* [22]: Recognized as the world's earliest monograph on medicinal cuisine, This work significantly contributed to the development of the "One Root of Medicine and Food" theory.

Modern TCM Literature. To bridge ancient wisdom with contemporary practice, we include recent scholarly works:

- *Shiwuzhongyao yu Bianfang (Food as Medicine and Handy Remedies)* [23]
- *Zhongguo Shiliao Xue (Chinese Dietary Therapy)* [24]
- *Zhongguo Yaoshan Xue (Chinese Medicinal Diets)* [25]

These modern texts provide updated interpretations and applications of the "One Root of Medicine and Food" principle, ensuring our knowledge base reflects current TCM practices.

Regulatory Documents and Research Papers. To align with contemporary standards and scientific advancements, we incorporate:

– Regulatory guidelines, such as *The List of Items that Can Be Used Both as Food and Drugs* [26], issued by relevant national departments.
– Modern research papers that explore the intersection of TCM principles and nutritional science.

Comprehensive Food and Herb Information. Our knowledge base includes detailed information on various foods and herbs, encompassing: flavors (e.g., sweet, bitter, sour), associated meridians, therapeutic effects, traditional and modern uses. For instance, ginger might be described as warm in nature, associated with the lung and stomach meridians, and effective for dispelling cold and alleviating nausea.

Knowledge Base Structure. To optimize retrieval efficiency, we segmented the collected documents into blocks using a sentence-level separator. This granular approach allows for precise information retrieval, crucial for generating accurate and context-specific dietary recommendations.

Our RAG knowledge base consists of a total of 1,012 documents. Figure 2 provides a statistical overview of these documents, categorized by source type.

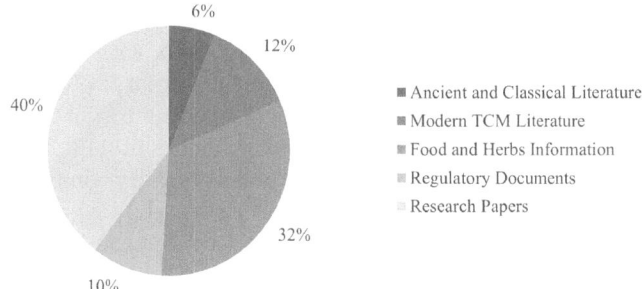

Fig. 2. Statistical Distribution of 1,012 Documents in the RAG Knowledge Base

This meticulously constructed knowledge base serves as the cornerstone of our system, enabling the generation of dietary recommendations that harmoniously blend ancient TCM wisdom with modern nutritional insights.

3.2   Comparison of LLMs

To identify the most suitable LLM for generating dietary recommendations based on the TCM principle of "One Root of Medicine and Food", we designed a unified set of prompts to evaluate the basic capabilities of several mainstream

LLMs before the introduction RAG. The models tested include GPT 4.0, Gemini [28], Qwen [29], ERNIE Bot [30], and HuatuoGPT-II [31]. GPT 4.0 and Gemini are representative of state-of-the-art general-purpose LLMs with strong cross-cultural adaptability, while Qwen and ERNIE Bot are optimized for Chinese linguistic understanding. HuatuoGPT-II is specifically fine-tuned for medical applications, ensuring it aligns well with the dietary and health guidance requirements essential in our study.

We selected the task of generating a daily meal plan as the testing scenario because it comprehensively demonstrates an LLM's ability to produce detailed dietary recommendations. The evaluation metrics for this test encompass several aspects: 1) whether a comprehensive daily meal plan is provided, 2) if each meal consists of more than one dish, offering variety, 3) does the model specify exact quantities for each ingredient, 4) when the prompt is run multiple times, does the model produce different dishes, indicating an ability to generate diverse recommendations? and finally 5) whether the rationale behind ingredient recommendations is explained from a TCM perspective.

To more accurately assess the performance of each model, we employed a manual evaluation method, assessing the models across four metrics: relevance of the answers, practicality of the answers, alignment with user preferences, and adherence to the TCM principle of "One Root of Medicine and Food". For the first three metrics, we adopted self-assessments by users who evaluated the meal plans based on their personal experiences and needs. For the fourth metric, we enlisted ten senior TCM practitioners, all holding the Physician Practice Certificate, to conduct professional scoring. Their expertise ensured that the evaluation accurately reflected the depth of TCM integration in the meal plans. Each metric was carefully scored on a scale from 0 to 5, with higher scores indicating better performance in the task of generating dietary recommendations.

This comprehensive evaluation approach allowed us to not only gauge the general capabilities of each LLM but also assess their suitability for generating dietary recommendations grounded in TCM philosophy. By combining quantitative scores with qualitative insights from both users and TCM professionals, we obtained a well-rounded understanding of each model's strengths and areas for improvement in this specialized application.

3.3   Retrieval Strategy

In knowledge retrieval, the process begins by extracting keywords from the user's queries using prompt engineering techniques. These keywords are crucial for tailoring personalized dietary recommendations based on the Traditional Chinese Medicine (TCM) principle of "One Root of Medicine and Food". The extracted keywords may include, but are not limited to, the user's constitution type (such as Yin deficiency or Yang deficiency), health status, dietary preferences, and restrictions (such as allergies or vegetarianism). An example of the prompt designed for keyword extraction is shown in Fig. 3.

Prompt =
You are an excellent keyword extractor for Traditional Chinese Medicine (TCM) dietary queries. You will receive an input text, and your task is to accurately identify and extract each keyword from the provided input text. The generated keywords must be in Chinese. The content of the keywords includes but is not limited to the user's TCM body constitution type (such as Yin deficiency, Yang deficiency), health condition, dietary preferences and restrictions (such as allergies, vegetarianism), the user's requirements (such as generating recipes, dietary advice, ingredient Q&A), etc.
Your response must be a list of keywords, with each element in the list corresponding to the keywords you have extracted, do not include content not mentioned in the text.
Input text: [Input Text].
Response format: [Keyword 1, Keyword 2, ...].
Generated keyword list:

Fig. 3. An Example Prompt for Extracting Keywords from User Queries.

For instance, if a user says, "I often feel cold and tired, and I prefer warm soups," the system would extract keywords such as *cold, tiredness, warm soups*, and may infer a constitution type of Yang deficiency.

After obtaining the list of keywords, we employ *Dense Retrieval* to search for relevant professional knowledge documents within our knowledge base. Dense retrieval is a modern information retrieval technique that represents both queries and documents as dense vectors in a continuous vector space using pre-trained language models. This method effectively captures semantic similarities, placing related information closer together in the vector space.

Typically, Dense Retrieval uses deep learning models, such as BERT [32] or other pre-trained language models, to encode text into fixed-dimensional vectors. The input query vector is compared with the vectors of all documents in the document pool to compute similarity scores. The top-k most relevant document blocks are then obtained by ranking based on cosine similarity.

Compared to traditional sparse retrieval methods, which rely on keyword matching and sparse representations (e.g., TF-IDF and BM25), Dense Retrieval can more comprehensively handle synonyms and contextual semantics, significantly improving retrieval accuracy. For example, it can recognize that "cold extremities" and "cold hands and feet" refer to the same symptom.

However, since BERT is not fine-tuned for the medical field, it may suffer from semantic discrepancies in representing medical texts, affecting the performance of Dense Retrieval in this domain. To address this issue, we replace the pre-trained language model used in Dense Retrieval with the domain-adapted *MedBERT* [33] model. MedBERT is a variant of BERT specifically optimized for medical corpora, capable of more effectively capturing the complex relationships between professional medical terminology and clinical concepts.

We utilize the *Dense Passage Retrieval (DPR)* [34] framework for our Dense Retrieval implementation. The core of DPR lies in its dual-tower architecture, where one tower encodes the query and the other encodes the documents, as illustrated in Fig. 1. Specifically, the MedBERT model is first used to transform the queries and candidate documents into dense vector representations. Then a contrastive learning strategy is employed to train the model by minimizing the distance between the query vector and the vectors of relevant documents while maximizing the distance from the vectors of irrelevant documents.

3.4 Retrieval Integration and Answer Generation

Retrieval integration refers to the process incorporating information retrieved from external knowledge sources into the generation phase of LLMs. In our proposed method, this integration is achieved through prompt engineering, where the top-k document blocks retrieved from the knowledge base are included as additional components within the prompts fed to the LLM.

Prompt engineering plays a crucial role in guiding LLMs to produce more relevant and accurate outputs. By carefully designing and optimizing the prompts, we can significantly impact the relevance and quality of the generated content, especially for complex tasks or specialized fields like TCM. A precise prompt helps the model to:

- **Focus on Specific Topics or Tasks**: Direct the model's attention to the relevant subject matter.
- **Reduce Generation Bias**: Mitigate unintended deviations in the output.
- **Improve Output Accuracy**: Enhance the correctness of the information provided.

Furthermore, providing specific background information or examples enhances the model's understanding of the task requirements.

During the answer generation phase, we construct a detailed prompt that includes:

- **The Patient's Question**: The original query posed by the user.
- **Task Requirements**: Specific instructions or objectives for the model.
- **Patient Information**: Relevant details about the user's condition.
- **Disease Descriptions**: Information about the health issues involved.
- **Background in TCM Theory**: Contextual knowledge extracted from the retrieved documents.

This comprehensive prompt clarifies the task objectives and guides the model to focus on TCM knowledge related to the principle of *"One Root of Medicine and Food"*. By doing so, we assist users in choosing appropriate foods based on their individual conditions, ensuring that the generated dietary recommendations are both professional and practical.

The prompt designed for retrieval integration during the answer generation stage of this study is illustrated in Fig. 4.

4   Experiments

In this section, we evaluate the performance of our retrieval and generation systems using several established metrics.

Prompt =
You are an expert in Traditional Chinese Medicine (TCM) dietary issues. Please, based on
the questions raised by the user and the retrieved document snippets, generate personalized
dietary recommendations in Chinese that incorporate the TCM concept of "One Root of
Medicine and Food." The suggestions may include but are not limited to: 1. Recommending
ingredients suitable for the user's constitution type. 2. Providing dietary recommendation
that helps treat the user's health conditions. 3. Adhering to the user's dietary preferences and
restrictions. 4. Based on TCM theory, offering specific food therapy methods and
precautions.
User Question: [User Question].
Retrieved Document Snippets: [Document 1], [Document 2], [Document 3]...
Generated Dietary Advice:

Fig. 4. Prompt for Retrieval Integration and Answer Generation.

4.1 Evaluation Metrics

In this section, we evaluate the performance of our retrieval and generation
systems using several established metrics.

Retriever Evaluation. For the retriever, we utilize the Recall@k and Mean
Reciprocal Rank (MRR@k) metrics. Recall@k measures the proportion of relevant documents among the top-k retrieval results for each query. It evaluates how
effectively the system retrieves relevant documents within a limited result set.
The Recall@k is calculated as:

$$\text{Recall@k} = \frac{|R \cap T_k|}{|R|}, \tag{1}$$

where R denotes the set of all relevant documents, and T_k represents the set of
top-k retrieved items.

Mean Reciprocal Rank (MRR@k) evaluates the average reciprocal rank of
the first relevant document across multiple queries. A higher MRR indicates that
relevant documents tend to appear in higher (more prominent) positions in the
retrieved results. MRR@k is caculated as:

$$\text{MRR@k} = \frac{1}{|Q|} \sum_{i=1}^{|Q|} \frac{1}{\text{rank}_i}, \tag{2}$$

where $|Q|$ is the total number of queries, and rank_i is the rank position of the
first relevant document retrieved for the i-th query.

Generation Evaluation. To assess the performance of the retrieval-augmented
generation (RAG) results, we employ two widely used metrics: *ROUGE-L* and
Accuracy. ROUGE-L is based on the Longest Common Subsequence (LCS) [35],
and it measures the similarity between the generated text and the reference

answer, capturing the semantic fidelity of the generated content. The ROUGE-L score is calculated using the following formula:

$$\text{ROUGE-L} = \frac{(1 + \beta^2) \cdot P \cdot R}{R + \beta^2 \cdot P} \tag{3}$$

where P and R represent the precision and recall of the LCS between the generated text X and the reference answer Y, defined as:

$$P = \frac{LCS(X,Y)}{|X|} \tag{4}$$

$$R = \frac{LCS(X,Y)}{|Y|} \tag{5}$$

Here, $LCS(X,Y)$ denotes the length of the longest common subsequence between X and Y, and $|X|$ and $|Y|$ are the lengths of the generated text and the reference answer, respectively. The parameter β balances the emphasis between precision and recall.

Accuracy assesses the overall correctness of the generated results, determining whether the generated text contains all the necessary content from the reference answer. It is defined as:

$$\text{Accuracy} = \frac{N_{\text{TG}}}{N_{\text{C}}} \tag{6}$$

where N_{TG} is the number of generated texts that contain the entire content of the reference answer, and N_{C} is the total number of instances evaluated.

4.2   Comparison Results of LLMs

Table 1 compares the capabilities of different LLMs in generating meal plans. Both Qwen and ERNIE Bot demonstrate outstanding performance across several metrics, including generating comprehensive daily meal plans with multiple dishes and providing detailed ingredient quantities. In contrast, GPT 4.0 and Gemini show weaker performance, particularly in providing precise ingredient quantities and maintaining consistency in the generated content. They also produce an average variety of dishes across multiple generations and fail to offer clear analyses from a Traditional Chinese Medicine (TCM) perspective. While HuatuoGPT-II offers recommendations based on TCM principles, it lacked consistency and variety in dish generation.

Table 2 presents the results of a manual evaluation of the LLMs. For the first three metrics, 300 users are each randomly evaluates a diet recommendation generated by one of the LLMs. For the fourth metric, each senior TCM practitioner evaluates 50 diet recommendations generated by each LLM. The scores for each model are then summed within each metric, resulting in a final score for every model on each metric. Overall, Qwen achieves the highest ratings, excelling in user preference alignment and answer relevance. It also shows a significant

Table 1. Comparative Evaluation of LLMs in Daily Meal Plan Generation

Model	Full-Day Menu	Multiple Dishes per Meal	Provides Ingredient Quantities	Dish Variety	TCM Analysis
GPT 4.0	Yes	Yes	No	General	No
Gemini	Yes	Yes	No	General	No
Qnwen	Yes	Yes	Yes	Richer	Yes
ERNIE Bot	Yes	Yes	Yes	Richer	Yes
HuatuoGPT-II	Yes	Yes	No	General	Yes

advantage over other models in adhering to the TCM concep of "One Root of Medicine and Food". However, all models show room for improvement regarding the *"Adherence to TCM Theory"* indicator, with scores lower than those for other indicators. Notably, models like GPT 4.0 and Gemini score relatively low in consistency of medicinal dietary principles and the practicality of their responses. This may be due to an insufficient understanding of TCM-specific corpus support. The complexity of TCM theory and its rich cultural background make it challenging for LLMs to fully grasp the concepts, affecting the accuracy and professionalism of their responses.

Table 2. Manual Evaluation Results of LLMs

Model	User Preference Alignment	Answer Relevance	Answer Practicality	Adherence to TCM Theory
GPT 4.0	221	233	207	1,263
Gemini	217	228	192	1,235
Qwen	**225**	236	**220**	**1,550**
ERNIE Bot	222	**237**	215	1,415
HuatuoGPT-II	212	226	209	1,486

Based on these results, we select Qwen as the base model for subsequent answer generation. To compensate for its shortcomings in TCM knowledge, we introduce Retrieval-Augmented Generation (RAG). By integrating retrieved professional documents from our TCM-spefic knowledge base, we aim to significantly enhance the model's understanding and performance in applying the principle of "One Root of Medicine and Food".

4.3 Results of RAG

The evaluation results of the retrievers are shown in Fig. 5. The traditional sparse retrieval method, BM25, performs the worst in Recall@100 and MRR@10. The scores improve with the TF-IDF model and are further enhanced with the introduction of the dense retriever DPR (BERT) model based on pre-trained language models. The domain-specialized DPR (MedBERT) model, trained with contrastive learning, achieves the best performance on these metrics, with Recall@100 and MRR@10 scores of 0.620 and 0.493, respectively. This

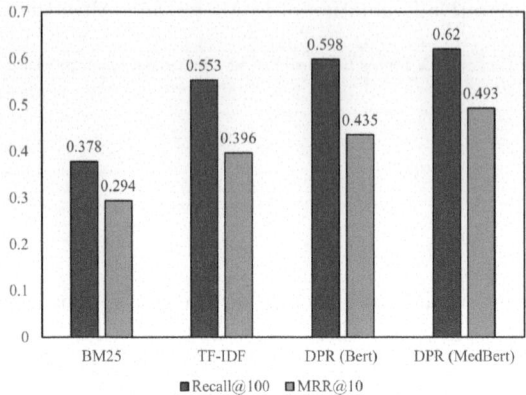

Fig. 5. Evaluation of Retriever Models

indicates that domain-specialized pre-trained models can effectively improve retrieval performance, especially in medical domain retrieval tasks.

Table 3 presents the comparative evaluation results before and after incorporating RAG. The performance of the generation models improves across both ROUGE-L and Accuracy metrics following the introduction of RAG. Specifically, the model that integrates Qwen with RAG significantly outperforms models without retrieval augmentation, with ROUGE-L increasing from 0.133 to 0.427 and Accuracy rising from 0.124 to 0.439. By utilizing Qwen as the base model alongside RAG, the model's ability to understand and respond to user queries is greatly enhanced, enabling it to provide more accurate answers and reasonable dietary recommendations.

Table 3. Evaluation Results with Retrieval-Augmented Generation

Model	ROUGE-L	Accuracy
Qwen + RAG	0.427	0.439
Qwen	0.294	0.315
GPT 4.0	0.271	0.283
Gemini	0.242	0.250
ERNIE Bot	0.291	0.299
HuatuoGPT-II	0.193	0.208

To further validate the model's performance in generating dietary recommendations consistent with TCM theory, we presents an actual case of dietary Q&A in Fig. 6.

In this example, the response without RAG provides a basic daily meal plan as requested, but each meal includes only one dish, leading to a monotonous

User's Question:
最近我工作压力很大，经常加班到深夜，感觉自己的精神状态越来越差，注意力也难以集中。能否根据我的情况推荐一个每日饮食计划？

User's Question (Translation):
I've been under a lot of work pressure lately, often working late into the night, and I feel my mental state is getting worse, with difficulty concentrating. Could you recommend a daily meal plan based on my condition?

Response without RAG:
根据你的症状，它们可能与心脾两虚有关。以下是一个简单的日常饮食计划，旨在改善你的健康状况：早餐：一碗燕麦粥，加入几颗红枣和一小把枸杞。午餐：红烧鸡腿（使用较为嫩的部位），搭配炒菠菜和一碗米饭。晚餐：瘦肉汤（用瘦猪肉或牛肉制作），加入当归和黄芪，还有清蒸鱼和炒青菜。

Response without RAG (Translation):
Based on your symptoms, they may be associated with Heart-Spleen Deficiency. Here is a simple daily meal plan designed to improve your health condition: Breakfast: A bowl of oatmeal with a few jujubes and a small handful of goji berries. Lunch: Braised chicken legs (using the more tender parts), paired with stir-fried spinach and a bowl of rice. Dinner: Lean meat soup (made from lean pork or beef), incorporating dang gui (Chinese angelica) and huang qi (astragalus), along with steamed fish and stir-fried green vegetables.

Response with RAG:
根据您的症状，中医认为是心脾两虚，以下是每日的饮食计划，旨在滋养心脏和脾脏，减轻压力，并改善您的精神状态：早餐：莲子百合粥：50克大米，30克莲子，20克百合。在中医中，莲子和百合被认为有安神健脾的功效。这道粥不仅为早晨提供能量，还有助于安抚心情。2个水煮蛋：高质量蛋白质有助于集中注意力和记忆。水果：1个苹果/梨，以补充维生素和纤维。午餐：黄芪党参炖鸡汤：1只鸡腿，15克黄芪，10克党参，适量生姜。黄芪和党参对于补气提神非常有益，而鸡肉则提供了修复身体组织所需的高质量蛋白质。炒菠菜：富含铁和维生素，养血安神。一碗白米饭：为日常活动提供能量。晚餐：瘦肉红枣枸杞汤：100克瘦猪肉或牛肉，10颗红枣，10克枸杞，几片生姜。红枣和枸杞具有养血安神的作用，瘦肉提供的高质量蛋白质有助于提高睡眠质量。清蒸鱼：选择一条新鲜的小鱼，如鲫鱼或海鲈鱼进行清蒸。鱼类富含高质量蛋白质和不饱和脂肪酸，有助于滋养身体和改善睡眠。炒白菜：白菜具有清热解毒、增进食欲和帮助消化的作用，保持良好的精神状态。请尝试上述饮食计划一段时间，并注意身体的变化。如果您的症状没有明显改善或者出现其他不适，建议及时寻求专业医疗意见。

Response with RAG (Translation):
Based on your symptoms, which suggest Heart-Spleen Deficiency in Traditional Chinese Medicine (TCM), here's a daily meal plan to nourish the heart and spleen, reduce stress, and improve your mental state: Breakfast: Lotus Seed & Lily Bulb Porridge: 50g rice, 30g lotus seeds, 20g lily bulbs. In TCM, lotus seeds and lily bulbs are known for their effects of calming the mind and tonifying the spleen. This porridge not only provides energy for the morning but also helps to soothe the mind. 2 Boiled Eggs: High-quality protein for focus and memory. Fruit: 1 Apple/Pear for vitamins and fiber. Lunch: Astragalus & Codonopsis Stewed Chicken Soup: 1 chicken leg, 15g astragalus, 10g codonopsis, and an appropriate amount of ginger. Astragalus and codonopsis are excellent for tonifying qi and boosting energy, while chicken provides high-quality protein to repair body tissues. Stir-Fried Spinach: Rich in iron and vitamins, nourishes blood, calms mind. 1 Bowl White Rice: Provides energy for daily activities. Dinner: Lean Meat & Jujube Goji Berry Soup: 100g lean pork or beef, 10 jujubes, 10g goji berries, and a few slices of ginger. Jujubes and goji berries have the effect of nourishing blood and calming the mind, while lean meat provides high-quality protein to improve sleep quality. Steamed Fish: Choose a fresh small fish, such as a crucian carp or sea bass, and steam it. Fish is rich in high-quality protein and unsaturated fatty acids, helping to nourish the body and improve sleep. Stir-Fried Bok Choy: Bok choy has the effect of clearing heat and detoxifying, promoting appetite, and aiding digestion, maintaining good mental state. Please try the above meal plan for some time and pay attention to any changes in your body. If there is no noticeable improvement in your symptoms or if other discomforts arise, it is advisable to seek professional medical advice promptly.

Fig. 6. An Actual Case of Dietary Q&A with RAG

and non-targeted nutritional intake. In contrast, the response enhanced by RAG not only includes multiple dishes for each meal, ensuring a balanced intake of nutrients, but also features a more diverse selection of ingredients, avoiding repetition. The dishes are combined with TCM theory, briefly explaining the effects of the ingredients, which helps users better understand the role of each component. Such a meal plan is not only more scientifically sound and reasonable but also easier for users to understand and implement.

5 Conclusion

This paper proposes a novel method for generating dietary recommendations that adhere to TCM's principle of "One Root of Medicine and Food" by using retrieval-augmented LLMs. Firstly, we conduct a comparative analysis of several widely used LLMs is conducted to evaluate their effectiveness in generating dietary suggestions from a TCM perspective. Among these, Qwen emerges as the best-performing model and is selected as the base model. By integrating RAG, we enhance the model's ability to extract pertinent knowledge from a specialized knowledge base. The experimental results demonstrate that this approach facilitates the development of personalized dietary recommendations that consider individual user conditions and preferences. It prioritizes a diverse range of ingredients and dishes while providing comprehensive explanations rooted in TCM principles.

In future work, we plan to continuously enrich and update the RAG knowledge base by incorporating more high-quality, up-to-date research findings to improve the model's accuracy and coverage. Additionally, we will explore enhancements to the retrieval strategies of RAG and investigate its broader applications in the field of TCM, thereby enhancing the reliability and usability of TCM-related information systems.

Acknowledgments. This paper is supported by the NSFC (Grant No. 82104786).

References

1. Feng, D., Luqi, H., Guo, J., et al.: History and development of "One Root of Medicine and Food". Life Sci. **27**(08), 1061–1069 (2015)
2. Shangshan, Y.: Huangdi Neijing Taisu. 1st edn. Wang, H, Beijing (2005)
3. Shuyu, Y.: Guidelines for the prevention and management of diabetes with traditional Chinese medicine at the grassroots level. J. Tradit. Chin. Med. **63**(24), 2397–2414 (2022)
4. Tang, X., Xie, G., Zhou, R., et al.: Development and Application of "One Root of Medicine and Food". Chin. Mod. Traditional Chin. Med. **22**(09), 1428–1433 (2020)
5. Introducing ChatGPT. https://openai.com/index/chatgpt, Accessed 20 Sep 2024
6. Thirunavukarasu, A.J., Ting, D.S.J., Elangovan, K., et al.: Large language models in medicine. Nat. Med. **29**(8), 1930–1940 (2023)
7. Fan, W., Ding, Y., Ning, L., et al.: A survey on rag meeting llms: towards retrieval-augmented large language models. In: Proceedings of the 30th ACM SIGKDD Conference on Knowledge Discovery and Data Mining, pp. 6491–6501 (2024)
8. Manoharan, S.: Patient diet recommendation system using K clique and deep learning classifiers. J. Artif. Intell. **2**(02), 121–130 (2020)
9. Chen, Y., Subburathinam, A., Chen, C. H., et al.: Personalized food recommendation as constrained question answering over a large-scale food knowledge graph. In: Proceedings of the 14th ACM International Conference on Web Search and Data Mining, pp. 544–552 (2021)
10. Tang, J., Huang, B., Xie, M.: Anticancer recipe recommendation based on cancer dietary knowledge graph. European J. Cancer Care (2023)
11. Chen, Y., Guo, Y., Fan, Q., et al.: Health-aware food recommendation based on knowledge graph and multi-task learning. Foods **12**(10) (2023)
12. Ma, W., Li, M., Dai, J., et al.: Nutrition-related knowledge graph neural network for food recommendation. Foods **13**(13), 2144 (2024)
13. Xu, Z., Gu, Y., Xu, X., et al.: Developing a personalized meal recommendation system for Chinese older adults: observational cohort study. JMIR Formative Res. **8**(1), e52170 (2024)
14. Jin, H., Lin, Q., Lu, J., et al.: Evaluating the effectiveness of a generative pretrained transformer-based dietary recommendation system in managing potassium intake for hemodialysis patients. J. Renal Nutrition (2024)

15. Sun, H., Zhang, K., Lan, W., et al.: An AI dietitian for type 2 diabetes mellitus management based on large language and image recognition models: preclinical concept validation study. J. Med. Internet Res. **25**(2) (2023)

16. Hannon, B., Kumar, Y., Li, J.J., et al.: Chef Dalle: transforming cooking with multi-model multimodal AI. Computers **13**(7) (2024)

17. Kopitar, L., Stiglic, G., Bedrac, L., et al.: Personalized meal planning in inpatient clinical dietetics using generative artificial intelligence: system description. In: 2024 IEEE 12th International Conference on Healthcare Informatics (ICHI), pp. 326–331 (2024)

18. Tang, X., Xie, G., Zhou, R., et al.: Development and Application of "One Root of Medicine and Food". Mod. Chin. Med. **22**(09), 1428–1433 (2020)

19. Tian, Y., Ding, Y., Shao, B., et al.: Interaction between homologous functional food Astragali Radix and intestinal flora. China J. Chin. Materia Medica **45**(11), 2486–2492 (2020). https://doi.org/10.19540/j.cnki.cjcmm.20200119.401

20. Liu, Y., Xiao, W., Qin, Z., et al.: Annotation of drug and food as the same origin and its realistic significance. Mod. Chin. Med. **17**(12), 1250–1252+1279 (2015). https://doi.org/10.13313/j.issn.1673-4890.2015.12.005

21. Anonymous.: Huangdi Neijing Suwen. 1st edn. Guangdong Science and Technology Publishing Co., Ltd, Guangzhou (2022)

22. Sun, X.: Academic achievements and modern applications of "Shiliao Bencao". New Chin. Med. **43**(5), 129–131 (2011)

23. Ye, J.: Shiwuzhongyao yu Bianfang, 1st edn. Jiangsu Science and Technology Press, Nanjing (1980)

24. Qian, B.: Zhongguo Shiliao Xue, 1st edn. Shanghai Science and Technology Press, Shanghai (1987)

25. Peng, M.: Zhongguo Yaoshan Xue, 1st edn. People's Medical Publishing House, Beijing (1985)

26. Que, L., Yang, G., Li, Y., et al.: Overview of the revision of the "list of substances that are both food and medicine". Chin. Pharm. J. **52**(07), 521–524 (2017)

27. Marvin, G., Hellen, N., Jjingo, D., et al.: Prompt engineering in large language models. In: International conference on data intelligence and cognitive informatics, pp. 387–402. Springer Nature Singapore, Singapore (2023). https://doi.org/10.1007/978-981-99-7962-2_30

28. Gemini. https://gemini.google.com, (Accessed 2024/09/20)

29. Qwen. https://tongyi.aliyun.com (Accessed 20 Sep 2024)

30. Wenxinyiyan. https://yiyan.baidu.com, (Accessed 20 Sep 2024)

31. Zhang, H., Chen, J., Jiang, F., et al.: Huatuogpt, towards taming language model to be a doctor. arXiv preprint arXiv:2305.15075 (2023)

32. Devlin, J.: Bert: Pre-training of deep bidirectional transformers for language understanding. arXiv preprint arXiv:1810.04805 (2018)

33. Yang, F.: Research on the BERT Model for Chinese Clinical Natural Language Processing. Peking Union Medical College (2021)

34. Karpukhin, V., Oguz, B., Min, S., et al.: Dense passage retrieval for open-domain question answering. In: Proceedings of the 2020 Conference on Empirical Methods in Natural Language Processing (EMNLP), pp. 6769–6781 (2020)

35. Lin, C. Y.: Rouge: A package for automatic evaluation of summaries. In: Text Summarization Branches Out, pp. 74–81 (2004)

OAGLLM: A Retrieval-Augmented Large Language Model for Medication Instructions

Wanqiu Cheng[1], Jintao Tang[1(✉)], Yuanyuan Sun[2], Ting Wang[1], Shasha Li[1], Xiang Liu[3], Ronghui Li[3], and Guoping Yang[2,4,5,6]

[1] National University of Defense Technology, Changsha 410073, China
tangjintao@nudt.edu.cn
[2] Center for Clinical Pharmacology, the Third Xiangya Hospital, Central South University, Changsha 410013, China
[3] Department of Clinical Pharmacy, Xiangtan Central Hospital, Xiangtan 411100, Hunan, China
[4] XiangYa School of Pharmaceutical Sciences, Central South University, Changsha 410013, China
[5] Hunan Key Laboratory of Diagnostic and Therapeutic Drug Research for Chronic Diseases, Central South University, Changsha 410013, China
[6] National-Local Joint Engineering Laboratory of Drug Clinical Evaluation Technology, Changsha 410013, China

Abstract. The precision of contextual information is crucial for the results of Large Language Models (LLMs). However, to achieve more precise results in the field of medication instructions, which are characterized by their specificity in covering multiple drug characteristics, it is necessary to refine these instructions. Additionally, most current methods for constructing indexes do not consider sentence-level semantic information, which can easily ignore important details. Therefore, we propose a retrieval enhancement method based on ontology subdivision for LLM(OAGLLM). In the domain of Medication Instructions, we propose an ontology-based subdivision approach for constructing a specialized ontology and systematically storing expert knowledge, accurately match various aspects of Medication Instructions. To capture sentence-level semantic information and improve retrieval accuracy, we have introduced a hierarchical construction indexing method, which is designed to enhance text relevance and coherence. Lastly, we develop a retrieval augmentation system that integrates the Medication Instructions ontology with the hierarchical database. To validate the effectiveness of OAGLLM, we constructed a dataset on medication instructions. Our experiments demonstrate that our method outperforms other models in overall performance and excels across various types of data.

Keywords: Medication Instructions · Ontology-based Subdivision · Hierarchical construction indexing method · Retrieval Augmented Method

© The Author(s), under exclusive license to Springer Nature Singapore Pte Ltd. 2025
Y. Zhang et al. (Eds.): CHIP 2024, CCIS 2433, pp. 268–284, 2025.
https://doi.org/10.1007/978-981-96-3752-2_16

1   Introduction

Medical Instructions is a vital component of patient education [1]. It refer to the clear written explanations provided by healthcare professionals regarding the usage, dosage, contraindications, and precautions of prescribed medications, ensuring that patients use their medications safely and effectively. However, with the development of the pharmaceutical industry and the increasing number of new drugs entering the market, the traditional model of extracting and paraphrasing medication instructions through manpower is facing significant challenges.

The development of Natural Language Processing (NLP), especially with Large Language Models (LLMs), provides a new solution for Medical Instructions. In recent years, these models have become a key focus in NLP research, demonstrating outstanding language understanding and knowledge mastery across various evaluation benchmarks, even exceeding human performance,e.g., The GPT series models [2], The ChatGLM series models [3], The LLama series models [4] and other LLMs. However, LLMs can encounter hallucination issues, as they may fail to provide accurate answers when handling specific or highly specialized queries due to a lack of factual knowledge.

Retrieval-Augmented Generation (RAG) technology can effectively address hallucination issues [5–7]. During the reasoning process, RAG dynamically retrieves information from external knowledge databases and uses the retrieved data as a reference for organizing answers, significantly enhancing the accuracy and relevance of the generated responses. Traditional retrieval-augmented methods, such as LangChain [8], are based on rules or pattern matching, segmenting text into indexed chunks to create a standard index. However, they overlook the semantic relationships within these text chunks, which can lead to incomplete information retrieval and affect the reasoning of generative models. Currently, some studies utilize knowledge graph indexing to account for semantic relationships, but they often operate at the document or paragraph level, ignoring finer-grained information at the sentence level. Additionally, while advancements have been made in the field of medical question-answering, these studies mainly focus on disease diagnosis and consultation, exemplified by Huato GPT [9] and Med-PaLM [10]. On the other hand, medication instructions constitute a specialized domain encompassing various facets of information such as indications, drug administration, drug dosage, and geriatric use. A systematic approach is essential to match each aspect of medication instructions for question-answering, rather than merely performing crude document retrieval.

To address the aforementioned limitations, we propose a new retrieval framework for Medication Instructions, whose innovations primarily stem from three methods within the framework:(i)**Ontology-based subdivision.** Medication Instructions need to cover various types of drug characteristics, including indications, contraindications, and others. To achieve this, we employ an ontology-based subdivision method for in-depth analysis across multiple drug characteristics, and systematically match the information in medication instructions with the corresponding queries related to various aspects. Additionally, we incor-

porate expert experience to design prompt templates for each drug characteristics, thereby enhancing the accuracy of retrieval and output. Ultimately, this
information is integrated into a structured ontology for Medication Instructions,
storing expert-guided knowledge.(ii)**Hierarchical construction indexing.**To
address the issue of existing methods neglecting sentence-level semantic information, we have adopted a novel hierarchical indexing approach. By employing an
adaptive segmentation algorithm, we are able to capture the semantic connections between sentences and segment information pertaining to different topics.
This ensures the richness of information within each text index while enhancing
the coherence of internal themes.(iii)**Retrieval Enhancer.**To integrate the drug
information ontology with the hierarchically constructed retrieval database, and
in consideration of the comprehensive nature of drug characteristics in medication instructions, we have developed a retrieval enhancer that utilizes a three-
tier search method. This enhancer accurately organizes and presents various drug
characteristic information, thereby optimizing the retrieval process. The method
gradually narrows the search scope, enhancing retrieval accuracy and enabling
quick location of medication instruction information related to specific drug
characteristics.

In conclusion, the main contributions of this paper are as follows:

1. We propose an Ontology-based segmentation method that incorporates multiple refinement dimensions to construct a comprehensive Medication Instructions framework. This approach combines expert templates and domain
   knowledge, resulting in a systematic Medication Instructions ontology that
   adequately addresses the need for medication instructions to encompass a
   wide range of drug characteristics.
2. We propose a new hierarchical construction indexing method that discards
   traditional rule-based and pattern-matching designs. Instead, it utilizes a
   novel adaptive segmentation algorithm to divide documents, ensuring both
   the richness of text chunks and the consistency of internal themes.
3. We have developed a retrieval enhancer component and designed a three-
   tier retrieval mechanism that integrates the medication explanation ontology with the retrieval database. This approach gradually narrows the search
   scope, enabling quick location of medication instruction information related
   to specific drug characteristics, significantly improving retrieval accuracy.
4. We constructed a Chinese dataset on medication instructions. Through experiments, we found that our retrieval framework achieved excellent results,
   with scores for ROUGE-1, ROUGE-2, ROUGE-L, and BLEU-4 increasing
   by 11.2%, 12.777%, 11.161%, and 11.52% respectively compared to the baseline model.

2   Related Work

In this section, we first review the relevant work on LLMs in the medical field,
and then summarize the current frameworks for retrieval enhancement as well
as the key technologies involved in various retrieval enhancement methods.

2.1 Developments in the Medical Field

In the medical field, the application of natural language processing technology has garnered widespread attention. "In the medical question-answering domain, Huatuo GPT [9] and Google's Med-PaLM [10] have fine-tuned their models on medical question-answering datasets to develop a medical dialogue system for online diagnosis and disease consultation. In the field of drug information, the FDA is interested in the automated detection of adverse drug reactions [11]. Its monitoring system, VAERS, which it helps manage, plays a crucial role in identifying vaccine-related adverse events [12]. AE-GPT [13] demonstrates the capability of customizing large language models (LLMs) for specific domain tasks through fine-tuning GPT-3 for adverse reaction entity extraction. Shi et al. [14] were the first to successfully apply BERT to solve the ADME semantic tagging task. PharmBERT [15] was specifically trained for the drug labeling domain, proving its superiority over standard BERT, ClinicalBERT, and BioBERT in various NLP tasks within this field. However, current research primarily focuses on medical disease diagnosis or drug information extraction, while studies in the area of Medication Instructions remain relatively insufficient.

2.2 Retrieval-Augmented Based on LLMs

Retrieval augmentation has gained significant attention due to the rapid development of large models [16–18]. This trend has prompted researchers to explore various optimization strategies. Generally, the optimization direction of retrieval augmentation can be divided into two categories: pre-retrieval and post-retrieval optimizations. Pre-retrieval optimization mainly focuses on the generation of data indices, with the goal of enhancing the quality of indexed content. Traditional indexing methods typically segment text into fixed blocks based on rules and pattern matching, which are then embedded and built into standard indices. Additionally, a chain structure expands to larger information through overlapping chunks and progressively extended chunks [8]. T-RAG introduces an entity tree that adds entity information to the original RAG framework [19]. However, both approaches overlook the semantic information of global context, which may result in incomplete information retrieval. To address this issue, researchers have proposed various optimized indexing methods. The LLaMA index possesses automatic evaluation capabilities for different chunking methods [4]. RET-LLM [20], SUGRE [21], and KnowledgeGPT [22] enhance the contextual relevance of retrieved text by establishing knowledge graph indices. However, knowledge graph indices are organized at the document or paragraph level, lacking more refined sentence-level indexing granularity. Moreover, due to preset patterns, they fail to resolve issues of semantic consistency despite differing expressions.At sentence level, Alibaba [23] has trained a large segmentation model using Wikipedia to divide documents into multiple text blocks. Meanwhile, Cai et al. [24] utilized clustering methods to aggregate multiple sentences into text blocks. However, pre-trained segmentation models are not suitable for specialized fields, and clustering methods tend to generate short text blocks, which can easily overlook information. In this context, the indexing construction methods still require further investigation.

3   Method

In this section, we describe the proposed retrieval augmentation framework and introduce the three key technologies involved.

3.1   Overall Framework

Our overall retrieval framework is divided into two phases: Retrieval Database Construction and LLMs + Refined Retrieval(see Fig. 1).

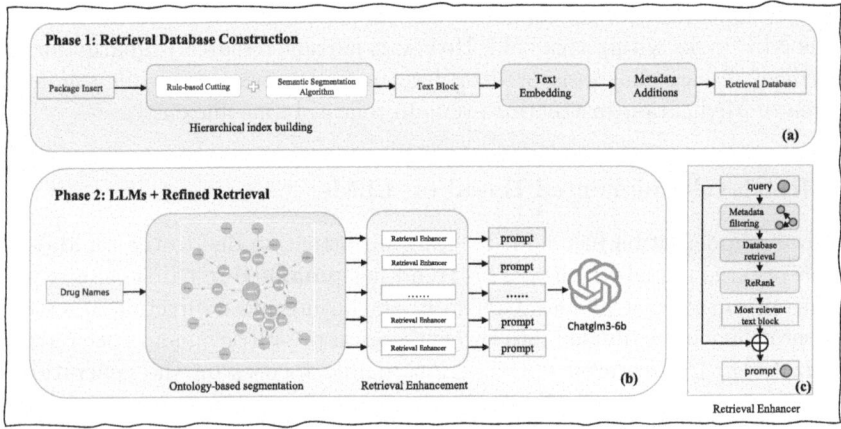

Fig. 1. Overall framework of Our OntologyRAGLLM. (a) represents phase 1 Retrieval Database Construction. (b) shows phase 2 LLMs + Refined Retrieval. (c) represents the retrieval enhancer.

Retrieval Database Construction. In this phase, we construct index using a hierarchical Approach to segment the documentation into text blocks. Based on this, we adding metadata information to each text block, ultimately saving them in the form of a FAISS database.

LLMs + Refined Retrieval. In this phase, we first perform ontology segmentation of medication instructions. This process involves classifying medication instructions according to different drug characteristics to provide more targeted retrieval and professional guidance. Next, Next, we designed a retrieval enhancer that offers personalized retrieval for each drug characteristics to ensure that the information obtained better aligns with ours needs.

The retrieval enhancer for a three-layer retrieval process:

1. **Metadata Filtering.** Utilize additional metadata information from text blocks along with ontological information for the first step of filtering;
2. **Database Retrieval.** After metadata filtering, relevant contextual information is retrieved from the database;
3. **Rerank.** Reordering the contextual information to obtain the most relevant data.

Finally, the most relevant information is integrated into the corresponding expert templates to form specific prompts, which are then input into the large model for reasoning. After processing by the model, we ultimately obtain accurate and effective answers.

3.2   Hierarchical Construction Indexing

In the database retrieval construction phase, we adopted a hierarchical indexing method to divide the instruction documents into text chunks. The hierarchical construction indexing method is based on the text_splitter component of the Langchain framework. The text_splitter is a tool in Langchain used for splitting long texts into manageable chunks. Traditional text-splitters utilize rules (such as symbols, punctuation, etc.) or pattern matching to convert documents into a collection of sentences.

However, merely relying on rules and pattern matching for chunking often overlooks the semantic information between sentences, failing to provide large models with sufficient contextual information. Therefore, based on traditional chunking methods, we designed a adaptive segmentation algorithm that divides the entire document into chunks based on different themes. The purpose of this approach is to ensure thematic consistency within the chunks while also guaranteeing the richness of the information contained within them.

Adaptive Segmentation Algorithm. Let the document be a collection of sentences (M_t), defined as follows,

$$M_t = \{S_t^i\} = \{S_t^0(v_t^0, index0), ..., S_t^{n-1}(v_t^{n-1}, index(n-1))\} \tag{1}$$

$$v_t^i = emb(s_t^i) \tag{2}$$

where S_t^i represents the (i)-th sentence in the (t)-th document, which includes an embedding vector v_t^i and a position index $index(i)$.

To avoid redundant calculations of the similarity between two neighboring embedding vectors in the algorithms, we set up a similarity matrix $A \in R^{1*n-1}$, defined as follows,

$$A_t = (a_t^0, a_t^1, ..., a_t^{n-1}) \tag{3}$$

$$a_t^i = \frac{v_t^i \cdot v_t^{i+1}}{\|v_t^i\| \times \|v_t^{i+1}\|} \tag{4}$$

where A_t represents the similarity matrix. a_t^i represents the cosine similarity between the (i)-th embedding vector and the ((i+1))-th embedding vector.

To ensure the richness of information within the chunks, we aim to retain longer texts as much as possible. Therefore, we set a maximum length, referred to as chunk_size, and assign it a value of k. When the length of the document exceeds k, we will find the minimum value a_t^p from A_t. based on this, we will proceed to segment the document,

$$
\begin{cases}
M_{t1} = \{s_t^0, ..., s_t^p\} \\
M_{t2} = \{s_t^{p+1}, ..., s_t^{n-1}\}
\end{cases}
\tag{5}
$$

where M_t1, M_t2 represent the two documents segmented at the boundary index p.

At this point, we obtain the two new documents and proceed to segment them again until each document's length is below the threshold k, at which point the algorithm terminates.

Retrieve Database. By hierarchically construct index, the drug package insert will be divided into a series of text blocks. We added metadata information to each text block. Through this metadata addition, the text blocks incorporated drug names and instruction labels, providing information sources for the first layer of the retrieval enhancer, namely metadata filtering. Ultimately, these text blocks were converted into a FAISS database to support efficient retrieval in subsequent framework.

3.3   Ontology-Based Categorization

The Medication Instructions itself involves multiple drug characteristics and requires fine-grained analysis. Furthermore, in the medical field, the process of Medication Instructions heavily relies on the guidance of expert knowledge. In this context, we closely collaborated with professionals to construct the Medication Instructions ontology. By employing an ontological categorization approach, we are able to analyze Medication Instructions from multiple dimensions and store expert knowledge in a structured format within the ontology. This method helps reduce the loss of important information, thereby ensuring the completeness and professionalism of the medication explanation. In the following sections, we will provide a detailed description of the Medication Instructions ontology based on Fig. 2 and its three core information.

The ontology of medication instructions includes three types (see Fig. 2). It consists of three types: medication instructions(red),drug characteristics (blue) and drug package insert labels (green). Drug characteristics are types that we have categorized based on ontology, comprising a total of 12 categories, such as indications, geriatric use, pediatric use, etc. drug package insert labels refer to the different components found in the drug's instructions, such as special populations, precautions, etc. The entire medication instructions ontology primarily encompasses three core pieces of information: Ontology Subdivision,Expert Knowledge, Expert Template. We will provide a detailed description of these three core information.

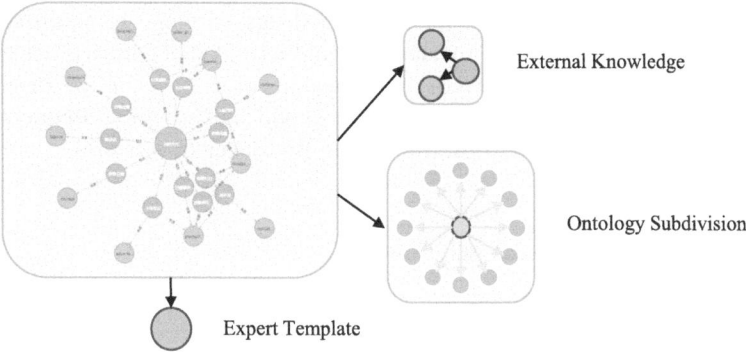

Fig. 2. Medication Instructions ontology. It consists of three types, two relationships, and two attributes, encompassing three core pieces of information internally.

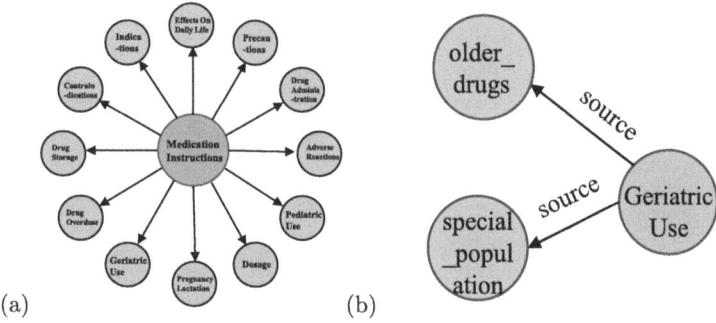

(a)   (b)

Fig. 3. Two core pieces of information:(a)Ontology Subdivision;(b)Expert Knowledge

Ontology Subdivision. The medication instructions for drugs, as a systematic whole, typically involve multi-dimensional and multi-attribute information. In this context(see Fig. 3(a)), we collaborated with professionals to construct the ontology of medication instructions and refined it into 12 different categories, such as indications, geriatric use, and pediatric use. The establishment of this knowledge classification system allows subsequent queries about medication instructions to avoid comprehensive inquiries into the entire drug information. Instead, we can start from these 12 subdivided types and conduct searches in a more granular and precise manner.

Expert Knowledge. Through the subdivision of the ontology, we categorized the medication instructions for drugs into 12 different drug characteristics. However, because the content covered by each drug characteristic varies, their retrieval locations in the drug package insert also differ. Experts provided information regarding the scope of sources for each drug characteristic. We stored this information in the 'source' relationship between the drug characteristic class and the drug package insert component class. As shown in Fig. 3(b), content related to 'geriatric use' will only appear in the 'older_drugs' and 'special_population' of the drug package insert. Therefore, the drug characteristic of geriatric use forms a 'source' relationship with the two drug package insert sections: 'older_drugs' and 'special_populations'.This 'source' relationship will be used in subsequent work to filter the metadata information during the first layer of retrieval.

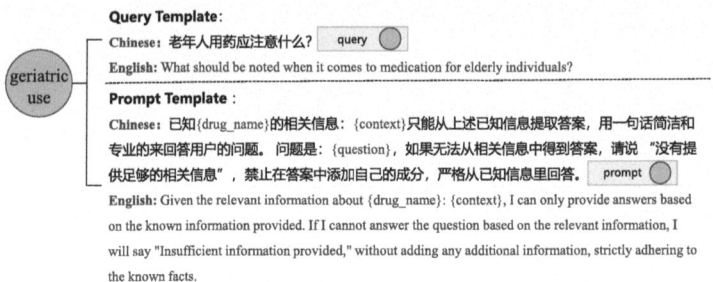

Fig. 4. External Knowledge. This paper is based on medication instructions in Chinese. therefore, our template is presented in Chinese. The figure illustrates a query template and prompt template for the characteristics of geriatric use.

Expert Template. Given the professionalism of medication instructions, the performance of different drug characteristics on their respective templates varies. Through collaborative efforts with professionals and multiple rounds of testing, this paper has designed a set of expert templates. These templates are optimized for each drug characteristic to ensure the accuracy and relevance of the information. The expert templates are divided into query templates and prompt templates. The former is used to generate a structured pattern for search queries. These templates help the model more effectively retrieve relevant information from external knowledge bases or documents, enhancing the quality of the generated content. The latter is used for prompt engineering, serving as a structured input format to guide the model in generating responses. By setting specific contexts or question frameworks, it helps the model better understand the task, resulting in more accurate and relevant outputs. As shown in Fig. 4, for the drug characteristic of geriatric use, we have developed specialized formats and guiding questions to enable professionals to input related information efficiently and accurately. We store these expert templates within the attributes of the drug characteristic class.

By constructing a Medication Instructions ontology, we embed expert guidance knowledge into the entire retrieval framework in a structured format. This structured information system enables us to more efficiently obtain comprehensive and accurate drug information, thereby enhancing the effectiveness of the retrieval process.

3.4   Retrieval Enhancer

The retrieval enhancer serves as the implementation module of the entire retrieval framework. Through the retrieval enhancer, we integrate the core information of the ontology with the retrieval database into the retrieval framework. The retrieval enhancer mainly consists of three layers of retrieval: metadata filtering, retrieval database, and rerank. This three-layer retrieval mechanism gradually narrows down the search scope, further improving retrieval accuracy.

Metadata Filtering. As described in the previous two sections, the process of metadata filtering involves utilizing the drug names and label information introduced through the metadata in text blocks. This information is then matched with the external knowledge of the ontology-specifically, determining whether the label information corresponds to a "source" relationship with the drug characteristics being queried at that stage. This strategy aims to narrow the search scope before formal retrieval, thereby enhancing the efficiency and relevance of the search process.

Retrieval Database. The second layer of retrieval enhancer employs the FAISS database's IndexFlatL2 index for searching, utilizing the most precise nearest neighbor search(NNS) method. This approach calculates the distances between the query vector and all other vectors, selecting the top k vectors with the highest similarity. In this process, we set k to a larger value to expand the range of text blocks covered by this layer of retrieval.

Rerank. In the retrieval database phase, the IndexFlatL2 retrieval we use calculates the Euclidean (L2) distance, which is defined as follows:

$$d(x, y) = \sqrt{\Sigma(x_i - y_i)^2} \tag{6}$$

The L2 distance is used to measure the absolute distance between two points in a multidimensional space; however, it is not suitable for distance measurement in high-dimensional vector data. Additionally, in the FAISS retrieval process, no minimum threshold is set, significantly increasing the likelihood of irrelevant information being introduced. To address this issue, we propose a reordering method based on the principles of LongLLMLingua [25] to recalculate the similarity between relevant texts and the query vector. Our reordering method primarily features two functions: (i) implementing a similarity reordering within a narrow range based on efficient large-scale retrieval using FAISS, employing cosine similarity to enhance contextual relevance; and (ii) setting a minimum threshold θ to reduce the introduction of irrelevant information.

4   Experiment

4.1   Setup

Dataset. Since Medication Instructions is a new field in computer applications, there currently exists no specific dataset for this purpose. In this context, we collaborated with the physicians from the Department of Clinical Pharmacy, Xiangtan Central Hospital. With their assistance, we selected authoritative drug package inserts to serve as the foundation for our retrieval database. Furthermore, we manually constructed a Chinese dataset specifically for medication instructions.

Drug Package Inserts Dataset. physician obtained the drug package inserts for relevant medications, along with their approval numbers, implementation standards, or national standards, from the official website. In cases where there were multiple drug package inserts for the same medication, we retained the latest version based on the timestamps of the approval numbers, implementation standards, and national standards. Ultimately, we obtained all the insert information for 68 medications. Each drug package insert contains 11 labels such as "special_populations," "precautions," and so on. The content within different labels is complex and abundant, with much overlapping information. It is unrealistic and impossible for patients to rely solely on lengthy inserts to understand their medications. We treated these drug package inserts as documents, performed adaptive segmentation on them, and stored them in a retrieval database.

Medication Instructions Dataset. The aim of our work is to summarize the characteristics of each drug by retrieving information from drug package inserts, and then derive medication instructions to help patients use medications safely and effectively. To validate the effectiveness of our model, we constructed a Chinese medication instruction dataset. Taking the individual characteristics of drugs as units, we applied a first-layer filter to obtain relevant content from the drug package inserts, which was then provided to physicians as context. Based on the information provided, physicians gave answers related to those drug characteristics. In summary, our constructed medication instruction dataset includes a total of 68 drugs, with each drug having 12 drug characteristics, resulting in 816 data entries. With the intention of assisting patients, our data is characterized by its brevity and effectiveness, striving to extract the most core content from lengthy drug package inserts and convert it into easily understandable text.

Evaluation Metrics. We use the widely adopted evaluation metrics for text generation tasks, namely the ROUGE series (ROUGE-1, ROUGE-2, ROUGE-L) and BLEU-4. The ROUGE series focuses more on the comprehensiveness and coverage of content, particularly the matching of vocabulary and phrases. In contrast, BLEU-4 emphasizes the quality and precision of the generated text, ensuring that it is consistent with the reference text.

4.2 Comparison of Overall Performance

We use full-text retrieval as the baseline, where full-text retrieval involves inputting the entire medication instruction into the model. Furthermore, to validate the effectiveness of our adaptive segmentation method, we compared it with other document segmentation methods, including langchain [8] rule-based and pattern-matching segmentation method, the K-means [24] method for continuously expanding blocks, and Alibaba open-source segmentation model [23]. Please note that we adhere to the principle of controlling variables; all segmentation algorithms are based on our entire retrieval framework, and the retrieval-enhanced three-layer retrieval mechanism continues to work on other segmentation methods.

Table 1. Overall Performance

segmentation method	Rouge-1	Rouge-2	Rouge-L	BLEU-4
Baseline	33.883	20.081	29.885	17.550
langchain	38.229	24.005	33.623	20.584
Kmeans	40.566	26.331	35.998	22.852
Alibaba	40.432	26.468	35.907	23.168
Ours	**45.113**	**32.858**	**41.046**	**29.067**

Quantitative Performance Comparison. According to the results in Table 1. We found that our method significantly outperforms other methods across four metrics. Whether in terms of content comprehensiveness and coverage or content accuracy and consistency, our method achieves optimal results.

Qualitative Performance Comparison. To further understand the reasons for the superiority of our method, we conducted a qualitative comparison, and the results are presented in Fig. 5. In comparison, we can observe that our adaptive segmentation method is able to capture more information, while the other three methods tend to focus on shorter texts, even though we have set the same maximum length k. Additionally, the rule-based and pattern-matching approach of Langchain, as well as the Alibaba segmentation model, are also affected by punctuation marks, which can result in incomplete sentences.

4.3 The Performance of Each Drug Characteristics

To further understand the comparison results of the 12 drug characteristic of data, we evaluated each of the 12 drug characteristics sequentially using BLEU-4, resulting in Table 2.

Drug_name: 盐酸二甲双胍肠溶片(Metformin Hydrochloride Enteric - Coated Tablets)   **Drug characteristic:** Contraindications

Manual Answer:

Chinese: 1.肾脏疾病或循环衰竭（休克）、急性心肌梗死和败血症引起的肾功能障碍 2.需要药物治疗的充血性心衰和其他严重心、肺疾患 3.严重感染和外伤、外科大手术、临床有低血压和缺氧等患者 4.已知对盐酸二甲双胍过敏 5.急性或慢性代谢性酸中毒，包括有或无昏迷的糖尿病酮症酸中毒，和糖尿病酮症酸中毒需要使用胰岛素治疗 6.酗酒者 7.接受血管内注射碘化造影剂者，应暂时停用本品 8.维生素B12，叶酸缺乏未纠正者。

English: 1.Renal dysfunction caused by kidney disease, circulatory failure (shock), acute myocardial infarction, and sepsis. 2. Congestive heart failure requiring drug therapy and other severe heart and lung diseases. 3. Patients with severe infections, trauma, major surgeries, clinical hypotension, and hypoxia. 4. allergy to metformin hydrochloride. 5. Acute or chronic metabolic acidosis, including diabetic ketoacidosis with or without coma, and diabetic ketoacidosis requiring insulin therapy. 6. Alcoholics. 7. Those undergoing intravascular injection of iodinated contrast agents should temporarily discontinue this product. 8. Individuals with unresolved deficiencies in vitamin B12 and folic acid.

---

langchain retrieve content:

Chinese: （1）禁忌症≥1。（2）禁忌症:严重感染和外伤、外科大手术、临床有低血压和缺氧等。（3）禁忌症:5毫克/分升（男性）。

English:(1)Tabos:≥1.(2) Tabos: Severe infections, trauma, major surgeries, clinical hypotension, and hypoxia.(3)Tabos: 5 mg/dL (male).

langchain answer:

Chinese: 盐酸二甲双胍肠溶片禁用于严重感染和外伤、外科大手术、临床有低血压和缺氧等情况。

English: Metformin hydrochloride enteric-coated tablets are contraindicated in cases of severe infections, trauma, major surgeries, clinical hypotension, and hypoxia.

Alibaba retrieve content:

Chinese: （1）禁忌症:严重感染和外伤、外科大手术、临床有低血压和缺氧等。（2）禁忌症:维生素B12，叶酸缺乏未纠正者。（3）禁忌症:5毫克/分升（男性）

English:(1)Tabos: Severe infections, trauma, major surgeries, clinical hypotension, and hypoxia.(2) Tabos: Tabos: Individuals with unresolved deficiencies in vitamin B12 and folic acid.(3) Tabos: 5 mg/dL (male).

Alibaba answer:

Chinese: 盐酸二甲双胍肠溶片禁用于严重感染和外伤、外科大手术、临床有低血压和缺氧情况下，以及维生素B12和叶酸缺乏未纠正者和5毫克/分升（男性）、≥1的情况。

English: Metformin hydrochloride enteric-coated tablets are contraindicated in cases of severe infections, trauma, major surgeries, clinical hypotension, and hypoxia. They are also contraindicated in individuals with unresolved deficiencies in vitamin B-12 and folic acid, as well as in those with serum creatinine levels of ≥5 mg/dL (males) or ≥1.4 mg/dL (females).

Kmeans retrieve content:

Chinese: （1）禁忌症:酗酒者。（2）禁忌症:接受血管内注射碘化造影剂者，应暂时停用本品。维生素B12，叶酸缺乏未纠正者。（3）禁忌症:肾脏疾病或下列情况禁用本品：循环衰竭（休克）、急性心肌梗死和败血症引起的肾功能障碍（血清肌酐水平≥1.5毫克/分升（男性）、≥1.4毫克/分升（女性）或肌酐清除异常）。

English:(1)Tabos: Alcoholics.(2)Tabos: Those undergoing intravascular injection of iodinated contrast agents should temporarily discontinue this product. Individuals with unresolved deficiencies in vitamin B12 and folic acid.(3)Tabos: This product is contraindicated in cases of kidney disease or the following conditions: renal impairment caused by circulatory failure (shock), acute myocardial infarction, and sepsis (serum creatinine level ≥1.5 mg/dL for males, ≥1.4 mg/dL for females, or abnormal creatinine clearance).

Kmeans answer:

Chinese: 禁用于酗酒者、接受血管内注射碘化造影剂者、维生素B12和叶酸缺乏者、肾脏疾病患者、严重感染和外伤、外科大手术、临床有低血压和缺氧等患者、对盐酸二甲双胍过敏者、急性或慢性代谢性酸中毒患者。

English: Contraindicated in alcoholics, those undergoing intravascular injec-tion of iodinated contrast agents, individuals with vitamin B12 and folic acid deficiencies, patients with kidney disease, severe infections an-d trauma, major surgeries, clinical hypotension and hypoxia, those aller-gic to metformin hydrochloride, and patients with acute or chronic me-tabolic acidosis.

Our retrieve content:

Chinese: 禁忌症:肾脏疾病或下列情况禁用本品：循环衰竭（休克）、急性心肌梗死和败血症引起的肾功能障碍（血清肌酐水平≥1.5毫克/分升（男性）、≥1.4毫克/分升（女性）或肌酐清除异常）。需要药物治疗的充血性心衰，和其他严重心、肺疾患。严重感染和外伤、外科大手术、临床有低血压和缺氧等。已知对盐酸二甲双胍过敏。急性或慢性代谢性酸中毒，包括有或无昏迷的糖尿病酮症酸中毒，和糖尿病酮症酸中毒需要使用胰岛素治疗。酗酒者。接受血管内注射碘化造影剂者，应暂时停用本品。维生素B12，叶酸缺乏未纠正者。

English: Tabos: Those undergoing intravascular injection of iodinated contrast agents should temporarily discontinue this product. Individuals with unresolved deficiencies in vitamin B12 and folic acid. Congestive heart failure requiring drug therapy, as well as other severe heart and lung diseases. Severe infections, trauma, major surgeries, clinical hypotension, and hypoxia. allergy to metformin hydrochloride. Acute or chronic metabolic acidosis, including diabetic keto-acidosis with or without coma, and diabetic ketoacidosis requiring treatment with insulin. Alcoholics. Those undergoing intravascular injection of iodinated contrast agents should temporarily discontinue this product. Individuals with unresolved deficiencies in vitamin B12 and folic acid.

Our answer:

Chinese: 禁用于以下情况：肾脏疾病或下列情况禁用本品：循环衰竭（休克）、急性心肌梗死和败血症引起的肾功能障碍（血清肌酐水平≥1.5毫克/分升（男性）、≥1.4毫克/分升（女性）或肌酐清除异常）。需要药物治疗的充血性心衰，和其他严重心、肺疾患。严重感染和外伤、外科大手术、临床有低血压和缺氧等。对盐酸二甲双胍过敏。急性或慢性代谢性酸中毒，包括有或无昏迷的糖尿病酮症酸中毒，和糖尿病酮症酸中毒需要使用胰岛素治疗。酗酒者。接受血管内注射碘化造影剂者，应暂时停用本品。维生素B12，叶酸缺乏未纠正者。

English: This medication is contraindicated in the following conditions: kidney disease or renal impairment caused by circulatory failure (shock), acute myo-cardial infarction, and sepsis (serum creatinine level ≥1.5 mg/dL for males, ≥1.4 mg/dL for females, or abnormal creatinine clearance). It should not be used in cases of congestive heart failure requiring drug therapy, as well as in other severe heart and lung diseases. Additionally, it is contraindicated in cases of severe infections, trauma, major surgeries, clinical hypotension, and hypoxia. Allergic reactions to metformin hydrochloride, acute or chronic metabolic acidosis, inclu-ding diabetic ketoacidosis with or without coma, and diabetic ketoacidosis requiring treatment with insulin, are also contraindications. Alcoholics and those undergoing intravascular injection of iodinated contrast agents should temporarily discontinue this medication. Furthermore, individuals with unresolved defic-iencies in vitamin B12 and folic acid should not use this medication.

Fig. 5. Qualitative Performance Comparison of Ours with three other segmentation methods based on our Chinese dataset,with 'Chinese' being our original answer and 'English' being the translated version.

Our model outperforms the baseline in every drug characteristic, further validating its ability to meet the requirements for medication instructions. In terms of Drug Storage, Dosage and Summary of Drug Effects on Daily Life, the performance shows only a slight improvement compared to the baseline. Through further investigation, we found that these medication characteristics with similar performance exhibit a centralized nature, meaning that the required text is concentrated within a single paragraph of the drug package insert, without the need for cross-paragraph retrieval and summarization. This somewhat mitigates the advantages of our model.

Table 2. The performance of each drug characteristic

Drug Characteristic	Ours	Baseline
Indications	**52.23**	47.59
Contraindications	**42.03**	17.58
Drug Storage	**29.54**	28.48
Drug Overdose	**39.67**	11.57
geriatric use	**34.85**	8.41
Medication During Pregnancy and Lactation	**14.28**	13.33
Dosage	**32.52**	29.66
Pediatric Use	**31.58**	8.29
Adverse Reactions	**26.60**	23.70
Summary of Drug Administration	**27.07**	20.66
Summary of Precautions	**21.15**	5.00
Summary of Drug Effects on Daily Life	**5.86**	4.54

4.4 Ablation Study

In this section, we explore the effectiveness of the three-layer retrieval mechanism of the retrieval enhancer. According to the results in Table 3, we found each layer of the retrieval mechanism contributes to the search results. According to the results, removing Metadata Filtering resulted in a significant decline in performance, with various metrics decreasing by 6 to 8% points. Meanwhile, removing Rerank or using only Metadata Filtering also led to a decrease of at least 3% points in all metrics. These results fully validate the effectiveness of our three-layer retrieval mechanism.

Table 3. Ablation Study. '-' represents the remove of this component.

segmentation method	Rouge-1	Rouge-2	Rouge-L	BLEU-4
- Metadata Filtering	39.386	25.359	35.039	21.940
- Rerank	41.176	27.098	36.734	23.649
Only Metadata Filtering	42.223	28.081	37.306	24.940
Ours	**45.113**	**32.858**	**41.046**	**29.067**

5   Conclusion

In this work, we propose OAGLLM, a retrieval-augmented large model for Medication Instructions. Medication Instructions necessitate further refinement due to their encompassing various drug characteristics. Our model addresses this limitation by applying subdivision to the medication instructions ontology, thereby refining it into match-and-answer queries tailored to individual drug characteristics. In addition, current indexing methods ignore fine-grained semantic information at the sentence level, potentially resulting in the omission of details. In contrast, our model employs an adaptive segmentation algorithm to hierarchically construct indexes based on the semantic relationships between sentences, thereby preserving sentence-level information. We have also designed a retrieval enhancer that integrates the subdivided ontology knowledge with the new index database through a three-tier retrieval mechanism. We have constructed a Chinese dataset for medication instructions and conducted comprehensive experimental evaluations. The results demonstrate that our OAGLLM outperforms other models and excels in various types of drug characteristics. Furthermore, we have conducted rigorous ablation studies to confirm the effectiveness of the three-tier retrieval mechanism in our retrieval augmenter. Looking ahead, Looking ahead, we are committed to exploring a wider range of medication instruction scenarios in order to provide more personalized support for healthcare professionals.

Acknowledgement. This work is partially supported by Department of Clinical Pharmacy, Xiangtan Central Hospital. They took on the manual construction of the dataset for this study, ensuring its professionalism and reliability.

References

1. Leep Hunderfund, A.N., Bartleson, J.D.: Patient education in neurology. Neurol. Clin. **28**(2), 517–536 (2010)
2. Achiam, J., et al.: Gpt-4 technical report. arXiv preprint arXiv:2303.08774 (2023)
3. GLM, T., et al.: Chatglm: A family of large language models from glm-130b to glm-4 all tools. arXiv preprint arXiv:2406.12793 (2024)
4. Touvron, H., et al.: Llama 2: Open foundation and fine-tuned chat models. arXiv preprint arXiv:2307.09288 (2023)

5. Izacard, G., et al.: Few-shot learning with retrieval augmented language models. arXiv preprint arXiv:2208.03299 **2**(3) (2022)
6. Zhu, Y., et al.: Large language models for information retrieval: a survey. arXiv preprint arXiv:2308.07107 (2023)
7. Rogers, A., Boyd-Graber, J., Okazaki, N.: Proceedings of the 61st annual meeting of the association for computational linguistics (volume 1: Long papers). In: Proceedings of the 61st Annual Meeting of the Association for Computational Linguistics (Volume 1: Long Papers) (2023)
8. Liu, Q., Song, J., Huang, Z., Zhang, Y., glide the, liunux4odoo: langchain-chatchat. https://github.com/chatchat-space/Langchain-Chatchat (2024)
9. Zhang, H., et al.: Huatuogpt, towards taming language model to be a doctor. arXiv preprint arXiv:2305.15075 (2023)
10. Singhal, K., et al.: Large language models encode clinical knowledge. Nature **620**(7972), 172–180 (2023)
11. Roberts, K., Demner-Fushman, D., Tonning, J.M.: Overview of the tac 2017 adverse reaction extraction from drug labels track. In: TAC (2017)
12. Gringeri, M., et al.: Herpes zoster and simplex reactivation following covid-19 vaccination: new insights from a vaccine adverse event reporting system (vaers) database analysis. Expert Rev. Vaccines **21**(5), 675–684 (2022)
13. Li, Y., Li, J., He, J., Tao, C.: Ae-gpt: using large language models to extract adverse events from surveillance reports-a use case with influenza vaccine adverse events. PLoS ONE **19**(3), e0300919 (2024)
14. Shi, Y., Wang, J., Ren, P., ValizadehAslani, T., Zhang, Y., Hu, M., Liang, H.: Fine-tuning bert for automatic adme semantic labeling in fda drug labeling to enhance product-specific guidance assessment. J. Biomed. Inform. **138**, 104285 (2023)
15. ValizadehAslani, T., et al.: Pharmbert: a domain-specific bert model for drug labels. Brief. Bioinform.**24**(4), bbad226 (2023)
16. Gao, Y., et al.: Retrieval-augmented generation for large language models: a survey. arXiv preprint arXiv:2312.10997 (2023)
17. Zhang, Y., et al.: Siren's song in the ai ocean: a survey on hallucination in large language models. arXiv preprint arXiv:2309.01219 (2023)
18. Kandpal, N., Deng, H., Roberts, A., Wallace, E., Raffel, C.: Large language models struggle to learn long-tail knowledge. In: International Conference on Machine Learning, pp. 15696–15707. PMLR (2023)
19. Fatehkia, M., Lucas, J.K., Chawla, S.: T-rag: lessons from the llm trenches. arXiv preprint arXiv:2402.07483 (2024)
20. Modarressi, A., Imani, A., Fayyaz, M., Schütze, H.: Ret-llm: Towards a general read-write memory for large language models. arXiv preprint arXiv:2305.14322 (2023)
21. Kang, M., Kwak, J.M., Baek, J., Hwang, S.J.: Knowledge graph-augmented language models for knowledge-grounded dialogue generation. arXiv preprint arXiv:2305.18846 (2023)
22. Wang, Y., Lipka, N., Rossi, R.A., Siu, A., Zhang, R., Derr, T.: Knowledge graph prompting for multi-document question answering. In: Proceedings of the AAAI Conference on Artificial Intelligence. vol. 38, pp. 19206–19214 (2024)
23. Zhang, Q., Chen, Q., Li, Y., Liu, J., Wang, W.: Sequence model with self-adaptive sliding window for efficient spoken document segmentation. In: IEEE Automatic Speech Recognition and Understanding Workshop, ASRU 2021, Cartagena, Colombia, December 13-17, 2021, pp. 411–418. IEEE (2021). https://doi.org/10.1109/ASRU51503.2021.9688078

24. yunsheng cai: Optimization of document segmentation method in langchain framework: Methods and applications. Computer Science and Application (2023). https://api.semanticscholar.org/CorpusID:266776021
25. Jiang, H., Wu, Q., Lin, C.Y., Yang, Y., Qiu, L.: Llmlingua: Compressing prompts for accelerated inference of large language models. arXiv preprint arXiv:2310.05736 (2023)

Author Index

© The Editor(s) (if applicable) and The Author(s), under exclusive license
to Springer Nature Singapore Pte Ltd. 2025
Y. Zhang et al. (Eds.): CHIP 2024, CCIS 2433, pp. 285–286, 2025.
https://doi.org/10.1007/978-981-96-3752-2